Behavioral Couples Therapy
for Alcoholism and Drug Abuse

BEHAVIORAL COUPLES THERAPY
for ALCOHOLISM and DRUG ABUSE

Timothy J. O'Farrell

William Fals-Stewart

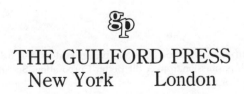

THE GUILFORD PRESS
New York   London

© 2006 The Guilford Press
A Division of Guilford Publications, Inc.
72 Spring Street, New York, NY 10012
www.guilford.com

Printed in Canada

This book is printed on acid-free paper.

Last digit is print number: 9 8 7 6 5 4 3 2 1

Library of Congress Cataloging-in-Publication Data

O'Farrell, Timothy J.
  Behavioral couples therapy for alcoholism and drug abuse / by Timothy J. O'Farrell, William Fals-Stewart.
     p. cm.
  Includes bibliographical references and index.
  ISBN-10: 1-59385-324-6   ISBN-13: 978-1-59385-324-2 (pbk.)
  1. Alcoholism—Treatment.   2. Marital psychotherapy.   3. Drug abuse—Treatment.   4. Marital psychotherapy.   I. Fals-Stewart, William.   II. Title.
  RC565.O34 2006
  616.86'106—dc22

                                                            2006006047

Screen Beans® clip art images in Figures 3.2, 6.1, 6.5, and 6.6; in Posters B.4, B.11, B.15, and B.17; and in Form C.10 are used with permission from A Bit Better Corporation. Screen Beans is a registered trademark of A Bit Better Corporation.

To Jayne and Colin
—T. J. O.

To my family—Leslie, Emily, and Will
—W. F. S.

About the Authors

Timothy J. O'Farrell, PhD, ABPP, is Professor of Psychology in the Department of Psychiatry at Harvard Medical School, and he directs the Families and Addiction Program and the Counseling for Alcoholics' Marriages (CALM) Project at the VA Boston Healthcare System. His clinical and research interests focus primarily on couple and family therapy in alcoholism and drug abuse treatment and various aspects of substance abusers' family relationships, including partner violence, child functioning, and sexual adjustment. Dr. O'Farrell's books include *Alcohol and Sexuality* (1983), *Treating Alcohol Problems: Marital and Family Interventions* (1993), and *Substance Abuse Program Accreditation Guide* (1997).

William Fals-Stewart, PhD, is a clinical psychologist, a principal scientist at RTI International in Research Triangle Park, North Carolina, and the Director of the Addiction and Family Research Group at RTI. His clinical and research interests include the effects of substance abuse on the family, partner- and family-involved treatments for alcoholism and drug abuse, and psychological assessment.

Preface

A 1974 report from the National Institute on Alcohol Abuse and Alcoholism (NIAAA) to the U.S. Congress called couple and family therapy "one of the most outstanding current advances in the area of psychotherapy of alcoholism."[1] Case reports and uncontrolled treatment studies that presented favorable results were the basis for this enthusiastic appraisal. NIAAA recommended that controlled outcome studies should be conducted to evaluate these promising treatment methods. This report came in the beginning years of NIAAA and the National Institute on Drug Abuse (NIDA), which were founded on the hope that science would improve treatment outcomes for patients with alcoholism and substance abuse.

Now over 30 years later, considerable research has confirmed the early enthusiasm for couple and family therapy, and family involvement in substance abuse treatment is generally accepted. However, evidence-based couple and family therapy methods are not widely practiced. Behavioral couples therapy (BCT), the subject of this book, is the most effective couple and family therapy method with by far the largest number of studies supporting its effectiveness in treating substance abuse among adults.[2] Studies show that BCT produces greater abstinence and better relationship functioning than typical individual-based treatment and reduces social costs, domestic violence, and emotional problems of the couple's children. BCT is cited as an empirically supported method by virtually all recent reviews of research on psychosocial treatments for alcoholism and drug abuse and by statements from both NIAAA and NIDA. Thus BCT is well known among substance abuse researchers. Unfortunately, BCT is virtually unknown and unused by practitioners.[3]

So why is there such a huge gap between research and practice where BCT is concerned? We have been asking ourselves this question more and more in recent years as we completed study after study demonstrating the efficacy of BCT but did not see any increased use of BCT in treatment centers around the country. We started our first study of BCT[4] in 1977 and there was a lot about BCT in scientific journal articles over many years, but there was no comprehensive guidebook and treatment manual available on BCT. We started to realize that we may be partly to blame for the research–practice gap in BCT. We concentrated so much on doing studies of BCT that we were not making available the tools counselors need to implement BCT. Once we realized we were part of the problem, we set out to create this book.

In this volume we offer a comprehensive guidebook on BCT for alcoholism and drug abuse. It includes an extensive practitioner guide to BCT with many case examples and consideration of problem cases and challenging clinical situations, plus a session-by-session BCT treatment manual. It shows you how, and provides forms and materials needed, to utilize each part of BCT. You will learn how to (1) engage couples to take part in BCT, (2) support abstinence with a "recovery contract" that involves both members of the couple in a daily ritual to reward abstinence, (3) improve the relationship with techniques for increasing positive activities and improving communication, and (4) plan for continuing recovery to prevent or minimize relapse. Each of these efforts helps BCT achieve its purpose: to build support for abstinence and to improve relationship functioning among married or cohabiting individuals seeking help for alcoholism or drug abuse.

Chapter 1 introduces the background, concepts, and procedures of BCT and provides a detailed preview of the book's contents. Chapters 2–11 describe how to implement the four parts of the BCT program, including recent developments combining BCT with parent training, partner violence prevention, and HIV risk reduction. The closing chapter considers practical issues in implementing BCT in day-to-day practice, such as getting administrative "buy-in" to start a BCT program and choosing between brief versus more extended and one-couple-at-a-time versus couples group BCT formats. Appendices include a session-by-session BCT treatment manual and reproducible checklists, forms, and client education posters that you may copy and use with your clients.

This book is intended to give you, the practitioner, the clinical tools you need to use BCT in your work with substance-abusing individuals and their spouses or domestic partners. Incorporating BCT into your practice should be relatively easy because BCT is readily compatible with 12-step approaches and other types of counseling. The ultimate value of this book will come from your own attempts to apply the methods presented here in your day-to-day work to help substance-abusing patients and their families.

NOTES

1. Keller (1974, p. 116).
2. Epstein and McCrady (1998).
3. Fals-Stewart and Birchler (2001).
4. O'Farrell and Cutter (1977a, 1977b).

Acknowledgments

We thank the many individuals who contributed to this book and to the work on which it is based. We acknowledge our debt to the pioneers in the field on whose work we built: Alan Hedberg, Peter Miller, Nathan Azrin, and Barbara McCrady for their early work on BCT with alcoholism; and Robert Liberman, John Gottman, and Richard Stuart for their work on BCT for marital conflict without substance abuse. A special note of appreciation goes to Gary Birchler who trained Bill Fals-Stewart in BCT, helped Bill launch the first study of BCT with drug abuse, introduced us to each other, and joined together in many collaborative studies of BCT. In addition, we thank Michael Feehan and Michelle Kelley for pushing us to look at the effects of BCT on children, which has now become a very important part of this programmatic line of research.

Tim O'Farrell thanks the following individuals who contributed to his work on BCT: Jane Alter, Judith Bayog, Alfredo Chan, Keith Choquette, Kevin Clancy, Henry Cutter, Marie Fairbanks, David Goodenough, Terence Keane, Fay Larkin, Steve Maisto, Robert McCarley, Jim McKay, Patrice Muchowski, Christopher Murphy, Marie Murphy, Leslie Reid, Rob Rotunda, and Dennis Upper.

Bill Fals-Stewart thanks the following individuals who contributed to his work on BCT: Elizabeth Barkley, David Beniamino, Cyndy Birke, Deborah Birke, Margaret Birke, Beth Bossler-Kogut, Cindy Byrne, Deborah Evans, James Golden, Sally Hayes, Mae Hodge, Todd Kashdan, Keith Klostermann, Timothy Logsdon, Jill Murray, Ellen Roche, Linda Walters, and Jamie Winters.

We gratefully acknowledge funding for our research on BCT that is the basis of this book from the National Institute on Alcohol Abuse and Alcoholism, the National Institute on Drug Abuse, the Department of Veterans Affairs, the Alpha Foundation, the Harry Frank Guggenheim Foundation, and the Smithers Foundation. We appreciate the outstanding work on this book by The Guilford Press, with special thanks to Jim Nageotte, who encouraged us to write this book and shepherded us through each step of the process; Barbara Watkins for her extremely helpful editing of our first draft; and Laura Specht Patchkofsky for her patience and skill in production. Finally, we thank our families for their love, support, and willingness to put up with our hectic work schedules.

Contents

1

An Introduction
to Behavioral Couples Therapy
for Alcoholism and Drug Abuse

Alcoholism and drug abuse have traditionally been viewed as individual problems best treated on an individual basis. However, it is now widely recognized that substance abuse affects not only the individual with the drug or alcohol problem, but also the family members with whom they live. In turn, use of family-involved treatments for alcoholism and drug abuse has become a staple of many substance abuse treatment programs, much to the benefit of the patients and their families.

Although there are several well-described family-based models of addictive behavior and its treatment, the family disease approach is the best known and most widely used family approach in substance abuse treatment programs.[1] Based on the 12-step programs of Alcoholics Anonymous (AA) and Al-Anon, this approach views alcoholism or drug abuse as an illness that affects both the substance abuser and the family. Family members are seen as reacting to the substance abuser with characteristic behavior patterns, such as enabling the addiction by protecting the substance abuser from the negative consequences of drinking or drug taking. This set of behaviors is often called "codependence." The substance abuser is said to suffer from the disease of addiction and the family members from the disease of codependence.

This approach traditionally uses separate parallel recovery programs for the substance abuser and for the family member. The substance abuser gets counseling plus Alcoholics Anonymous (AA) or Narcotics Anonymous (NA). The spouse or family member gets education or counseling plus Al-Anon or Nar-Anon, which involves separate treatment for family members without the substance-abusing patient present. Treatment for the spouse or family member often consists of (1) psychoeducational groups that provide information about the disease concept of addiction and codependency, (2) individual or group therapy to address various psychological issues, and (3) referral to Al-Anon or Nar-Anon. In the recently developed method of Al-

1

Anon facilitation therapy, the family member meets with a counselor, who uses a systematic strategy to encourage involvement in this 12-step program for families of alcoholics.[2]

The family disease approach urges the spouse or family member to give up attempts to influence the substance-abusing patient's drinking or drug use. Family members are told to detach themselves from the patient's substance use in a loving way, accept that they are powerless to control the substance abuser, and seek support from other Al-Anon or Nar-Anon members. They are instructed to focus on themselves in order to reduce their own emotional distress and improve their own coping. This approach puts a primary emphasis on increasing the well-being and serenity of the spouse or family member. It does not focus directly or extensively on supporting the substance abuser's abstinence or on improving couple or family relationships.

Recent studies have shown that family members of alcoholics who were referred to Al-Anon or took part in Al-Anon facilitation therapy reduced their emotional distress and improved their coping more than counterparts in a wait-list control group.[3] An advantage of the family disease approach is that the individual programs of recovery help the substance abuser and the family member to focus strongly on what each of them needs to do to improve his or her life, which has been torn by addiction.

However, the family disease approach does not deal directly with relationship issues, and it may neglect the need for relationship repair and recovery. Family conflicts that are not dealt with constructively can precipitate relapse. Many relationships break up after the substance abuser gets help. Although precise statistics are lacking, one frequently hears in 12-step circles that many marriages and relationships break up in the first year of recovery. Even when the drinking and drugging are gone, intense conflicts may continue, spouses may have grown apart, or one spouse may be unwilling to set aside the past hurts.

All of this would seem to suggest that, to be most effective, family-involved treatments need to address not only drinking and drug use but also relationship and family issues. Behavioral couples therapy (BCT) is an approach that explicitly focuses on both substance use and relationship issues, and it is readily compatible with self-help groups and other counseling.

WHAT IS BCT?

BCT is designed for married or cohabiting individuals seeking help for alcoholism or drug abuse. BCT sees the substance-abusing patient together with the spouse or live-in partner. Its purposes are to build support for abstinence and to improve relationship functioning. BCT pro-

---

TABLE 1.1. BCT for Alcoholism and Drug Abuse

- The purpose of BCT is to support abstinence and improve relationship functioning.
- The Recovery Contract supports abstinence.
- BCT increases positive activities and improves communication.
- BCT fits well with self-help groups, recovery medications, and other counseling.

---

motes abstinence with a "Recovery Contract" that involves both members of the couple in a daily ritual to reward abstinence. BCT improves the relationship with techniques for increasing positive activities and improving communication. Table 1.1 notes key aspects of BCT. Before considering the specific methods used in BCT, we examine some of the ideas behind it.

Ideas behind BCT

THEORETICAL RATIONALE

The causal connections between substance abuse and relationship discord are complex and reciprocal. Couples in which one partner abuses drugs or alcohol usually also have extensive relationship problems, with increased risk of separation or divorce, verbal and physical abuse, and adjustment problems for the couple's children. The negative effects of substance abuse (e.g., lying to cover up substance use, job and legal problems) create relationship problems. Stress from relationship problems, in turn, becomes one more trigger for substance abuse. Thus, as shown in the top half of Figure 1.1, substance abuse and relationship problems create a destructive cycle in which each induces the other.

In the perpetuation of this cycle, couple and family problems (e.g., poor communication and problem solving, habitual arguing, financial stressors) often set the stage for excessive drinking or drug use. There are many ways in which family responses to the substance abuse may then inadvertently promote subsequent abuse. In many instances, for example, drinking or drug use serve relationship needs (at least, in the short term), as when it elicits the expression of emotion and affection through caretaking of a partner suffering from a hangover. Finally, even when recovery from the alcohol or drug problem has begun, couple and family conflicts may often lead to relapse.

This strong interrelationship between substance abuse and relationship issues is largely ignored by standard treatments for substance abuse, which focus mainly on the individual substance-abusing patient. Recognizing these interrelationships, BCT has three primary objectives:

- To eliminate abusive drinking and drug abuse;
- To engage the family's support for the patient's efforts to change; and
- To change couple and family interaction patterns in ways conducive to long-term, stable abstinence and a happier, more stable relationship.

As shown in the bottom half of Figure 1.1, BCT attempts to create a constructive cycle between substance use recovery and improved relationship functioning through interventions that address both sets of issues at the same time.

CLINICAL STANCE

BCT encourages a good-faith–individual-responsibility approach in which each member of the couple freely chooses to make needed changes in his or her behavior independent of whether or not the partner makes corresponding changes in behavior. Thus, we ask each partner to volunteer to make changes that are needed to help the patient stay abstinent and to improve the

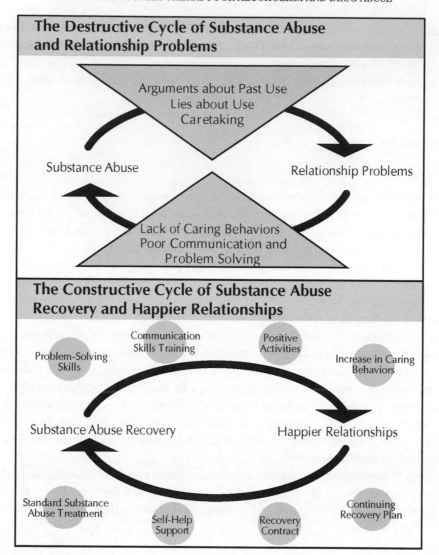

FIGURE 1.1. Reversing a destructive cycle through BCT. From "Behavioral Couples Therapy for Substance Abuse: Rationale, Methods, and Findings," by W. Fals-Stewart, T. J. O'Farrell, and G. R. Birchler, 2004, *Science and Practice Perspectives*, 2, p. 32. Adapted from original, which is in the public domain.

couple's relationship. In BCT we emphasize abstinence as a primary goal that must be achieved before lasting change in couple and other problems is possible. It is only human nature that each member of the couple will want the other to change first and also will want to stop his or her own efforts if the partner does not seem to be making a serious effort to change. The counselor can help both partners understand that really giving their relationship a good chance to improve by changing how they act with each other requires risk and vulnerability—but there is no other way.

BCT does not assume that substance abuse is a symptom of underlying couple dynamics or that, if the couple's dynamics are changed, then the substance-abusing member will no longer need to abuse drugs. Although some early family therapists believed this notion, it no longer has much acceptance because it was not supported by clinical experience. For example, many a family therapist has apparently resolved a couple's relationship problems successfully, only to find that the couple returns to bitter conflict when the substance-abusing member returns to drinking or drug use. From the perspective of BCT, substance abuse is a complex biopsychosocial problem, arising from an individual's vulnerabilities and choices, which is expressed in a social context that includes the couple relationship. In BCT the spouse supports the patient's abstinence and the couple works together to make a happier relationship. BCT is based on the patient's commitment to and pursuit of abstinence and each partner's good-faith commitment to do what they can to improve the relationship.

BCT and 12-Step Concepts

An important strength of BCT is that it can be easily integrated into other intervention services provided by substance abuse treatment programs (e.g., individual counseling, group therapy). The underlying philosophy of, and methods used in, BCT are consistent with the 12-step treatment model that is used in the vast majority of community-based treatment programs. As summarized in Table 1.2, BCT and 12-step work well together. BCT counselors and self-help group members usually share the same treatment goal of abstinence, and both use behavioral and cognitive techniques to achieve their goals. BCT tries to increase and reward behaviors that support abstinence and long-term recovery. Participation in AA and NA are actions that support abstinence and a changed lifestyle conducive to long-term recovery. So it is practical and relatively easy to encourage self-help group involvement and integrate it into BCT. Participation in AA or NA for patients and Al-Anon or Nar-Anon for partners is strongly encouraged in BCT. For those who choose them, these commitments are reviewed at each BCT session, and the counselor reinforces not only attendance at meetings but also the actions of getting a sponsor, speaking at meetings, and so forth. Moreover, when completing a "continuing recovery plan" toward the end of weekly BCT sessions, continued participation in self-help groups is encouraged to help prevent relapse.

TABLE 1.2. BCT and 12-Step Work Well Together

- Both have abstinence as goal.
- BCT rewards behaviors that support abstinence and long-term recovery.
- 12-step supports recovery.
- BCT Recovery Contract often includes 12-step participation.
- Many BCT studies were done in settings with 12-step orientation.
- Many counselors in BCT studies were 12-step proponents.

Most of our studies of BCT were done in settings with a strong 12-step orientation, and nearly all the BCT counselors were proponents of the disease model of addiction. Thus, in our experience, BCT and the disease model of treatment can be easily integrated.

Overview of BCT Methods

Thus far, we have provided a theoretical overview of BCT and a discussion of its easy integration into existing intervention services provided in community-based treatment programs. Yet this begs the question "What is involved in delivering and using BCT with alcoholic and drug-abusing couples?" Although much of this book is devoted to answering this very question, here is a brief preview.

Generally BCT consists of 12–20 weekly couple sessions, each of which lasts 50–60 minutes. Sessions tend to be moderately to highly structured, with the counselor setting the agenda at the outset of each meeting. Typically, the first few BCT sessions focus on establishing a Recovery Contract to support abstinence for the patient and to decrease couple conflicts about past or possible future substance abuse. This contract decreases tension about substance use and builds good will. When abstinence and attendance at BCT sessions have stabilized, the counselor adds relationship-focused interventions to increase positive activities and improve communication. Finally, when abstinence has been maintained for 3–6 months, the counselor plans for continuing recovery to prevent or minimize relapse and reduces BCT sessions from weekly to less frequent sessions.

Table 1.3 lists the main methods used to achieve the four key objectives of BCT: (1) engaging the couple, (2) supporting abstinence, (3) improving the relationship, and (4) continuing recovery. We discuss briefly how BCT supports abstinence and improves the relationship next. Remaining chapters give more details about these and other aspects of BCT.

ENGAGING THE COUPLE AND STARTING BCT

Generally we have run our BCT programs as part of larger substance abuse treatment centers. In such settings the alcoholic and drug-abusing patients have already sought help and begun treatment for themselves. The challenge for the BCT counselor is to get the patient and the spouse to attend an initial session together as a couple. Many substance abuse counselors have had experiences in which they were unsuccessful at engaging the patient and spouse together. We have found it is not that difficult if the counselor follows a few simple steps.

To engage the spouse and the patient together in BCT, first the counselor must get the substance-abusing patient's permission to contact the spouse. Next, the counselor talks directly to the spouse to invite him or her for a joint interview with the patient. Then the counselor takes small steps to gain the couple's commitment to trying BCT. In the joint couple interview, an initial couple session that does not assume further meetings as a couple, the counselor aims to establish rapport and determine if the couple is interested in, and appropriate for, BCT.

If the couple decides to try BCT, it starts in earnest at the second couple session. In this session the couple makes four promises (e.g., not to threaten separation or violence) designed to launch BCT on a positive note. The rest of the second couple session involves negotiating the Recovery Contract to support abstinence, as described next.

TABLE 1.3. Therapeutic Tasks and Specific Procedures in BCT for Alcoholism and Drug Abuse

Engaging the couple for initial sessions

1. Engagement
2. Initial interviews
3. Assessment for BCT
4. Gaining commitment and starting BCT

Supporting abstinence

- Recovery Contract
  1. Daily Trust Discussion
  2. Self-help involvement
  3. Urine drug screens
  4. Medication to aid recovery

- Other support for abstinence
  1. Review substance use or urges to use
  2. Decrease exposure to alcohol and drugs
  3. Address stressful life problems
  4. Decrease behaviors that reward use

Improving the relationship

- Increasing positive activities
  1. "Catch Your Partner Doing Something Nice"
  2. Shared Rewarding Activities
  3. Caring Days

- Improving communication
  1. Communication Sessions
  2. Listening skills
  3. Expressing feelings directly
  4. Negotiating for requests
  5. Conflict resolution
  6. Problem solving

Continuing recovery

1. Continuing Recovery Plan
2. Action plan to prevent or minimize relapse
3. Check-up visits for continuing contact
4. Relapse prevention sessions
5. Couple and family issues in long-term recovery

HOW BCT SUPPORTS ABSTINENCE

Dynamics of the Early Recovery Period

Before the substance abuser seeks help, the substance problem often becomes the focus of much of the couple's interactions. The negative effects of substance abuse lead the couple into an intense, hostile struggle in which the spouse tries desperately to control the substance abuse. In turn the substance abuser, although at times promising to reform or staying abstinent for short periods, continues to drink or use drugs. Such repeated unkept promises to change, and the problems cased by the substance abuser's continued use, lead to a high level of distrust and anger in the spouse.

Frequently by the time the substance abuser seeks help, the couple's interactions have become so intensely focused on substance abuse that although drinking and drug use may have stopped, it is by no means forgotten. The spouse has considerable resentment about past drinking and drug use and fear and distrust about the possible return of substance abuse in the future. The substance abuser, although feeling guilty about problems caused by past drinking or drug use, wants the spouse to recognize his or her efforts to change.

This atmosphere of distrust and conflict often leads to arguments about past or possible future substance abuse—and such conflicts can trigger relapse. In addition, the spouse may complain about past substance abuse, ignore current sober behavior, and question the amount of time that recovery meetings take away from the family. These behaviors are understandable because generally, the spouse has suffered considerable stress from the substance abuse. Nonetheless, the early recovery period is a time when the substance abuser needs support for a new way of life that emphasizes abstinence and a lifestyle that is conducive to abstinence.

The Recovery Contract

COMPONENTS OF THE BCT RECOVERY CONTRACT

The BCT Recovery Contract addresses the issues and dynamics of the early recovery period. It specifies behaviors that each member of the couple can do to reduce distrust and conflict about substance abuse and to reward abstinence and actions leading toward abstinence. The Recovery Contract starts with the "trust discussion" in which the patient states his or her intent not to drink or use drugs that day, the spouse expresses support for the patient's efforts to stay abstinent, and the patient thanks the spouse for the encouragement and support. For patients taking a recovery-related medication (e.g., disulfiram, naltrexone), daily medication ingestion is witnessed and verbally reinforced by the spouse during the trust discussion. Self-help meetings and drug urine screens are part of the contract for most patients. The spouse records performance of the discussion on a calendar, which is provided. Performance of other recovery activities (self-help meetings, drug screens, medication) also is marked on the calendar. The couple agrees not to discuss substance-related conflicts that can trigger relapse, reserving these discussions for the counseling sessions.

DEVELOPMENT AND EVOLUTION OF THE BCT RECOVERY CONTRACT

The BCT Recovery Contract developed from behavioral contracts used to maintain disulfiram (Antabuse) ingestion among alcoholic patients. Disulfiram is a drug that produces extreme nausea and sickness if the person taking it ingests alcohol. Traditional disulfiram therapy often is not effective because the drinker stops taking it when he or she wants to drink. The disulfiram contract was designed to maintain disulfiram and abstinence by having a spouse or significant other witness the medication taking each day. Two slightly different versions of the disulfiram contract appeared in the literature at about the same time.

The BCT version, first described by Peter Miller,[4] included the following elements:

1. Observed ingestion of disulfiram, with mutual thanking by alcoholic and spouse;
2. An early warning system for couple to call if contract was missed 2 days in a row;
3. An established length of time for observing the contract; and
4. Commitment to refrain from discussions about the alcoholic's drinking.

Like all disulfiram contracts, the BCT version seeks to maintain disulfiram ingestion and abstinence. The BCT version also seeks to restructure the couple's relationship to reduce conflicts about past drinking or likelihood of future drinking and to decrease the spouse's anxiety, distrust, and need to control the alcoholic. Such conflicts can lead to relapse.[5] The BCT version tries to deal with these presumed relationship dynamics of the early sobriety period in order to increase support for abstinence and reduce the risk of relapse.

The community reinforcement approach (CRA) version derives from Azrin's[6] attempt to augment the effectiveness of his CRA approach to alcoholism treatment by adding a disulfiram component to it. The CRA version of the disulfiram contract is identical to the BCT version, except that CRA does not include the item restricting discussions about drinking. Multiple outcome studies show that disulfiram contracts in combination with BCT and with CRA increase medication compliance and reduce drinking and alcohol-related problems.[7]

Disulfiram contracts have certain limitations, however. They cannot be used with alcoholic patients who are unwilling or not medically cleared to take disulfiram. They do not apply to most patients who have a primary drug abuse problem. Many treatment programs do not use this medication. The solution to this problem was the Sobriety Trust Contract, first used by Daniel Kivlahan and Elizabeth Shapiro[8] with alcoholic patients who were not taking disulfiram. This procedure is very similar to the trust discussion we currently use in the BCT Recovery Contract, as described above. The trust discussion was a major advance. Although we began using it as a way to include alcoholic patients in BCT who were not taking disulfiram, the clinical response led us to use it with all our BCT patients. Couples responded very favorably to the trust discussion, often embellishing it in highly personal and meaningful ways (e.g., adding a prayer or a hug). It also led to very productive research on BCT with drug-abusing patients.

The most recent evolution over the past decade has involved adding self-help meetings and urine drug screens to the contract. We had always used these with many of our patients but had not integrated them into the contract or recorded them on the contract calendar. We added these components to the contract as we expanded the goals to broadly support abstinence and behaviors leading to abstinence. Couples and clinicians liked these additions, so we have continued them.

Other Support for Abstinence

The Recovery Contract is a major source of support for abstinence. BCT also uses four other methods to promote abstinence, which we describe next.

REVIEWING SUBSTANCE USE OR URGES TO USE

Reviewing substance use or urges to use is part of each BCT session. Discussing situations, thoughts, and feeling associated with urges helps identify potential triggers for alcohol or drug use. Such discussions also can identify successful coping strategies the patient used to resist an urge. If substance use has occurred, crisis intervention is important. BCT works best if the counselor intervenes before the substance use goes on for too long a period. The counselor should help the patient stop using and see the couple as soon as possible to use the relapse as a learning experience. While each BCT session reviews urges or use, time spent on the remaining supports for abstinence depends on the needs of the couple.

DECREASING EXPOSURE TO ALCOHOL AND DRUGS

Exposure to situations where alcohol or drugs are available or others are using such substances is a high risk for relapse among individuals in treatment for substance abuse. BCT sessions can reduce the risk of relapse by discussing how the patient and spouse will deal with such situations. The BCT counselor helps each couple develop their own plan for dealing with common exposure situations, such as whether to have alcohol in the house.

ADDRESSING STRESSFUL LIFE PROBLEMS

Stress caused by unresolved life problems can be a trigger for relapse. Using BCT sessions to help couples resolve or work on life problems, such as financial or legal issues, reduces relapse risk and makes abstinence more rewarding. It also strengthens the therapeutic relationship because the couple comes to view the counselor as someone who cares about their broader life concerns, not just the patient's recovery.

DECREASING PARTNER BEHAVIORS THAT TRIGGER OR REWARD USE

Partners try many ways to cope with their loved one's substance abuse, but some of these coping behaviors can unintentionally trigger or reward substance use. Common examples are giving the user money to buy alcohol or drugs, and lying to others to protect the user. BCT helps the couple identify and stop such behaviors.

HOW BCT IMPROVES RELATIONSHIPS

Relationship Tension in Early Recovery

Once the Recovery Contract is going smoothly, the counselor can focus on improving couple and family relationships. As noted, spouses often experience resentment about past substance abuse and fear and distrust about its return in the future. The patient often experiences guilt and a desire for recognition of current improved behavior. These differing feelings experienced by the patient and spouse often lead to an atmosphere of tension and unhappiness in couple and family relationships.

Problems caused by substance use (e.g., bills, legal charges) need to be resolved. In addition, often there is a backlog of unresolved couple and family problems. Everyday relationship problems typically pile up because the couple's anger and focus on the substance abuse prevent effective communication to resolve the problems. Often the problems are blamed on the substance abuse with the expectation that the problems would resolve with abstinence. However, a woman whose life has revolved around drinking for the past 5 years does not immediately become an attentive, caring wife and mother just because she gets sober. Similarly, a man who has been marginally employed for a number of years due to drug abuse does not become a responsible provider and father overnight just because he becomes abstinent.

Couples frequently lack the mutual positive feelings and communication skills needed to resolve these relationship problems. As a result, many marriages and families break up during the first 1 or 2 years of the patient's recovery. In other cases, couple and family conflicts trigger relapse and a return to substance abuse. Even for couples who do not have serious relationship problems, abstinence can produce temporary tension and role readjustment even as it also provides an opportunity to stabilize and enrich couple and family relationships.

Joan Jackson's pioneering work, based on interviews with women attending Al-Anon, described the stages in the adjustment of the family to the crisis of alcoholism.[9] She described how wives took on more and more family roles as their husbands' alcoholism got worse. The wife took on the main responsibility for parenting, for financial decision making, and often for financial support of the family because the alcoholic husband could not be depended on to carry out these roles. Steinglass also has written about similar adaptations that families and spouses make to maintain (rather than dissolve) the marital and family relationship in the face of continued alcoholism.[10]

When the substance-abusing individual enters treatment and becomes abstinent, the couple often experiences a period of tension and role readjustment. The patient wants to regain some of the roles in the family that were lost. The spouse is reluctant to let go of the roles that have been assumed for fear that abstinence will not last and the patient will cause further problems. In BCT the focus on increasing positives reduces some of the negative feelings over possibly shifting roles. BCT work on communication helps the couple negotiate a shift in roles back to greater trust and responsibility for the patient as abstinence progresses.

BCT relationship-focused interventions have two major goals: (1) to increase positive couple and family activities in order to enhance positive feelings, goodwill, and commitment to the relationship; and (2) to teach communication skills to help the couple resolve conflicts, problems, and desires for relationship change. The general sequence in helping couples increase positive activities and improve communication is (1) therapist instruction and modeling, (2) couple practice (under the counselor's supervision), (3) homework assignment, and (4) review of homework and further practice.

Increasing Positive Activities

BCT uses a number of methods to increase positive couple and family activities. "Catch Your Partner Doing Something Nice" asks each person to notice and acknowledge one nice thing each day that their partner did. "Caring day" involves each person planning ahead to surprise their partner with some special activity to show their caring. "Shared rewarding activities" cultivates fun, either by themselves or with their children or other couples, and can bring the couple closer together.

Improving Communication

Inadequate communication is a major problem for alcoholism and drug abuse patients and their spouses.[11] Once the patient is abstinent, inability to resolve conflicts and problems can cause substance abuse and relationship tensions to recur. Teaching couples how to resolve conflicts and problems can reduce family stress and decrease risk of relapse. BCT includes basic communication skills of effective listening and speaking, and use of planned communication sessions. Couples also learn more advanced skills of conflict resolution, negotiating agreements for desired changes, and problem-solving skills.

These relationship-focused procedures were based on BCT methods developed for couples without alcohol or drug problems by BCT pioneers Robert Liberman, John Gottman, Robert Weiss, Gary Birchler, and Richard Stuart.[12] O'Farrell adapted these procedures for use with alcoholic patients,[13] Fals-Stewart applied the procedures to drug-abusing patients,[14] and together we updated the procedures for use in a series of collaborative studies of BCT in alcoholism and drug abuse.[15]

CONTINUING RECOVERY IN BCT

Most couples who attend BCT sessions faithfully show substantial improvement. However, when the structure of the weekly BCT sessions ends, there is a natural tendency for backsliding. Therefore it is critical to help couples maintain the gains they made in BCT and prevent or minimize relapse. Near the end of weekly sessions, the BCT counselor helps the couple make (1) a Continuing Recovery Plan that specifies which aspects of BCT (e.g., trust discussion) they wish to continue, and (2) an Action Plan of steps to prevent or minimize relapse. Couple "checkup" visits every few months for an extended period can encourage continued progress. Finally, those with more severe problems may benefit from periodic couple relapse prevention sessions in the year after weekly BCT ends.

WHO ARE APPROPRIATE CLIENTS FOR BCT?

BCT works directly to increase relationship factors conducive to abstinence. A behavioral approach assumes that family members can reward abstinence—and that alcoholic and drug-abusing patients from happier, more cohesive relationships with better communication have a lower risk of relapse. Typically, the substance-abusing patient and the spouse are seen together in BCT for 12–20 weekly outpatient couple sessions over a 3- to 6-month period, followed by periodic maintenance contacts. BCT can be an adjunct to individual counseling or it can be the only substance abuse counseling the patient receives. To reiterate: BCT fits well with recovery-related medications and with Alcoholics Anonymous, Al-Anon, and other self-help groups. The couple starts BCT soon after the substance abuser seeks help. BCT can start immediately after detoxification or a short-term intensive rehab program or when the substance abuser seeks outpatient counseling.

Definitely Suitable Cases

Generally, "definitely suitable" couples have been married or cohabiting for at least a year and are living together when they start BCT. Only one member of the couple has a current problem with alcoholism or drug abuse. He or she accepts at least temporary abstinence as a goal. Both partners are willing to work together to see if their substance abuse and relationship problems can be improved. Neither member of the couple has a history of a psychotic disorder. These definitely suitable cases represent the majority of couples counselors will see in a typical substance abuse treatment setting. They are the cases for which BCT has been shown to be effective in outcome studies. Other possibly suitable cases are addressed briefly next.

Cases Possibly Suitable for BCT

• *Separated couples* generally cannot be together frequently enough to provide the daily support that is critical to the success of BCT. Often the counselor can see the couple for some initial sessions to negotiate a return to living together. Once the couple has reunited, BCT proceeds as with other couples.

• *"Dual couples"*—couples in which both the male and female member have a current substance abuse problem—may benefit from BCT only under certain circumstances. If both members want to stop drinking and drugging when they first see the counselor, or if this mutual decision to seek abstinence can be attained during the first few couple sessions, then BCT generally is workable. However, when only one member of the couple wants to change, this person should get individual counseling; BCT is not advised.

• *Couples with severe emotional problems* in the substance abuser or the spouse often may not benefit from BCT. Nonetheless, our clinical experience suggests that at times BCT may be effective with such cases, when it is used along with appropriate individual therapy and psychotropic medication for the emotionally troubled person. In such cases, BCT sessions proceed slowly and are carefully tailored to the special needs of such clients.

• *Couples seen outside a substance abuse treatment setting* may present challenges for BCT. Studies showing BCT effectiveness were conducted in substance abuse treatment settings and research projects. In such settings, participants recognize the substance problem and are ready to address it, at least to some degree. In other settings, such as typical office practice of psychotherapy or marriage and family counseling, clients often are not ready to address the substance problem. Therefore, in other settings, BCT may work only if a client has, or can be helped to develop, the needed readiness for change.

Cases Definitely Not Suitable for BCT

Contraindications for BCT relate to legal and safety issues. Couples in which there is a court-issued restraining order for the spouses not to have contact with each other should not be seen together in therapy until the restraining order is lifted or modified to allow contact in counseling. Some situations present concerns for the safety of participants in BCT. If the clinical assessment indicates that there is an active and acute risk for very severe domestic violence (i.e., could cause serious injury or be potentially life-threatening), then it is better not to use BCT. As described in more detail in Chapter 10, couples are excluded from BCT if very severe violence (defined as resulting in injury requiring medical attention or hospitalization) has occurred in the past 2 years, or if one or both members of the couple fear that taking part in couples treatment may stimulate violence. Although domestic violence is quite common among substance-abusing patients, most of this violence is not so severe that it precludes BCT. In our experience fewer than 2% of couples seeking BCT are excluded from treatment due to very severe violence or fears of couples therapy. The best plan in most cases is to address the violence in BCT sessions. Research reviewed below shows that violence is substantially reduced after BCT and virtually eliminated for patients who stay abstinent. Table 1.4 summarizes key points about who are appropriate clients for BCT.

HOW TO BE AN EFFECTIVE BCT COUNSELOR

Address Substance Abuse First

Certain counselor attributes and behaviors are important for successful BCT with alcoholic and drug-abusing patients. From the outset, the counselor must structure BCT sessions so that abstinence from alcohol and illicit drugs is the first priority, before attempting to help the couple with other problems. Many of our clients have had previous unsuccessful experiences with couple and family therapists who saw the couple without dealing with the substance abuse problem. The hope that reducing relationship problems will lead to improvement in the sub-

---

TABLE 1.4. Suitability of Cases for BCT

Definitely suitable cases

- Married or cohabiting couples
- Reside together (i.e., not separated)
- Only one has current substance problem
- Both partners accept the need for temporary abstinence at least
- Both partners are willing to work on problems
- Neither partner has history of psychosis
- Start after detox, rehab, or no prior treatment

Possibly suitable cases

- Separated couples
- Both partners have current substance problems
- One partner has severe emotional problems
- Not in a substance abuse treatment setting

Definitely not suitable cases

- High risk of injurious/lethal violence
- Restraining order prohibiting contact

---

stance abuse problem rarely is fulfilled. More typically, recurrent substance-related incidents undermine whatever gains have been made in couple and family relationships.

Deal Effectively with Anger

The counselor needs to be able to tolerate and deal effectively with strong anger in early sessions and at later times of crisis. The counselor can use empathic listening to help each person feel that he or she has been heard, and the counselor can insist that only one person speak at a time. Helping the couple defuse their intense anger is very important because failure to do so often leads to a poor outcome.

Structure and Control Sessions

The counselor also needs to structure and take control of treatment sessions, especially the early assessment and therapy phase and at later times of crisis (e.g., episodes of drinking or intense family conflict). Structured therapy sessions with a directive, active counselor are more effective than is a less structured mode of therapy. Many counselors' errors involve difficulty establishing and maintaining control of the sessions and responding to the myriad forms of resistance and noncompliance presented by couples. The counselor needs to steer a middle course between lack of structure and being overly controlling and punitive in response to noncompliance. The counselor needs to clearly establish and enforce the rules of treatment and also acknowledge approximation to desired behavior despite significant shortcomings.

Empathize Readily with Both Partners

Other counselor qualities can promote successful BCT. The counselor needs to empathize with each person and not take sides, favoring one over the other on a consistent basis, or join the spouse in scapegoating the substance abuser. Using humor constructively can contribute to patients' feeling comfortable. Practical knowledge of financial and legal issues commonly faced by substance abusers and their families also can help. A further helpful stance, often used by counselors in BCT, is to act as educator or "coach" by teaching behavioral techniques to deal with substance use (e.g., monitoring urges to drink) or relationship issues (e.g., communication skills).

Do Not Impose Your Own Beliefs on Couple

Counselors also need to be aware of their own beliefs and experiences regarding relationships and recovery. If a counselor's divorce led to a happier second marriage, he or she may naturally be more inclined to see separation as a positive option for clients than would a counselor who stayed with a difficult relationship that improved over time. The important point is that counselors should try not to impose their own beliefs on patients. Patients and their partners need to make their own decisions based on their own values and experiences. Similarly, counselors who are recovering themselves might tend to think their patients should do what worked for them. Of course, just because the counselor did "90 meetings in 90 days" does not mean everyone should.

Avoid Blame and Maintain Contact

The counselor needs to take a long-term view of the course of change. Both the alcohol or drug problem and associated relationship problems may be helped substantially only by repeated efforts, including some failed attempts. Such a long-term view may help the counselor encounter relapse without becoming overly discouraged or engaging in blaming and recriminations with the substance abuser and spouse. The counselor also should maintain contact with the couple long after the problems apparently have stabilized. Leaving such contacts to the couple usually means that no follow-up contacts occur until they are back in a major crisis again.

Forge a Strong Therapeutic Relationship

A strong therapeutic relationship can keep the patient and spouse coming to therapy, especially early in treatment when risk for dropout is high. Patients and spouses are likely to continue in therapy if they consider the counselor a knowledgeable and helpful guide to the process of substance abuse and relationship recovery. As described above, counselors who develop successful relationships with their patients have the ability (1) to put "first things first" by giving priority to the substance use problem, (2) to defuse and manage anger, (3) to be fair and show evenhanded understanding of each person's viewpoint, and (4) to steer a steady course through the confusing emotions and family conflicts encountered in substance abuse recovery. The therapeutic relationship is strengthened when the counselor takes an active role to help clients deal with the everyday problems that arise between sessions in coping with recovery, relapse, and relationships. Finally, whenever possible, it helps to have clients leave therapy sessions on a positive note, feeling as good as, or better than, when they arrived. This improvement will make them want to return for the next session and promote continued treatment.

Background and Training Needed

Ideally a counselor conducting BCT with substance abuse patients would have a master's degree or higher in psychology, social work, or counseling. Training should include courses on the nature and treatment of both substance abuse and marital and family problems, and supervised clinical experiences providing individual, couple, and family counseling for patients with alcohol and drug problems. Counselors also need training in basic cognitive-behavioral methods for treating substance abuse.

Clearly this level of training is an ideal that often is not a practical reality. Most graduate programs and internships do not provide training in substance abuse or in family problems of substance abuse patients. Many counselors in substance abuse settings learn on the job. In our projects, experienced substance abuse counselors have become proficient in BCT. In fact, we trained bachelor's level counselors to deliver BCT,[16] but they received intensive, ongoing supervision in BCT that is not available in most settings. On the other hand, we have noticed that a couple or family therapist with little substance abuse experience may have some difficulty learning BCT. Such therapists often do not give the necessary priority to the substance abuse problem and the substance-focused parts of BCT.

Table 1.5 summarizes key counselor attributes and behaviors that are important for successful BCT.

TABLE 1.5. How To Be An Effective BCT Counselor

- Address substance abuse problem first.
- Tolerate and defuse strong anger.
- Structure and control sessions.
- Empathize readily with both partners.
- Do not impose your own beliefs.
- Use positive approach with humor.
- Know common legal and money problems.
- Avoid blame and hopelessness.
- Maintain long-term contact with couples.
- Forge a strong therapeutic relationship.

EFFECTIVENESS OF BCT

Randomized studies show that family-involved treatment in alcoholism and drug abuse results in more abstinence than does individual treatment.[17] BCT is the family therapy method with the strongest research support for its effectiveness in treating substance abuse among adults.[18] BCT produces greater abstinence and better relationship functioning than typical individual-based treatment and reduces social costs, domestic violence, and the emotional problems of couples' children.

Primary Clinical Outcomes: Abstinence and Relationship Functioning

Studies comparing substance abuse and relationship outcomes for substance-abusing patients treated with BCT or individual counseling show a fairly consistent pattern of results. Substance-abusing patients who receive BCT have more abstinence and fewer substance-related problems, happier relationships, and lower risk of couple separation and divorce than those who receive only typical individual-based treatment. These results come from studies with mostly male alcoholic[19] and drug-abusing[20] patients. Two studies (one in alcoholism and one in drug abuse) show the same pattern of results with female patients.[21] Drug abuse patients for which BCT had better outcomes than individual treatment include heterogeneous samples (mostly cocaine and heroin), methadone maintenance patients, and heroin patients taking naltrexone. These BCT studies have included diverse patient populations, with: (1) income levels ranging from public assistance to solidly middle class, (2) minority group representation from almost none to over half African American, and (3) gay and lesbian patients and their same-sex partners.[22]

Reduced Social Costs

The social costs of substance abuse include treatment, substance-related crimes, and public assistance. Studies have examined whether BCT reduced these costs. In three studies (two in alcoholism and one in drug abuse),[23] the average social costs per case decreased substantially in the 1–2 years after, as compared to the year before, BCT. Cost savings averaged $5,000–$6,500 per case. The costs saved by BCT was more than five times the cost of delivering it, producing a benefit-to-cost ratio greater than 5:1. For every dollar spent in delivering BCT, $5 in social costs are saved. In addition, BCT was more cost-effective when compared with individual treatment for drug abuse and when compared with interactional couples therapy for alcoholism.

Reduced Domestic Violence

Two studies reported that male-to-female partner violence was significantly reduced in the first and second year after BCT, and it was nearly eliminated with abstinence.[24] In two other studies, BCT reduced partner violence and couple conflicts better than individual treatment.[25] These results suggest that couples learn to handle their conflicts with less hostility and aggression in BCT.

Impact of BCT on the Children of Couples

Kelley and Fals-Stewart[26] conducted two studies (one in alcoholism, one in drug abuse) to find out whether BCT for a substance-abusing parent also has beneficial effects for the children in the family. Results were the same for children of male alcoholic and male drug-abusing fathers. BCT improved children's functioning in the year after the parents' treatment more than did individual-based treatment or couple psychoeducation. Only BCT couples showed reduction in the number of children with clinically significant impairment.

Increased Compliance with Recovery-Related Medication

BCT has been used to increase compliance with recovery-related medications. Male BCT patients stopping opioid use had better naltrexone (Trexan) compliance compared with their individually treated counterparts. The better compliance led to greater abstinence and fewer substance-related problems.[27] Another study found that BCT produced better compliance with HIV medications among HIV-positive drug abusers in an outpatient treatment program than did treatment as usual.[28] BCT also has improved compliance of alcoholic patients with disulfiram (Antabuse)[29] and with naltrexone (ReVia).[30]

Evidence Supports Wider Use of BCT

Table 1.6 summarizes key points about the effectiveness of BCT, an approach that needs wider application by counselors so that patients and their families can benefit from this evidence-based method of treating alcoholism and drug abuse. A major obstacle to this wider application has been that, until now, there has been no guide showing how to implement BCT.

PREVIEW OF THIS BOOK

This book is written as a clinical guide for counselors who want to use BCT with patients seeking outpatient treatment for alcoholism or drug abuse. It also is a resource for marriage and family counselors who treat couples with substance abuse problems. Chapters 2–8 describe how to implement the BCT program outlined in Table 1.3. First, the counselor engages the

TABLE 1.6. What Studies of BCT Show

- BCT produces more abstinence, happier relationships, and fewer separations than individual treatment.
- Benefit-to-cost ratio for BCT is greater than 5 to 1.
- Domestic violence is greatly reduced after BCT.
- BCT helps a couple's children more than individual treatment for the substance-abusing parent.
- BCT improves compliance with recovery medications (e.g., disulfiram, naltrexone).
- Evidence supports wider use of BCT.

patient and spouse for initial couple sessions in which the counselor assesses substance abuse and relationship functioning and gains commitment to starting BCT (as shown in Chapter 2). BCT begins with the Recovery Contract and other substance-focused interventions that continue throughout the therapy to promote abstinence (as shown in Chapters 3 and 4). The next step in BCT is to add relationship-focused interventions to increase positive activities (Chapter 5) and improve communication (Chapters 6 and 7). Finally, when the couple has progressed and it is time to stop weekly BCT sessions, the counselor helps them plan for continuing recovery to prevent or minimize relapse (as shown in Chapter 8). Chapters 2–8 cover BCT with what we call *definitely suitable cases*: married or cohabiting couples with one substance-abusing member and without very severe violence or psychosis. As noted, such cases constitute the majority of couples counselors will see and those for which BCT has been shown effective.

Chapters 9–11 cover challenges and enhancements to BCT. Chapter 9 shows how to use BCT with potentially suitable couples who are separated or where both members have a current substance problem. Chapter 10 takes a detailed look at partner violence among couples treated in BCT. Earlier chapters give the standard BCT approach to partner violence: Assess violence history, exclude the very small number of couples with histories of very severe violence, monitor commitment to nonviolence, teach communication and conflict resolution skills, and coach nonusing spouses on how to stay safe if relapse occurs. Chapter 10 provides an in-depth rationale for using BCT with couples who have experienced violence and gives extended case examples. Chapter 10 also recaps solutions to common challenges in BCT (e.g., noncompliance with homework). (Another good place to look for answers to BCT challenges are the frequently asked questions at the end of each chapter.) Chapter 11 shows how we enhanced BCT outcomes by adding parent training and an HIV-risk reduction module, and by expanding BCT to family members other than a spouse. Although these enhancements have not been fully researched, we included them because they appear promising.

The closing chapter considers practical issues in implementing BCT in day-to-day practice in substance abuse treatment centers and other settings. It has suggestions for counselors who want to get started with BCT and for those who want to establish an ongoing BCT program. For example, we suggest that counselors start using BCT with couples who are likely to benefit (i.e., definitely suitable couples) to build their skill and confidence in BCT before moving on to more difficult situations. Chapter 12 also considers the various formats in which BCT has been delivered. Most often we have used BCT with one couple at a time, but we also have used a BCT couples group format. Typically BCT has ranged from 12 weekly sessions to a flexible length program of 20 sessions or more. We have used BCT in many different community-based substance abuse treatment programs, where BCT was combined with individual-based treatment for the patient that included 12-step, cognitive-behavioral, or treatment as usual provided in individual or group counseling.

This book describes a set of BCT procedures that counselors can use flexibly with their patients, basing the timing of interventions on their judgement of patients' needs. Counselors also may find helpful a session-by-session treatment manual they can follow. Appendix A contains a 12-session BCT treatment manual. Each session includes a therapist checklist and an outline. Once familiar with BCT, a counselor can use the checklist to guide his or her implementation of the session. Appendix B contains posters that we often use to convey key points to couples receiving BCT. These posters can be enlarged and kept in the counselor's office for use in BCT sessions. Appendix C contains BCT-related forms that can be copied by counselors for use with their own couples.

Sequence of Interventions in BCT

Table 1.7 shows how the therapeutic tasks and interventions of BCT unfold over the sequence of couple sessions. The table shows a 12-session weekly format of core BCT sessions preceded by initial couple engagement sessions and followed by elective periodic maintenance sessions. Sessions are also broken into "early," "middle," and "later" phases of BCT for flexible expansion to BCT formats with more than 12 sessions. As shown in the table, assessment and commitment interventions that begin before BCT may continue for the first few core BCT sessions in some cases. The sequence of interventions in the core BCT sessions is described as follows.

RECOVERY CONTRACT

The couple starts doing the daily trust discussion in the first BCT session and continues this practice through all sessions. Depending on the couple's needs and willingness, other components (i.e., 12-step meetings, drug screens, medication) may be part of the Recovery Contract. If so, these other components usually start in the first few BCT sessions and continue to the end of the therapy.

OTHER SUPPORT FOR ABSTINENCE

Review of substance use and urges is part of every session. Other components (i.e., decreasing substance exposure, stressful problems, enabling) are first addressed in early sessions if needed by the couple. Most couples need some attention given to stressful problems and substance exposure. Whether these other components are continued in subsequent sessions is based on the particular needs of the couple.

INCREASING POSITIVE ACTIVITIES

"Catch Your Partner Doing Something Nice" may start as early as the first BCT session. Other components (shared rewarding activities and caring days) are phased in during the early sessions. Starting with the middle sessions and continuing to the end of BCT, the couple picks at least one of the three assignments to carry out each week.

TABLE 1.7. Sequence of Therapeutic Tasks and Sessions in BCT for Alcoholism and Drug Abuse

Therapeutic tasks	Before core BCT sessions	Early sessions 1	2	3	4	Middle sessions 5	6	7	8	Later sessions 9	10	11	12	After core BCT sessions
Initial couple sessions														
1. Engagement	X													
2. Initial interview	X													
3. Assessment for BCT	X	(X)	(X)											
4. Gaining commitment and starting BCT	X	(X)												
Supporting abstinence														
• Recovery Contract														
1. Daily Trust Discussion		X	X	X	X	X	X	X	X	X	X	X	X	C
2. Self-help involvement		(X)1	(X)1	(X)1	(X)1	(X)1	(X)1	(X)1	(X)1	(X)1	(X)1	(X)1	(X) 1	C
3. Urine drug screens		(X)1	(X)1	(X)1	(X)1	(X)1	(X)1	(X)1	(X)1	(X)1	(X)1	(X)1	(X)1	C
4. Medication to aid recovery		(X)1	(X)1	(X)1	(X)	(X)1	(X)1	(X)1	(X)1	(X)1	(X)1	(X)1	(X)1	C
• Other Support for Abstinence														
1. Review substance use or urges to use		X	X	X	X	X	X	X	X	X	X	X	X	C
2. Decrease exposure to alcohol and drugs			X	X	X	(X)	(X)	(X)	(X)	(X)	(X)	(X)	(X)	C
3. Address stressful life problems			X	X	X	(X)	(X)	(X)	(X)	(X)	(X)	(X)	(X)	C
4. Decrease behaviors that reward use					(X)	(X)	(X)	(X)	(X)	(X)	(X)	(X)	(X)	C
Improving the relationship														
• Increasing Positive Activities														
1. "Catch Your Partner Doing Something Nice" (and tell him or her)		X	X			(X)2	(X)2	(X)2	(X)2	(X)2	(X)2	(X)2	(X)2	C
2. Shared Rewarding Activities				X	X	(X)2	(X)2	(X)2	(X)2	(X)2	(X)2	(X)2	(X)2	C
3. Caring Days				X	X	(X)2	(X)2	(X)2	(X)2	(X)2	(X)2	(X)2	(X)2	C

(continued)

21

TABLE 1.7. (continued)

Therapeutic tasks	Before core BCT sessions	Core BCT sessions												After core BCT sessions
		Early sessions				Middle sessions				Later sessions				
		1	2	3	4	5	6	7	8	9	10	11	12	
● Improving Communication														
1. Communication sessions					X	X	X	X	X	X	X	X	X	C
2. Listening skills						X	X	X	X	X	X	X	X	C
3. Expressing feelings directly							X	X	X	X	X	X	X	C
4. Negotiating for requests								X	X	(X)	(X)	(X)	(X)	C
5. Conflict resolution									X	X	(X)	(X)	(X)	C
6. Problem solving										X	X	(X)	(X)	C
Continuing Recovery														
1. Continuing Recovery Plan											X	X	X	C
2. Action Plan to prevent or minimize relapse												X	X	C
3. Checkup visits for continuing contact														(X)
4. Relapse prevention sessions														(X)
5. Couple and family issues in long-term recovery														(X)

Note. X = This task is part of this session for all or nearly all couples; (X) = this task *may be* part of this session, depending on the couple's needs and choices and the counselor's recommendation; 1 = if part of couple's treatment, this task is part of all BCT sessions; 2 = couple picks at least one of the three positive activities to do for this session; C = partners may choose to continue this procedure after weekly core BCT sessions end, as part of their own self-directed Continuing Recovery Plan or as part of additional checkup visits or relapse prevention sessions conducted by the counselor.

22

IMPROVING COMMUNICATION

Basic skills of effective listening and speaking and use of planned communication sessions are introduced starting at the end of the early sessions. These basic skills are part of all subsequent sessions because they are used in all the more advanced communication skills (i.e., negotiating requests, resolving conflicts, problem solving). Each of these more advanced skills is introduced for two sessions starting toward the end of the middle sessions, and may be continued in later sessions, depending on the particular needs of the couple.

CONTINUING RECOVERY

In the last three BCT sessions, couples focus on their Continuing Recovery Plan of activities to continue after BCT and their Action Plan to prevent or minimize relapse. Finally, depending on the couple's needs and willingness, the counselor may schedule additional checkup visits or relapse prevention sessions after the weekly core BCT sessions end.

A Note on Terminology

As we end this introductory chapter, a note on the terminology used throughout the book may be helpful. We use the term "substance-abusing patient" or just "patient" to indicate generically the alcoholic or drug-abusing member of a couple. Similarly, we use the term "substance abuse" generically to refer to problems with either alcohol or drugs or both. If a specific substance (e.g., alcohol, cocaine) is at issue, it is referred to specifically. We use the term "spouse" or "partner" interchangeably to indicate the non-substance-abusing spouse or unmarried live-in partner who is in a couple relationship with the patient. These terms refer to couples in which only one member has a current substance problem (the majority of the couples described in this book). When we refer to couples in which both members have a substance problem, this is indicated. Each case example we present in this book is a composite case with individual identities disguised to protect the privacy and anonymity of the couples with whom we have worked. Finally, starting with frequently asked questions below and continuing throughout the book, we address our comments in the form of a dialogue with you, the reader, our colleague and potential BCT counselor.

FREQUENTLY ASKED QUESTIONS

- *Question 1*: You advocate starting BCT right after the patient leaves detox, during the early recovery period. I thought you were not supposed to do couple or family counseling until the substance-abusing patient has had at least a year of abstinence. The patient needs to focus on him- or herself. Couples therapy may lead to relapse because it distracts the patient from the priority of staying abstinent, or it stirs up negative emotions that the patient isn't ready to deal with.
- *Answer*: This was a popular belief for many years. However, as described above, studies do not support this belief. After more than 30 years of research on couples therapy during the early recovery period, outcome data show that patients who get BCT are *less likely* to relapse than patients who get only individual substance abuse counseling. As you will see in later chapters, BCT helps the patient stay focused on abstinence, and it helps the couple deal construc-

tively with strong anger and resentments without breaking up—or the patient breaking out. The belief that couples counseling should be delayed may come from advice in AA that it is unwise to make major changes in the first year of abstinence. This advice, which is particularly strong against starting a new relationship or ending an existing one, seems like pretty good advice for many people. The early recovery period is a good time to "take it easy" and not make impulsive choices on major life decisions. However, extending this advice to prohibit couple and family counseling seems like an overgeneralization.

- *Question 2*: If a substance-abusing patient has serious relationship problems that interfere with his or her recovery, BCT might make sense. But you seem to be advocating BCT for nearly all patients with a spouse or live-in partner. If relationship problems or issues are not interfering with the patient's recovery, why should the patient get BCT? How would BCT help such patients?

- *Answer*: When we started in the field over 25 years ago, we assumed that all, or nearly all, alcoholism and drug abuse patients had serious relationship problems and could benefit from therapy to address these problems. Two things have changed over the years. First, although studies show that most substance abuse patients do have relationship problems, the problem severity varies considerably; some have very serious problems, whereas others score in the nonproblem range on relationship adjustment measures.[31] Second, we have changed our focus from one of couples therapy to alleviate relationship distress to one of BCT with the dual goals of helping the patient stay abstinent and helping the couple get along better. Even patients without serious relationship problems can benefit from BCT to help them stay abstinent. BCT should not be reserved for substance abuse patients who have serious relationship problems secondary to, preceding, or coexisting with the substance abuse problem. Couples with less serious problems often are better able to work together to help the patient stay abstinent and to enrich their relationship, which has been strained by substance-related stressors. Further, even when couple factors do not play an important role in triggering or maintaining the substance abuse, involving the spouse in BCT may help the patient stay abstinent while learning how to deal with triggers for substance use that are outside the relationship. In addition, BCT can help support healthier activities (e.g., involvement with children and spouse) that are incompatible with substance abuse.

- *Question 3*: You said that BCT can be an adjunct to individual counseling, or it can be the only substance abuse counseling the patient receives. When can BCT be the only counseling the patient receives?

- *Answer*: Our answer is based solely on clinical experience because research has not examined this question. BCT is frequently delivered as part of a comprehensive treatment package that includes individual and group therapy for the identified substance-abusing patient. However, some patients can benefit from BCT without other ongoing counseling. Patients with less severe problems may benefit from BCT alone. Patients who have a strong commitment to a 12-step self-help program and make this part of their BCT Recovery Contract may not need individual counseling. Alcoholic patients who take Antabuse or opioid-dependent patients who take naltrexone often do well with BCT alone, because they tend to stay on these medications as part of the BCT daily Recovery Contract. Patients who have had prior successful treatment, accept they have an addiction, and know what they need to do to stay abstinent (but need support to do it) benefit from the structure of BCT and the monitoring of the Recovery Contract. Patients who are likely to need both BCT and individual counseling include those with more severe substance abuse problems, those with comorbid psychiatric problems, and those who are new to substance abuse treatment or very ambivalent about abstinence.

SUMMARY

- The 12-step Al-Anon family disease approach is the most widely used approach for dealing with family issues in recovery. It emphasizes separate individual programs for the patient and the spouse. Al-Anon helps reduce family members' emotional distress, but it does not deal directly with relationship issues. So BCT may have a role to play in recovery programs.

- This chapter introduced you to behavioral couples therapy (BCT), in which a substance-abusing patient and his or her spouse work together each day to support abstinence and improve their relationship. BCT promotes abstinence with a "Recovery Contract" that involves both members of the couple in a daily ritual to reward abstinence. BCT improves the relationship by implementing techniques that increase positive activities and improve communication.

- Couples are "definitely suitable" for BCT if (1) they are married or living together, (2) one member has a current substance problem and accepts the need for at least temporary abstinence, (3) both are willing to work together for improvement, and (4) there is no acute risk of very severe partner violence or a history of psychosis. "Possibly suitable" cases already mentioned are considered further in Chapters 9 and 10.

- Successful BCT counselors have the ability (1) to put "first things first" by giving priority to the substance use problem, (2) to defuse and manage anger, (3) to be fair and show even-handed understanding of each person's viewpoint, and (4) to steer a steady course through the confusing emotions and family conflicts encountered in substance abuse recovery.

- Research has shown that BCT produces greater abstinence and better relationship functioning than more typical individual-based treatment, and it reduces social costs, domestic violence, and emotional problems of couples' children.

- Although some believe that 6–12 months of abstinence are needed before couples counseling is advised, we advocate starting BCT when the patient leaves detox. Concerns that couples therapy may lead to relapse by distracting patients from the priority of staying abstinent or stirring up negative emotions have not been borne out. Over 30 years of research show that patients who get BCT in the early recovery period are *less likely* to relapse than patients who get only individual counseling.

- BCT has dual goals of helping the patient stay abstinent and the couple get along better. Even patients without serious relationship problems can benefit from BCT to help them stay abstinent. Therefore, BCT should be provided for all couples, not just those who have serious relationship problems.

- BCT is frequently part of a comprehensive treatment program that includes individual and group therapy for the substance-abusing patient. However, some patients can benefit from BCT without other ongoing counseling if they have less severe problems, a strong commitment to AA or NA, take recovery medication, have had prior successful treatment, and accept they have an addiction.

- Starting in the next chapter, this book provides "how to" instructions to counselors who want to use BCT with patients seeking outpatient treatment for alcoholism or drug abuse.

NOTES

1. For more information on the family disease approach, see (a) program information from Al-Anon (e.g., Al-Anon Family Groups, 1981), (b) Nowinski's (1999) therapist manual for Al-Anon facilitation, (c) Laundergan and Williams (1993) on the family psychoeducational program at Hazelden, (d) Dittrich (1993) on group therapy for wives of alcoholic men, and (e) O'Farrell and Fals-Stewart (2003).
2. A therapist manual for Al-Anon facilitation therapy is available (Nowinski, 1999).
3. O'Farrell and Fals-Stewart (2003).
4. Miller (1976); Miller and Hersen (1975).
5. Maisto, McKay, and O'Farrell (1995); Maisto, O'Farrell, Connors, McKay, and Pelcovits (1988).
6. Azrin (1976).
7. For a review of the use of BCT to increase compliance with disulfiram, see O'Farrell, Allen, and Litten (1995).
8. Personal communication, May 18, 1984.
9. Jackson (1955).
10. Steinglass, Bennett, Wolin, and Reiss (1987).
11. O'Farrell and Birchler (1987).
12. Gottman, Notarius, Gonso, and Markman (1976); Liberman, Wheeler, DeVisser, Keuhnel, and Keuhnel (1980); Stuart (1980); Weiss, Birchler, and Vincent (1974).
13. O'Farrell and Cutter (1984a).
14. Fals-Stewart, Birchler, and O'Farrell (1996).
15. O'Farrell and Fals-Stewart (2000).
16. Fals-Stewart and Birchler (2002).
17. O'Farrell and Fals-Stewart (2001); Stanton and Shadish (1997).
18. Epstein and McCrady (1998).
19. Azrin, Sisson, Meyers, and Godley (1982); Bowers and Al-Redha, (1990); Chick et al. (1992); Fals-Stewart, Klosterman, Yates, O'Farrell, and Birchler (2005); Fals-Stewart and O'Farrell (2002); Hedberg and Campbell (1974); Kelley and Fals-Stewart (2002); McCrady, Stout, Noel, Abrams, and Nelson (1991); O'Farrell, Cutter, Choquette, Floyd, and Bayog (1992).
20. Fals-Stewart et al. (1996); Fals-Stewart and O'Farrell (2003); Fals-Stewart, O'Farrell, and Birchler (2001a, 2001b); Kelley and Fals-Stewart (2002).
21. Fals-Stewart, Birchler, and Kelley (in press); Winters, Fals-Stewart, O'Farrell, Birchler, and Kelley (2002).
22. Hequembourg, Hoebbel, Fals-Stewart, O'Farrell, and Birchler (2004).
23. Fals-Stewart, O'Farrell, and Birchler (1997); O'Farrell, Choquette, Cutter, Brown, et al. (1996); O'Farrell, Choquette, Cutter, Floyd, et al. (1996).
24. O'Farrell and Murphy (1995); O'Farrell, Murphy, Stephan, Fals-Stewart, and Murphy (2004).
25. Birchler and Fals-Stewart (2001); Fals-Stewart, Kashdan, O'Farrell, and Birchler (2002).
26. Kelley and Fals-Stewart (2002).
27. Fals-Stewart and O'Farrell (2003).
28. Fals-Stewart, O'Farrell, and Martin (2002).
29. Azrin et al. (1982); Chick et al. (1992); O'Farrell et al. (1992).
30. Fals-Stewart and O'Farrell (2002).
31. Fals-Stewart, Birchler, and O'Farrell (1999); O'Farrell and Birchler (1987).

2

Engaging the Couple
Initial Couple Sessions

This chapter describes how to get both the substance-abusing patient and his or her spouse to your office, how to conduct the initial couple session to explore the possibility of starting BCT, and how to get the couple started in BCT. Depending on the couple's initial interest and readiness for BCT, there may be one or two initial couple sessions before the couple starts the core BCT program.

GETTING THE PATIENT AND SPOUSE TO AN INITIAL COUPLE MEETING

As noted, we have run our BCT programs as part of larger substance abuse treatment centers. These centers have included inpatient and residential programs for detoxification and rehabilitation and outpatient programs for intensive outpatient and weekly counseling. We assume that most of you reading this book work in similar settings. In such settings the alcoholic and drug-abusing patients have already sought help and begun treatment for themselves. The challenge for the BCT counselor is to get the patient and the spouse to attend an initial meeting together as a couple. We routinely place posters, brochures, and other information about the BCT program in highly visible locations in the treatment center. We also regularly inform treatment center staff about the availability and benefits of BCT. In response to this information, a small number of patients will seek out, or be referred to, BCT. Usually, these are cases in which the couple has already separated, the spouse is making serious threats of separation or divorce, or there is other evidence of severe relationship problems.

How do you engage the rest of the patients who do not seek out BCT? This is one of the most frequently asked questions at workshops we conduct on BCT. Many substance abuse counselors have had experiences in which they were unsuccessful at engaging the patient and spouse together. We have found that it is not difficult if you follow a few simple steps. Table 2.1 summarizes these steps, which are described next.

TABLE 2.1. Engaging Patient and Spouse in BCT

- Use a nonthreatening, positive approach to get patient's permission to contact spouse.
- Deal with common fears about spouse contact.
- Talk directly to spouse to engage him or her for a joint interview with patient.
- Take small steps to gain couple's commitment.
    - Have a treatment planning meeting with patient and spouse in which BCT is presented as an option.
    - Conduct a couple session to explore possibility of starting BCT if couple expresses interest in it.

Obtain the Patient's Consent to Contact the Spouse

First, get the substance-abusing patient's permission to contact the spouse. A nonthreatening, positive approach works best. You may have to deal with common fears that patients have about addiction center staff contacting the spouse. Patients often fear that staff will tell spouses to leave them or to treat them with "tough love." Patients also often fear that spouses will tell staff things they had not yet revealed about the severity of their substance abuse problem and its effect on the family. Patients may know that their spouse is angry and want to "lie low" for a while in the hopes that the spouse will gradually get over being upset. Patients often avoid taking responsibility for life problems, instead dealing indirectly with them, including their relationship problems, because they fear that dealing directly will only make things worse.

If the patient raises any of these issues, you can reassure the patient that these fears are shared by many patients but that spouses usually respond positively to hearing from treatment center staff. It makes the spouse feel included rather than ignored and gives him or her hope that something is being done to address the substance abuse problem. Most patients do not raise these issues directly, however, so usually we say that contacting the family member with whom the patient lives is a routine part of the treatment program. We want to tell the spouse what an important step the patient has taken by entering the treatment program. We also want to invite the spouse to a joint interview with the patient to help finalize the patient's treatment plan so that the good start the patient has made by seeking treatment can be continued. Most patients will consent to contact their spouse when this contact is described as routine and it is presented in a positive manner.

If the patient refuses consent to contact the spouse, accept the refusal gracefully and move on to other matters. Do not get into a struggle with the patient over permission to contact the spouse because this is generally fruitless. With some reluctant patients, if you ask them again at a later time, after they have gotten to know you better and developed some trust, they may be willing to permit spouse contact.

Talk Directly to the Spouse to Arrange a Joint Interview

Second, once the patient has consented, talk directly to the spouse to invite him or her for a conjoint interview with the patient. When possible, call the spouse in the patient's presence; doing so lets the patient hear exactly what you say to his or her spouse. It also facilitates scheduling the conjoint interview because all parties are included in the call. Talking directly to the spouse is probably our most important suggestion for successfully engaging couples. Many patients offer to call their spouse to request that he or she attend the conjoint interview. Unfortunately, this tactic seldom works. The patient "forgets" to call or presents the request for a conjoint interview in such a way that the spouse refuses. What you say to the spouse depends on whether the patient has already expressed an initial interest in the BCT program. In cases where there is an interest in BCT, invite the spouse to meet with you and the patient once to learn more about the BCT program and whether it might be helpful to them. In most cases in which there is no initial interest in BCT, invite the spouse to meet with you and the patient for a joint treatment planning meeting in which they can share their insights about the substance problem and give their input to the treatment plan.

Take Small Steps to Gain the Couple's Commitment

Third, take small steps to gain the couple's commitment. This general strategy has already been described in the above suggestion that you start with a joint meeting to get the spouse's input into the patient's treatment plan. In the joint treatment planning interview with the patient and spouse, you can discuss the BCT program as one of the treatment options available. Do not require the couple to admit they have serious relationship problems in order for them to be a candidate for the BCT program. Admitting such problems can be threatening for some couples. Some couples also get along fine when the patient is not abusing substances, just as they claim. Of course, many couples readily admit that their relationship is in trouble because of the stress caused by substance-related problems and other relationship issues. Tell couples that BCT is a way to work together to promote abstinence in the patient, something that will benefit everyone in the family. BCT also helps repair the relationship if it is damaged or enriches a basically sound relationship that has been strained by the substance abuse.

Once a couple expresses interest in learning more about the BCT program, schedule a couple session to discuss the BCT program in more detail. This approach works best when the counselor who does the treatment planning interview with the couple is the same person the couple will see if they choose to schedule a couple session to explore the possibility of starting BCT. Make clear that the couple session to explore BCT does not obligate the couple to enroll in the BCT program. In this exploratory session the couple learns about the program in detail, and the counselor learns more about the patient and spouse so that they can make a decision about whether to take part in BCT.

THE INITIAL COUPLE SESSION TO EXPLORE
THE POSSIBILITY OF STARTING BCT

Starting the Initial Couple Session to Explore BCT

The initial couple session to explore BCT aims to (1) establish rapport with both members of the couple; (2) gather initial assessment information on key domains relevant to BCT; (3) orient the couple to the BCT program; (4) determine if the couple is interested in, and appropriate for, BCT; and (5) find out if crisis intervention or referral to other treatment is needed before, or instead of, BCT.

We usually begin this session by stating our understanding of the purpose of the meeting and confirming that this is also the couple's understanding. It goes something like this:

"As I understand it, we are meeting so that I can find out more about you, and you can learn more about the BCT program, so we can decide if this program would be a good fit for you both. At the end of the meeting, if you think you might be interested, I will make another appointment when you can let me know your final decision. If this program is not for you, then I will help you find another type of help that fits your needs better. . . . Is that your understanding also? . . . Is that agreeable to both of you?"

Once a common purpose has been confirmed, you can ask for some simple demographic information, including ages, where they live, employment situation, whether married or cohabiting and for how long, and children's names and ages, if any.

Move next to consider in some detail why they are seeking help now. As you listen to the couple's story of events leading to help seeking, you often will learn, or find opportunities to ask questions about, many of the things you need to know. You will need information about key domains relevant to BCT, described below; gather initial information about these domains in this session. You can get more detailed information in subsequent sessions. By connecting many questions about key domains to the help-seeking story, the interview flows better than would a linear question-and-answer session. An outline of domains to cover, such as that given in Table 2.2, can ensure that key areas are covered and also serve as an outline for the progress note written in the patient's clinical record after this session.

Domains Evaluated in the Initial Couple Session to Explore BCT

Demographics and reason for seeking help now have already been mentioned. The other key domains you need to cover in this initial couple session to explore BCT are discussed in the following material.

TABLE 2.2. Tasks of the Initial Couple Session to Explore BCT

- Establish rapport with both members of couple
- Assess the following key domains:
  - Demographics
  - Reasons for seeking help now
  - Alcohol and drug use by patient and spouse
  - Relationship stability and commitment
  - Relationship violence
  - Suicide and dangerousness
  - Children in need of services
  - Crises or major stressors
- Orient couple to BCT program, including limits to confidentiality
- Determine if couple is interested in, and suitable for, BCT
- Determine if crisis intervention or other treatment is needed before, or instead of, BCT

ALCOHOL AND DRUG USE BY PATIENT AND SPOUSE

You need to assess substance use by both partners, starting with the person who appears to have the more severe problem. Ask about recent types, quantities, and frequencies of substances used and which one the individual thinks is the most important substance of abuse. Determine whether the extent of physical dependence on alcohol or other drugs requires detoxification before starting BCT. Review outcomes of prior efforts to seek help and duration of abstinent periods to determine what helped the person to stay abstinent and what led to relapses. Evaluate the effect of substance use on the spouse and other family members. Review medical, legal, financial, employment, psychological, and social problems related to the substance abuse. Finally, examine whether the couple's goal is to reduce substance use or to abstain either temporarily or permanently.

Next assess the spouse's history of alcohol and drug problems, if any. If both members of a couple have a current active substance abuse problem and both want abstinence, then you can treat them in BCT. If both have a current problem but only one wants to stop, you can conduct a few exploratory couple or individual sessions to see if the reluctant party becomes ready to stop. If so, then you can start BCT. If not, then treat the one who wants to stop in individual treatment and leave the door open to BCT in the future, should things change. Chapter 9 provides more details on treating such "dual problem" couples.

Two other issues related to substance abuse can delay or prevent starting BCT. Some patients who want to stop substance use need detoxification to prevent withdrawal before starting BCT. Other patients will not be suitable for BCT because they do not want to stop substance use or they want to pursue a goal of reduced use rather than abstinence. To be suitable for BCT, the patient needs to be willing to try to abstain at least temporarily while taking part in BCT.

RELATIONSHIP STABILITY AND COMMITMENT

Assess the stability and commitment to the relationship for both members of the couple. Ask about recent or past separations and the manner of reconciliation. Ask whether the couple has discussed splitting up, and whether either partner has frequent thoughts of separation or divorce or has taken actions (e.g., asking others for advice, seeing an attorney) leading in that direction. What specific changes are desired to make the relationship viable? Spouses frequently state that their partner stopping substance use is necessary for the relationship to improve. Many couples enter BCT as a "last chance" to save their relationship. For some couples, one partner may be uncertain about whether sobriety or other changes will make a difference. Too much damage may have been done to the relationship for it to continue.

The minimum level of commitment needed is for both parties to be willing to live together and devote time and effort in BCT to see if substance abuse and relationship problems can be improved to a point where both are committed to the relationship. If the couple is separated at time of the initial session or if one member of the couple is not sure he or she wants to work on improving the relationship, then BCT is not appropriate. Exploratory sessions to clarify what, if anything, could lead to a reconciliation or a mutual willingness to work on the relationship often lead to starting BCT at a later date. For couples who are currently separated, you will need to know if there is a restraining order that prohibits contact. If so, it will have to be removed or modified to permit counseling before further couple sessions can occur. Chapter 9 has more details about working with separated couples.

RELATIONSHIP VIOLENCE

Find out if the couple has a history of partner violence. Begin this assessment by asking about the couple's arguments. Ask them specifically about physical conflicts if they do not mention any in response to your initial question.

> "When couples struggle with substance abuse, arguments can get pretty intense. Can you tell me what your conflicts are like? . . . [If no violence is revealed, ask more explicitly] . . . It is not uncommon for conflicts to get physical with pushing, grabbing, or hitting. What experiences like this have you had in your relationship?"

A history of partner violence is defined as pushing, grabbing, shoving, hitting, slapping, kicking, biting, choking, or using weapons by either the male or female partner. Also consider whether threats of violence or throwing or breaking objects has occurred. Do not be surprised to discover that many couples have experienced such violence. Studies show that 50–60% or more of both male and female substance abuse patients have been violent toward their relationship partner in the year before treatment.[1] Although partner violence is frequently detected among substance abuse patients, in our experience, most of this violence is not so severe that it precludes BCT.

For couples with a history of partner violence, determine the extent of current risk of lethal or physically injurious violence. The BCT counselor determines whether very severe violence has ever occurred, how long ago the last incident was, and whether there have been recent threats of such violence. The circumstances of violent incidents are reviewed, including whether the police were called, the couple separated, and the extent to which violence was perpetrated only by the male. The counselor also inquires whether either member of the couple, particularly the female victim, fears that such violence may occur in the near future. The presence or availability of weapons is also questioned. Finally, it is important to determine whether the violence occurred only or mostly when the substance-abusing patient was under the influence of alcohol or drugs. If so, then the patient's willingness to use methods such as Antabuse or regular AA attendance to deal with the substance abuse may reduce some of the couple's and the counselor's concerns about immediate risks of violence.

If your assessment reveals an active and acute risk for very severe partner violence that could cause serious injury or be potentially life-threatening, do not proceed with BCT. In such cases it is better to treat the substance abuser and the partner separately rather than together. This treatment includes making a safety plan to prevent violence to the potential victim. As noted, couples are excluded from BCT if very severe violence (defined as resulting in injury requiring medical attention or hospitalization) has occurred in the past 2 years or if one or both members of the couple fear that taking part in couples treatment may stimulate violence. In our experience fewer than 2% of couples seeking BCT are excluded from BCT due to very severe violence or fears of couples therapy. In couples with a history of violence but without an acute risk of very severe violence, you can proceed with BCT and make conflict containment an explicit goal of the sessions from the outset. Chapter 10 provides more details about working with couples in which there is violence.

SUICIDALITY AND DANGEROUSNESS FOR BOTH PARTNERS

Assessment of this domain proceeds as it would in any initial counseling session for substance abuse or mental health problems. Ask about current suicidal thoughts, intentions, and plans and review history of past attempts, gestures, plans, and thoughts of suicide for both the substance abuser and the spouse. Do the same for thoughts and actions related to harming others. Of course, if your assessment reveals substantial risk in either area, reducing this risk takes precedence over everything else.

CHILDREN POSSIBLY IN NEED OF SERVICES

If the couple has children, you can ask about their functioning in the first session if you have time or in a subsequent session. Discuss each child with the couple to see if they have any concerns about the child's functioning at home, with peers, or at school. We know that children's emotional problems improve after their parents receive BCT,[2] but children with obvious adjustment problems may benefit from additional specialized services. You can assist the parents in finding help for such a child. You also can use later BCT sessions to help the parents improve their joint parenting approaches. Chapter 11 provides more details on adding parent training to BCT to further improve children's functioning.

SUBSTANCE-RELATED OR OTHER CRISES OR MAJOR STRESSORS

Finally, determine whether there are any substance-abuse-related or other crises that require immediate attention. Crisis intervention is necessary for cases in which violence or divorce seems a likely result of delayed action, or for cases in which the patient is ready to stop substance use but needs immediate hospitalization for detoxification. Couple sessions can focus on the crisis, transitioning to BCT after it has been resolved. In addition to crises that require immediate attention, most couples face major stressors and problems that may include actual, impending, or threatened loss of job or home or other major legal or financial problems. Ongoing medical or psychiatric problems, parenting concerns, family-related stressors, and work-related problems also are common. Identifying these problems and stressors is important in order to help the couple deal with them in future BCT sessions.

Instruments to Assess Substance Abuse and Relationship Functioning

We use clinical interviews to assess substance abuse and relationship functioning in the initial and subsequent couple sessions, as just described. Generally, these interviews provide sufficient information to guide BCT sessions with a couple. However, when you want more detailed information for clinical or research purposes, specific instruments can be used for a more comprehensive assessment, as we have described in more detail elsewhere.[3]

To gather more detailed information about the substance abuse problem, we recommend certain instruments. The Time-Line Follow-Back Interview is a structured interview that uses a calendar and specialized interviewing methods.[4] You can use it to reconstruct the quantity and frequency of the substance abuser's drinking and drug use behavior during the prior 6–12 months. An alcohol breath test and a drug urine screen can detect any very recent substance use. Finally, to measure problems due to alcohol and drug abuse, we suggest the Drinker Inventory of Consequences and the Addiction Severity Index, respectively.[5]

To gather more detailed information about couple relationships, we use the following instruments. The Dyadic Adjustment Scale determines the overall level of satisfaction experienced in the relationship.[6] The Conflict Tactics Scale assesses the extent of verbal and physical abuse during the past year and in the life of the relationship.[7] The Marital Status Inventory evaluates thoughts, plans, and actions concerned with separation and divorce.[8] The Areas of Change Questionnaire measures specific changes desired in the relationship.[9] The Sexual Adjustment Questionnaire examines sexual functioning.[10] Finally, you can assess a couple's communication skills by making an audiotape or videotape of the couple talking about conflicts and problems.[3]

A more comprehensive assessment using these instruments generally takes three sessions to complete. It ends with a "feedback session," in which the couple and the counselor discuss the results of the assessment. Then BCT begins at the fourth session, if the couple agrees. We used this comprehensive assessment method in most of our earlier research studies and clinical work.

More recently we have used the method described above, in which assessment is done via interview in an initial couple session to explore BCT and BCT starts at the following session. This shift occurred because the community-based settings in which we began to work cut the number of outpatient sessions typically given and did not have students or research assistants to collect and score assessment data. The newer settings also had fewer court-ordered or coerced patients than in our original settings, so the risk of dropout also increased by delaying the start of BCT.

Another option combines both approaches. You do the initial clinical interview assessment in the initial couple session to explore BCT and start BCT in the following session. Then you conduct a more comprehensive instrument-based assessment in tandem with ongoing BCT sessions. This approach, when feasible, combines the advantages of starting BCT quickly with those of a rich assessment base to guide further sessions.

The Role of Assessment in BCT

A few words about the role of assessment in BCT may be useful. First, a major goal of the initial couple session to explore BCT is to determine if the couple is suitable for this treatment. You want to be sure that there is sufficient commitment to recovery and to the relationship and that there are no obvious barriers to BCT (e.g., lack of interest by patient or spouse, serious risk of very severe violence). Second, another function of the initial session is to gather preliminary information about specific content that should be addressed in BCT. For example, discovering what life problems and stressors the patient and spouse face can help guide the counselor in choosing which stressful life problems to help the couple address as part of providing support for abstinence (see Chapter 4).

Finally, those new to BCT occasionally ask how assessment findings collected in the first BCT session or in subsequent more structured assessment lead to an individualized plan of treatment in BCT. BCT is a fairly standardized treatment in which each couple receives roughly the same main interventions. Individualizing BCT occurs because different couples bring different life situations and content to the counseling. Individualization also occurs in relation to which aspects of BCT get more emphasis than others. Sometimes the initial assessment suggests that certain aspects of BCT should be given more emphasis than others. For example, all couples must promise to refrain from violence or threats of violence and learn conflict management and communication skills to defuse hostility. However, we emphasize these activities to a greater degree for a couple that has a history of partner violence and recurring heated arguments than for a couple who tends to avoid conflict and has no violence history. Similarly, all couples are helped to increase positive couple and family activities, but we might emphasize this aspect of BCT more for a very disengaged couple than for a couple that routinely spends time together and says that the relationship is happy except for the substance abuse.

Concluding the Initial Couple Session to Explore BCT

By the middle of this session, you should have a pretty good idea whether the couple is appropriate for BCT. As already mentioned, couples are likely to benefit from BCT if (1) they are married or living together, (2) one member of the couple has a current substance abuse problem and accepts at least temporary abstinence as a goal, (3) both partners are willing to work together to see if substance abuse and relationship problems can be improved, and (4) there is not an acute risk of very severe partner violence or a history of psychosis. Most of the following chapters describe how to use BCT to treat couples who meet these criteria. Again, as already mentioned, couples who do not meet all of these criteria may possibly be treated in BCT, but they require special methods to meet their needs, as described in Chapters 9 and 10. If the couple is not appropriate for BCT, then you will need to arrange other treatment.

ORIENT COUPLE TO BCT

Assuming the couple is appropriate for BCT, you will need to spend a few minutes toward the end of the session describing BCT and answering any questions. Indicate that the purpose of BCT is to support abstinence and to improve the relationship. Emphasize that the first priority is creating a Recovery Contract to support abstinence. As part of the contract, self-help meetings are suggested for most patients. Drug urine screens are required if a patient has a current drug problem. A recovery-related medication (e.g., disulfiram, naltrexone) may be suggested. To improve the relationship, BCT increases positive couple and family activities and teaches communication for dealing with areas of conflict and changes desired. Stress that completing assignments between sessions is a key part of the therapy. Highlight that BCT is a positive approach that emphasizes managing and reducing conflict. You may also want to mention briefly some of the benefits of BCT, as documented in research studies. These include: Patients who receive BCT, compared to those who receive typical individual counseling, have more abstinence, lower risk of separation and divorce, and fewer emotional problems in their children.

DETERMINE LEVEL OF INTEREST IN BCT

Finally, determine if the couple is interested in starting BCT. If not, then arrange for other treatment. If yes, then schedule another couple session at which time the couple is expected to give their final decision about whether or not they wish to start BCT. In our experience, the level of rapport you develop with the couple in the initial couple session to explore BCT will be a major factor determining whether the couple is interested in scheduling another session. Many couples will definitely want to start BCT. For other couples, at least one member will have some level of uncertainty. For all couples, we stress that, rather than rush into a commitment to BCT, it is better to think about it and return in a week with a final decision. BCT is a demanding form of counseling that is likely to help them if they attend the BCT sessions faithfully and follow through on recommended actions between sessions. In other words, to get the most from BCT, both members of the couple need to be committed to participating fully in it.

GAINING COMMITMENT AND STARTING BCT

Starting the First BCT Session

Generally a week or so after the initial couple session to explore BCT, the couple returns to begin their first BCT session in earnest.

FINALIZE DECISION TO START BCT

After welcoming the couple, ask what reactions, thoughts, or discussions they had about the initial couple session to explore BCT. Often couples will share positive reactions about wanting to start the BCT program or about the ease they felt in talking with the counselor. Sometimes reactions to the initial couple session to explore BCT reveal ambivalence by one member of the couple about the BCT program or continued bad feeling about something that was said at the initial couple meeting. You can address these initial reactions by examining the reluctant partner's concerns about BCT or by clarifying that future sessions would try to avoid negative carryover from the session to life at home.

After getting initial reactions, ask explicitly if they have decided whether to start BCT or if they have remaining questions or concerns that you can address. Once they have agreed to start BCT, congratulate them for making a good decision. Express your hope that this new beginning will lead to a better future for each of them and their family. Indicate that couples who attend the BCT sessions faithfully and try recommended changes usually experience increased abstinence and a more satisfying relationship.

Now that the couple has decided to start BCT, this is the time to give a detailed rationale and preview of the BCT sessions, review guidelines for getting the most out of BCT, and consider confidentiality policies.

GIVE RATIONALE FOR BCT

Figure 2.1 (a copy of which is Poster B.1 in Appendix B) is a poster we review with the couple when we explain the rationale for BCT. We briefly review each section of this table and get reactions from the patient and spouse about how the material presented applies to their own experiences. The message conveyed by the material in the first column of this table is that an active substance abuse problem interferes with relationship happiness and communication and contributes to relationship problems. Material in the second column indicates that, to the surprise of many couples, relationship happiness does not automatically return when the patient stops using. The third column shows that BCT has a number of components, each of which is

Why BCT?

	Active Drinking and Drug Use	**Recovery**	**BCT**
Alcohol or Drug Use	Alcohol and drug use become main focus of relationship	Gone but not forgotten Tension, nagging, arguments, fear, distrust	✓ Recovery Contract ✓ Continuing Recovery Plan
Love and Daily Caring	Anger and resentment replace love and caring; take over relationship	Anger and resentment continue; hard to remember what relationship was like without drugs and alcohol	Caring Behaviors ✓ Catch and Tell ✓ Caring Days
Fun Together	Time spent drinking, using drugs, arguing, or doing things without one another	Time spent trying to solve problems caused by drinking and drugging instead of doing things together	Shared Rewarding Activities
Problems	Too many problems caused by substance use (bills, job losses, etc.) Everyday relationship problems and differences pile up Problems go unresolved and often unrecognized	Problems caused by substance use can still be overwhelming and even worse Relationship problems becoming obvious Blame game: No good will or skills to solve problems and differences	Communication Skills Training ✓ Effective listening ✓ Effective speaking ✓ Communication sessions ✓ Problem solving ✓ Relationship agreements ✓ Conflict resolution

FIGURE 2.1. Rationale for BCT.

designed to deal with specific challenges faced by couples who want to pursue recovery for the substance-abusing patient and for the relationship.

REVIEW GUIDELINES FOR GETTING THE MOST OUT OF BCT

Review the following guidelines with couples.

1. It is important to show up on time for scheduled appointments. Patient and spouse are responsible to participate fully in sessions. There is much to cover in each scheduled appointment.

2. Regular attendance is critically important. Emphasize that different topics and exercises are covered in each session. Additionally, sessions tend to build on each other and cannot be easily skipped. This is a good point to establish a regular meeting time when both members of the couple will be able to attend faithfully in the weeks to come.

3. However, missing a session may be unavoidable (e.g., family emergencies, illness). Encourage the couple to call as soon as they know they will be missing a session. Emphasize

that they should not miss a session because they are having problems that week; at such times it is better to have only one person come than for both to miss the session.

4. The first month of BCT is critical. Those who attend faithfully, abstain, and follow recommendations during this period are most likely to benefit in the long run. For patients with prior treatment failures based on lack of consistent attendance at counseling sessions, you may want to make attendance and evidence of effort during the first month a condition for continuing BCT thereafter.

5. Although BCT is a positive approach, there will be times when the patient or spouse will be upset about statements made during a couple session. Emphasize that it is better not to argue at home about such upsets, but rather to discuss them in the session.

6. Finally, emphasize that patience and honesty are important. Recovery from serious substance abuse and relationship problems takes time, hard work, and patience. Months may go by before both partners feel a lot better, and it may take a few years before abstinence and relationship functioning feel stable to both. Honesty is an important part of recovery. Although concealing problems such as strong urges or substance use may be easier in the short run, revealing these problems so that they can be addressed lays a better foundation for long term success.

EXPLAIN CONFIDENTIALITY POLICY AND LIMITS

As part of orienting the couple about what to expect in BCT, you need to explain the nature and limits of confidentiality, as the policy is followed in BCT. This issue is important because there may be times during BCT when you talk with one member of the couple alone to gather assessment information, to deal with a crisis, or for other reasons. Before describing the confidentiality policy used in BCT when talking with one of the partners in a one-to-one situation, we briefly review different approaches to confidentiality.

Strict confidentiality is the first. In this model, the content of the one-to-one conversation with one partner is kept confidential from the other partner. Strict confidentiality evolved in the context of, and is best suited to, one-to-one therapy. It has drawbacks in the context of BCT with substance-abusing couples who commonly keep secrets from each other. Also, partners often don't talk directly to each other about ongoing problems but share their concerns, often in the form of secrets, with others. A strict confidentiality model can involve the counselor in this dysfunctional communication pattern, where he or she is now holding secrets of one or both partners. Over time, secret keeping may erode the fundamental principle of open and honest communication and block progress.

The *open confidentiality* model is a competing approach recommended by many couple and family therapists. Any contact with the partners, whether together or separately, is considered part of the counselor's work with the couple. Thus, all communication with either partner is treated as if the other partner were present. Partners are informed that they should not tell the therapist anything that they would not say to their partner. This model has many advantages over the strict confidentiality model for couples. It puts the focus of the counseling on the couple as a unit, not the individual partners. It prevents the counselor from getting drawn into dysfunctional, secret-keeping communication that can arise in the strict confidentiality model. We view this as a viable model, and it is clearly the foundation for the approach we use. However, the open confidentiality model requires the counselor to share all information, even when, in the counselor's professional judgement, doing so may cause serious harm to one or both partners (e.g., an old affair or plans to leave the relationship to escape abuse).

Limited confidentiality, the model we use in BCT, is closely akin to the open confidentiality model but with some important exceptions. In particular, strict confidentiality with a partner can be maintained if the issue being discussed, in the professional opinion of the counselor, might cause undue harm to a partner or the couple as a whole if disclosed. Thus, the counselor maintains a general stance of open confidentiality but explicitly states to the couple that he or she retains the right to use his or her professional judgment to keep strict confidentiality with a partner in certain circumstances. We call this a "No Secrets Policy" to stress our general rule that the BCT counselor will not keep secrets and also reserves the right to disclose, or not disclose, information from individual sessions as he or she professionally see fit. If the counselor thinks some information should be shared, he or she should discuss this fact with the confiding partner and give this partner the option of bringing up the issue or letting the counselor do so.

Of course, you also have to inform the couple about legally mandated limits on confidentiality related to dangerousness and child or elder abuse. You might want to introduce the "No Secrets Policy" and other limits to confidentiality in the following manner:

"Along with our couple sessions, there also may be times when I meet with each of you separately. Because I may be talking with you individually, I would like to introduce what we call our 'No Secrets Policy.' This means that if one of you tells me something that I believe is important to your relationship, I retain the option of whether, when, and to what extent I will discuss this in a joint session. Usually, I will first give the person who shared the information the chance to bring the issue up in a joint session before I do.

"I will not disclose any information to an outside party unless mandated by law or with your written consent. The law mandates that counselors report information when a person discloses an intent to harm him- or herself or someone else, or if there is a disclosure of abuse against a child or an elderly or disabled person.

"Holding information that one of you shares with me can be considered taking sides, and that goes against what we are trying to do here.

"This 'no secrets policy' may seem strange to you and lead you to keep certain information to yourself. Although I don't want to encourage that, I also want to make our time together most effective, and secret keeping may hurt that process.

"Are there any questions about this?"

Most couples do not express concerns about this policy, and confidentiality issues do not cause a problem in most of the couples treated in BCT. In terms of the limits on confidentiality (other than legal mandates), we do not give specifics to the couple in advance about what we will, and will not, disclose. There are only a few situations in which we routinely consider keeping information strictly confidential with a partner. These include some cases of marital infidelity and cases in which the information reveals an acute risk of very severe intimate partner violence.

If either partner discloses infidelity, and the affair is not active and is in the past, we do not require disclosure to the other partner. If it is not an issue now and does not appear to be an issue going forward, we encourage disclosure for health reasons but do not make it a requirement for continued BCT treatment. However, if a person reports being actively involved in an affair or has a competing love interest, we will not treat the couple in BCT. Either the person has to end the affair immediately or tell his or her partner immediately, or we discontinue

BCT. If the affair stops, we strongly encourage disclosure but do not make it a requirement. Early in our experience doing BCT, we tried disclosing past extramarital sex during couples therapy sessions in a few cases, but the couples stopped therapy.

If either partner describes dangerous episodes of very severe partner violence that have occurred recently, the counselor may need to maintain strict confidentiality while helping the victim develop and implement a safety plan. This plan might include making a referral to a shelter, a domestic violence counselor, and so forth. In such a case, the woman might confide that her male partner has threatened to kill her and that she fears for her life. Sharing her revelation with the male partner could increase the risk to the woman. As noted, such very severe, current violence situations are rare among substance abuse patients who seek BCT. Chapter 10 presents a case in which the counselor kept secret the female partner's revelation of violence, helped her plan for her safety, got the male partner into residential treatment, and discontinued BCT.

Four Promises

Next we ask the couple to make the four commitments shown in Figure 2.2 (a copy of which is Poster B.2 in Appendix B). Reviewing these promises, displayed as a poster, helps familiarize them with the BCT framework and shapes treatment expectations. We call these the "Four Promises." You can introduce these promises in the following manner:

> "I have four promises I would like you to consider. These promises embody the spirit of this new beginning you are making. If you agree, you will make these four promises just for the next week, until our next session. At our next session I will ask you to consider making these promises for the time you are attending these couple sessions."

Promises

➢ No Threats of Divorce or Separation

➢ No Violence or Threats of Violence (no angry touching)

➢ Focus on the Present and Future—Not on the Past

➢ Actively Participate in All Sessions and Do Homework Assignments

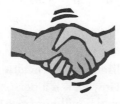

FIGURE 2.2. Four promises.

No Threats of Separation or Divorce

First, the couple promises to live together, at least for the initial course of therapy, and not to threaten separation or divorce, even when in a heated argument. This commitment discourages the use of threats as ammunition during conflict or out of frustration. It also reinforces the idea that both partners can work to repair the relationship without fear of abrupt decisions to separate. When one partner makes such a threat, it is disruptive to the process of relationship recovery. It takes time to pull back from such threats and move ahead on a positive tack. BCT helps couples learn to express their feelings directly and confront their problems without resorting to such threats. This promise does not require a lifelong commitment to the relationship. It does not mean that spouses will stop considering separation. It may take a number of months of abstinence before the thoughts of separation subside. Rather, the promise is to stop discussing separation at home. If separation remains or becomes a serious possibility, couples are instructed to discuss it in the BCT session, where the counselor can help them deal with this ongoing concern.

No Violence or Threats of Violence

Second, couples agree to refrain from violence or threats of violence. This promise is particularly important for couples who have a history of partner violence. You need to emphasize that violence and threatening or intimidating behavior are not acceptable. You also need to review what is meant by violence: that it includes pushing, shoving, grabbing, and throwing things as well as more severe forms of violence. Sometimes we use the term "angry touching" to refer to some of these milder forms of violence in order to be sure couples understand that these are included. Stress that each person is responsible for controlling his or her own emotions and actions. One partner blaming the other's actions for making him or her violent is not acceptable. Closely monitoring compliance with this promise at each BCT session can help prevent violence in most cases. For couples with a significant violence history, you also can ask if there were any situations in the past week when either person was concerned that anger might escalate to threats or violence. This focus helps identify factors that can trigger violence and provides an opportunity to teach the couple more constructive communication methods.

A Focus on Present and Future

Third, the couple agrees to do their best to focus on the present and future, and not on past substance abuse or negative events. The core promise is to refrain from bringing up the past in anger at home. Such charged discussions generally lead to bad feelings, often increase the risk of relapse, and do not help the process of relationship recovery. This commitment is usually kept by the patient because there is natural motivation to avoid the guilt and shame aroused by processing unsuccessful efforts to stay abstinent and the painful consequences caused by the substance abuse. However, the burden of this agreement falls on the spouse, who struggles to contain his or her anger and frustration with the patient's past behavior. You can empathize with the spouse's resentment, agreeing that he or she has a right to his or her feelings and that most spouses feel the same way. It also helps to ask that the couple discuss their substance-abuse-related past only in the safer context of BCT sessions, where the counselor can help them discuss these issues with a minimum of destructiveness. Thus, although critical incidents and reminders of the past may demand clarification and ongoing management, the message made explicit to the couple emphasizes their current responsibilities and potential to make their relationship better, rather than becoming mired in mutual blaming.

COMPLETION OF AGREED-TO ASSIGNMENTS

Fourth, the couple promises to complete whatever homework assignments they agree to do. Explain that assignments will be things they can do to help recovery or the relationship. A typical assignment, for example, might be to attend an AA meeting or to plan something fun to do together as a couple. Stress that partners will have a choice whether or not to accept an assignment, and that you would rather they refused an assignment or agreed to do less than suggested than to agree and then not follow through. The rationale given is that BCT is action-oriented and focused on behavior change. Emphasis is placed on helping couples renew their relationship in a more positive way by changing behaviors first and then assessing changes in feelings, rather than waiting to feel more positively toward each other before initiating changes in their own behavior.

GAINING COMMITMENT TO THE FOUR PROMISES

Conclude your review of the four promises by asking each member of the couple whether they are willing to make these promises for the coming week. Get a specific commitment from each person for each of the promises. Emphasize that each person is responsible for their own behavior. If one partner does not keep a promise, it does not relieve the other person of the responsibility to keep his or her own promise. Indicate that you will ask them at the next session about their success in keeping their promises and whether they will continue the promises for the duration of the BCT sessions.

TYPICAL SEQUENCE AND STRUCTURE OF BCT SESSIONS

After getting commitments to the four promises, the next steps are to explain the typical structure of BCT sessions (see below) and to start negotiating the Recovery Contract (see Chapter 3). Generally BCT consists of 12–20 weekly couple sessions, each of which lasts 50–60 minutes. The first few BCT sessions focus on establishing a Recovery Contract to support abstinence for the patient and to decrease couple conflicts about substance use. This contract decreases tension about substance use and builds goodwill. When abstinence and attendance at BCT sessions have stabilized for a few weeks, you add relationship-focused interventions to increase positive activities and improve communication. Toward the end of weekly sessions, you plan for continuing recovery and relapse prevention. Table 1.7 (in Chapter 1) provides more details on the sequence of interventions in BCT.

Table 2.3 summarizes key points about the structure of a typical BCT session. Appendix B contains a simpler version (see Poster B.3) that we typically use as a poster when telling a couple what to expect in BCT sessions. Sessions tend to be moderately to highly structured, with the counselor setting the agenda at the outset of each meeting. Each BCT session follows a predictable sequence of events. Although the content of BCT changes as sessions progress, the structure of most sessions follows this outline of a typical BCT session:

TABLE 2.3. Outline of a Typical BCT Session

- Session opening procedures.
  - Greet and welcome couple to session.
  - Ask for urine screen if patient has drug problem.
  - Review urges or use in past week.
  - Review use of promises in past week.
  - Note problems of past week and defer discussion.
- Review Recovery Contract in past week.
  - Review trust discussion and recovery calendar of past week.
  - Have couple practice trust discussion in session.
  - Review other parts of Recovery Contract.
- Review last session and home practice from past week.
- Deal with current problems.
  - Discuss problem mentioned earlier in session or an ongoing concern.
  - Consider the problem and begin to resolve it.
- Cover new material.
  - Explain skill and why it is important.
  - Model the skill for the couple.
  - Ask couple to practice the skill in the session.
- Assign home practice for next week.

---

1. *Greet and welcome couple to the session.*

2. *Urine screen.* If the patient has a drug problem, ask him or her to provide a urine sample for drug screening. Review results of urine screen taken at prior session later in session, when you discuss Recovery Contract compliance.

3. *Review urges or use in past week.* Ask if the patient has had any urges to use or has used in the past week. Chapter 4 explains how to conduct this review.

4. *Review of promises.* Ask if each member of the couple kept the four promises in the past week.

5. *Review relationship problems or other concerns of past week.* Ask if the couple has had any problems in the past week. Note any problems and defer in-depth discussion until after you review home practice (below). This lets partners know that you will address their concerns and, at the same time, keep the structure of the session intact.

6. *Review Recovery Contract in past week.* Review trust discussion (with medication, if taking it) and recovery calendar of past week. Couple practices doing trust discussion in session (with medication if taking it) with therapist feedback. Review self-help meetings, last week's urine screen results, and any other parts of Recovery Contract. Chapter 3 explains how to conduct this review.

7. *Review last session and home practice from past week.* Briefly review new material from the last session and answer any questions. Then review home practice assigned last session to find out extent and quality of follow-through on assignments. Often this portion includes more in-session practice of the skill assigned the preceding week for home practice.

8. *Deal with current problems.* After reviewing homework from the last session, you consider important events of the past week and address any problems identified earlier in the session. Or you may address an ongoing problem noted during the assessment in the first session. The point is to pay attention to the problem and to resolve, or begin to resolve, it.

9. *Cover new material (instruction and in-session practice)*. Each week new skills are introduced. The therapist explains the skill and why it is important, models the skill for the couple, and then asks the couple to practice the skill within the session. Finally, home practice of the skill may be assigned.

10. *Assign home practice for next week*. BCT includes weekly home practice assignments related to the topics discussed and practiced in the session. Home practice is a crucial part of BCT that is strongly encouraged. Home practice helps the couple apply skills learned in BCT sessions to their daily lives. Practicing the new behaviors at home allows the couple to see change and progress. To get the most benefit from BCT, the couple must do the home practice each week and come to the next session ready to discuss it.

When they first start doing BCT, many counselors feel a little overwhelmed by how much they need to cover in a session and how active they have to be. However, with more experience doing BCT, most counselors become more comfortable as they learn how to manage the couple sessions and see the benefit couples are experiencing. In addition, structuring the sessions gets easier; after a few sessions the couple learns what to expect and follows the order of the session you have taught them. Finally, many couples who take part in BCT report that the structured sessions and activity-based homework exercises are a welcome change from their chaotic lifestyles.

FREQUENTLY ASKED QUESTIONS

• *Question 1*: You advocate using BCT with couples that have a history of partner violence. Some states explicitly forbid the use of couples therapy with court-mandated batterers. BCT could increase women's risk of abuse. Couple sessions may provoke anger that could lead to abusive incidents. Treating violence in couple sessions also implies that women are to blame for violence—or at least that is the way some women will interpret it. Women who blame themselves are likely to be revictimized.

• *Answer*: We agree that couples with very severe violence should not be treated in BCT. Such couples are screened out of BCT. The couples we see are drawn from patients seeking substance abuse treatment. Although some of the cases we have seen in BCT were court-mandated to substance abuse treatment after a domestic abuse incident, most of our patients are not court-mandated for partner violence violations. In our clinical experience, we have not had problems with couple sessions leading to violence. As noted earlier, BCT strongly emphasizes that each person is responsible for controlling his or her own emotions and actions. One partner blaming the other's actions for making him or her violent is not acceptable in BCT. If we eliminated patients who had any recent partner violence history from BCT, it would prevent most patients from getting help. Sixty percent or more of couples starting BCT have experienced partner violence in the past year. Although it is a popular belief that couples with violence should not be treated together, the data on BCT for substance abuse do not support this belief. Four studies, which included over 500 substance abuse patients, show clearly that violence decreases after BCT.[11] Finally, we are not advocating BCT as a primary treatment for partner violence in batterer clinic patients. Most batterer clinic patients will have more severe violence than the alcoholic patients with whom we have used BCT successfully to reduce partner violence. Chapter 10 covers partner violence and BCT in considerable detail.

- *Question 2*: For the most part, the promises seem like good ideas, but they also seem kind of simplistic. Is it realistic to expect that making these promises will change entrenched patterns of behavior and get people to do the homework required in BCT?
- *Answer*: We do not expect that simply making these promises will produce consistent behavior change. We certainly do not expect, and we do not find, that homework compliance is guaranteed by gaining promises to do so. In our view, the promises establish positive expectations of making a new beginning, making specific changes, and each person being responsible for his or her own behavior. The promises get BCT off to a positive start. The real work is done week by week. Reviewing individual's successes and challenges with keeping these promises each week and helping them increase their faithfulness to the promises does, in fact, often lead to important changes.

- *Question 3*: Promising to stay together and not to threaten separation or divorce might not be in the best interest of many spouses. Women in partner violence situations might need these options to leave for safety reasons alone. Women also may need these options to set limits on their partner's behavior, especially regarding violence and abuse. This promise seems like it could trap a woman in an unsatisfying or abusive relationship that is not good for her.
- *Answer*: BCT participants need to be willing to work to see if the relationship can be improved, and they need to agree to refrain from threatening separation or divorce in anger. BCT participants do not need to have an open-ended commitment to maintaining the relationship. In fact, many couples enter BCT as a "last chance" to salvage their relationship; often the nonaddicted spouse makes it clear that if violence or serious substance use recurs, then the relationship is over. Couples do promise not to make threats of separation or divorce, in the heat of anger at home, because such threats usually sabotage progress and often lead to heightened anger than can escalate to violence or substance use. However, they also agree to discuss any serious thoughts they may have about possible separation or divorce during BCT sessions, where they can get help from the counselor in dealing with this issue. If separation becomes necessary due to recurrent serious violence, levels of substance abuse that are unacceptable to the spouse, or irreconcilable differences, then the BCT counselor tries to help the couple separate in the least destructive way possible. Dealing with couple separations that occur during BCT is considered in more detail in Chapter 9.

SUMMARY

- To engage the patient and spouse in BCT, get the patient's permission to contact the spouse, and then talk directly to the spouse to engage him or her for a joint interview with the patient. Take small steps to gain the couple's commitment to trying BCT.

- The initial couple session to explore the possibility of starting BCT aims to (1) establish rapport, (2) assess key domains relevant to BCT, (3) orient the couple to BCT, (4) determine if the couple is interested in, and appropriate for, BCT, and (5) schedule the first BCT session, if appropriate.

- Couples with very severe violence should not be treated in BCT; most violence seen in substance abuse patients is mild to moderate in severity. Data on BCT do not support the popular belief that couples with a history of violence should not be treated together. Four studies of over 500 substance abuse patients show that violence decreases after BCT. Chapter 10 covers partner violence and BCT in detail.

- The first BCT session begins with the couple promising (1) to refrain from threatening separation or violence, (2) to refrain from violence or threats of violence, (3) to focus on the present and future, and (4) to complete agreed-to assignments.

- The four promises get BCT off to a positive start. They establish positive expectations of making a new beginning, making specific changes, and each person being responsible for his or her own behavior. Reviewing the promises each week often does lead to important changes.

- Couples promise not to make threats of separation or divorce in the heat of anger, but they do not promise to stay together no matter what happens. If separation becomes necessary due to continuing unresolved problems or irreconcilable differences, then the BCT counselor tries to help the couple separate in the least destructive way possible, as described in more detail in Chapter 9.

- The rest of the first BCT session involves starting the daily Recovery Contract, as described in the next chapter. Although the content of BCT changes as sessions progress, most sessions have a similar structure. Sessions begin with reviewing substance use or urges and home practice assignments of the past week, move on to teaching and practicing a new skill, and end by assigning home practice for the coming week.

NOTES

1. Chase, O'Farrell, Murphy, Fals-Stewart, and Murphy (2003); Fals-Stewart, O'Farrell, and Birchler (1995); O'Farrell, Fals-Stewart, Murphy, and Murphy (2003); O'Farrell and Murphy (1995).
2. Kelley and Fals-Stewart (2002).
3. Fals-Stewart, Birchler, and Ellis (1999).
4. For the Time-Line Follow-Back method, see Fals-Stewart, O'Farrell, Freitas, McFarlin, and Rutigliano (2000), and Sobell and Sobell (1996).
5. For the Drinker Inventory of Consequences, see Miller, Tonigan, and Longabaugh (1995), and for the Addiction Severity Index, see McLellan et al. (1985).
6. For the Dyadic Adjustment Scale, see Busby, Crane, Larson, and Christensen (1995) and Spanier (1976).
7. For the Conflict Tactics Scale, see Straus (1979).
8. For the Marital Status Inventory, see Weiss and Cerreto (1980).
9. For the Areas of Change Questionnaire, see Margolin, Talovic, and Weinstein (1983), and Weiss and Birchler (1975).
10. For the Sexual Adjustment Questionnaire, see O'Farrell, Kleinke, and Cutter (1997).
11. Fals-Stewart, Kashdan, O'Farrell, and Birchler (2002); O'Farrell, Feehan, Murphy, and Fals-Stewart (1999); O'Farrell and Murphy (1995); O'Farrell, Murphy, Stephan, Fals-Stewart, and Murphy (2004).

3

Building Support for Abstinence
The Daily Recovery Contract

As we begin this chapter, imagine that you are meeting with a substance-abusing patient and spouse for their first BCT session. They have completed an initial couple meeting to explore BCT, they have decided to start the therapy, and they have committed themselves to the four promises for the coming week. You have stressed the importance of session attendance and honesty. Now you are ready to begin the process of creating the Recovery Contract, arguably the most important part of BCT. This chapter presents the Recovery Contract in detail, case examples of successful use of the procedure, and problems commonly encountered. We start with a case example to illustrate the contract concretely before going into the step-by-step details of how to set up and maintain it.

RECOVERY CONTRACT CASE EXAMPLE

Figure 3.1 presents the Recovery Contract and calendar for Mary Smith and her husband Jack. Forms for the Recovery Contract and calendar are in Appendix C (see Form C.1 for contract and Form C.2 for calendar). Mary was a 29-year-old teacher's aide in an elementary school who had a serious drinking problem and also smoked marijuana daily. She was admitted to a detoxification unit at a community hospital after being caught drinking at work and being suspended from her job. Her husband, Jack, worked in a local warehouse and was a light drinker with no drug involvement. Mary and Jack had been married 4 years and Jack was considering leaving the marriage when the staff at the detoxification unit referred them to the BCT program.

The counselor developed a Recovery Contract in which Mary agreed to a daily "trust discussion" in which she stated to Jack her intent to stay "clean and sober" for the next 24 hours and Jack thanked her for her commitment to sobriety. The couple practiced this ritual in the counselor's office until it felt comfortable, and then also performed the discussion at each weekly therapy session on Wednesday evening. As the calendar in Figure 3.1 shows, they did

RECOVERY CONTRACT

In order to help (patient) _Mary_ with his/her recovery and to bring peace of mind to (partner) _Jack_, we commit to the following.

Patient's Responsibilities	Partner's Responsibilities
☒ DAILY TRUST DISCUSSION (with medication _NA_ if taking it)	
• States his or her intention to stay substance free that day (and takes medication, if applicable). • Thanks partner for supporting his or her recovery.	• Records that the intention was shared (and medication taken, if applicable) on calendar. • Thanks patient for his or her recovery efforts.
☒ FOCUS ON PRESENT AND FUTURE, NOT PAST	
• If necessary, requests that partner not mention past or possible future substance abuse outside of counseling sessions.	• Agrees not to mention past substance abuse or fears of future substance abuse outside of counseling sessions.
☒ WEEKLY SELF-HELP MEETINGS	
• Commitment to 12-step meetings: _AA mtgs_ _7pm Tues at church_ _10am Sat at hospital_	• Commitment to 12-step meetings: _Al-Anon_ _mtg 7pm Tues at church_
☒ URINE DRUG SCREENS	
• Urine Drug Screens: _Weekly at counseling sessions_	☐ OTHER RECOVERY SUPPORT •

EARLY WARNING SYSTEM
If, at any time, the trust discussion (with medication, if taking it) does not take place for 2 days in a row, we will contact (therapist/phone #: _Dr. Tim OFarrell 123-456-7899_) immediately.

LENGTH OF CONTRACT
This agreement covers the time from today until the end of weekly therapy sessions, when it can be renewed. It cannot be changed unless all of those signing below discuss the changes together.

Mary Smith   Patient   _Jack Smith_   Partner

Tim OFarrell PhD   Therapist   _9 / 12 / xx_   Date

RECOVERY CONTRACT CALENDAR

☒ ✓ = Trust Discussion Done   ☒ N = Al-Anon or Nar-Anon
☐ ⊘ = Trust Discussion with   ☒ D = Drug Urine + or –
    Medication (_____)   ☐ O = Other (_____)
☒ A = AA or NA Meeting

Mo & Yr: _September, 20XX_

S	M	T	W	T	F	S
						✓ 1
✓A 2	3	✓ 4	✓D+ 5	6	✓ 7	8
✓ 9	✓ 10	11	✓D+ 12	13	✓A 14	15
✓ 16	17	✓A 18	✓D+ 19	20	✓A 21	✓A 22
✓AN 23	24	✓ 25	✓D– 26	27	✓A 28	29
30						

Mo & Yr: _October, 20XX_

S	M	T	W	T	F	S
	1	✓AN 2	✓D– 3	4	✓ 5	✓A 6
✓ 7	✓AN 8	✓ 9	✓D– 10	11	✓ 12	✓A 13
14	15	✓ 16	✓D– 17	18	✓ 19	✓A 20
21	22	✓AN 23	✓D– 24	25	✓ 26	✓A 27
28	29	✓AN 30	✓D– 31			

Mo & Yr: _November, 20XX_

S	M	T	W	T	F	S
				1	✓ 2	✓A 3
✓ 4	✓ 5	✓AN 6	✓D– 7	✓ 8	✓ 9	A 10
✓ 11	✓ 12	✓AN 13	✓D– 14	✓ 15	✓ 16	✓A 17
✓ 18	✓ 19	✓AN 20	✓D– 21	✓ 22	✓ 23	24
✓ 25	26	✓AN 27	✓D– 28	✓ 29	✓ 30	

Mo & Yr: _December, 20XX_

S	M	T	W	T	F	S
						✓A 1
✓ 2	✓ 3	✓A 4	✓D– 5	✓ 6	✓ 7	✓A 8
✓ 9	✓ 10	✓AN 11	✓D– 12	✓ 13	✓ 14	✓A 15
✓ 16	✓ 17	✓AN 18	✓D– 19	✓ 20	✓ 21	✓A 22
✓ 23	✓ 24	✓AN 25	✓D– 26	✓ 27	✓ 28	✓A 29
✓ 30	✓ 31					

FIGURE 3.1. Contract and calendar for Mary and Jack.

this part of the contract nearly every day, missing only on an occasional Saturday because their schedule was different that day and sometimes they forgot. Mary agreed to attend at least two AA meetings each week and actually attended three meetings per week for the first 2 months.

Jack was pleased to see Mary not drinking and going to AA. However, he was upset that weekly drug urine screens were positive for marijuana for the first few weeks, taking this as evidence that his wife was still smoking marijuana, even though she denied it. The counselor explained that marijuana can remain in the system for some time, particularly in someone who had been a daily pot smoker. He also acknowledged that there was no way to know whether Mary was telling the truth. The counselor suggested that Jack go to Al-Anon to help him deal with his distress over his wife's suspected drug use. After a few weeks, the drug screens were negative for marijuana—and they stayed that way—lending further credence to Mary's daily statement of intent. Jack found Al-Anon helpful, so the couple added another recovery-related activity to their contract: One night a week they would go together to a local church where Mary could attend an AA meeting and Jack could go to an Al-Anon meeting.

Figure 3.1 shows their Recovery Contract calendar through the first 4 months of weekly BCT sessions. Mary and Jack continued weekly BCT sessions for another month, then monthly sessions through Mary's 1-year anniversary of abstinence, and then quarterly for 2 more years. Drug urine screens stopped when weekly sessions stopped. Mary and Jack continued their daily trust discussions, and Mary attended two or three 12-step meetings per week for the first 2 years, then weekly meetings thereafter. When seen by the counselor for a yearly check-up at 3 years of sobriety, Mary had been reinstated in her job and was pregnant with the couple's first child.

Implementing BCT went more smoothly with Mary and Jack than it does typically. They complied with the contract almost completely from the beginning. Mary accepted, without complaint, weekly drug urine screens and recommendations to attend 12-step meetings. Although their relationship was in crisis at the start of BCT, they did not have serious conflicts other than those related to the substance abuse. As a relatively younger couple who still had strong positive feelings for each other, they were able to work together fairly easily with the counselor's guidance. Many other patients and their spouses will present considerably greater challenges; still, a skilled BCT counselor ultimately may prove successful. The rest of this chapter discusses the steps in implementing the Recovery Contract in some detail to help you master this procedure for use with a wide variety of cases.

COMPONENTS OF THE RECOVERY CONTRACT

Table 3.1 summarizes the six typical components of the Recovery Contract: the trust discussion, medication to aid recovery, self-help involvement, urine screens, other weekly activities to support recovery, and a calendar to record progress. The trust discussion and calendar are always included in the contract. The other components may be included, based on the needs and willingness of the patient and spouse.

The first part of the daily Recovery Contract is the "trust discussion." Each day, at a specified time, the patient initiates this brief discussion. In it, the patient states his or her intent not to drink or use drugs that day (in the tradition of "one day at a time"), the spouse expresses support for the patient's efforts to stay abstinent, and the patient thanks the spouse for the encouragement and support. For patients taking a recovery-related medication (e.g., disulfiram,

TABLE 3.1. Components of Recovery Contract

- Daily Trust Discussion
  - Alcohol/drug abuser states intention to stay abstinent *that day*.
  - Spouse thanks alcohol/drug abuser for efforts to stay abstinent.
  - Patient thanks spouse for support.
  - Partners do not argue about past or future substance use.
- Medication to aid recovery.
- Self-help involvement.
- Weekly urine drug screens.
- Other weekly activities to support recovery.
- Progress recorded on calendar.

naltrexone), medication ingestion is witnessed and verbally reinforced by the spouse as part of the trust discussion. The spouse records the performance of the daily contract on a calendar that is on the back of the contract form you provide. To prevent substance-related conflicts that can trigger relapse, both partners agree not to discuss past or possible future substance use; these discussions are reserved for the therapy sessions. Finally, the couple agrees to a specific length of time during which the contract will be in effect and to call the counselor if the trust discussion does not take place for 2 days in a row.

At the start of each BCT session, once the contract is in place, you will review the Recovery Contract calendar to see how well each person has done his or her part. The couple also will do the trust discussion (and medication taking, if applicable) in each session to highlight its importance and to let you see how they do it. Twelve-step or other self-help meetings are a routine part of BCT for all patients who are willing. Urine drug screens taken at each BCT session are included for all patients with a current drug problem. Other weekly activities to support recovery can be chosen by the couple in order to personalize the contract so it meets their needs. Activities can vary as long as they aid in substance abuse and relationship recovery. Examples are group or individual counseling, exercise, reading from the AA Big Book, meditation, spiritual counseling, and so forth. If the Recovery Contract includes 12-step meetings, urine drug screens, or other weekly activities, these are also marked on the calendar and reviewed. The calendar provides an ongoing record of progress that you reward verbally at each session.

SPECIFIC STEPS TO ESTABLISH THE RECOVERY CONTRACT

Remember that when they start BCT many couples will be having very little contact with each other and/or frequent arguments. The contract asks them to talk together in a positive way every day about staying abstinent and to avoid negative interactions. The contract represents a big change, and they will need a lot of help from you to succeed.

Although the Recovery Contract seems simple enough, once introduced, it generally takes three or more BCT sessions before all goes smoothly. Table 3.2 lists the steps you follow to establish the contract. Introduction of the contract typically happens in the first BCT session, but the timing can vary somewhat. Sometimes, when the couple is cooperative and sure that they want to start BCT, you can introduce the contract at the end of the initial couple session to

---

TABLE 3.2. Steps to a Recovery Contract

- Introduce Recovery Contract in first BCT session.
  - Explain contract.
  - Have couple do trust discussion (with medication, if taking it) in session.
  - Couple agrees to try out contract for a week.
- Establish Recovery Contract in second BCT session.
  - Review performance of contract behaviors and any problems or discomfort.
  - Have couple do trust discussion (with medication, if taking it) in session.
  - Sign contract, if couple is ready.
- Maintain Recovery Contract in third BCT session and beyond.
  - Review contract since last session.
  - Have couple do trust discussion (with medication, if taking it) in each session.
  - Discuss how to get more benefits (e.g., add self-help group or, if going to AA, join a group or get a sponsor).

---

explore BCT and assign the trust discussion for home practice in the following week. Other times, for chaotic couples or those unsure about whether they want to commit to BCT, the contract may not be introduced until the second BCT session. The point is that, once introduced, the procedures of the contract take about three sessions to become fully established.

Introduce Recovery Contract in the First BCT Session

Table 3.3 shows the therapist checklist for introducing the trust discussion and Recovery Contract (from the checklist for session 1 of the 12-session BCT manual contained in Appendix A). Next we describe how the counselor completes each of these steps.

In establishing the Recovery Contract, you start with the daily trust discussion. For patients who are taking a recovery-related medication, taking the medication can be added to the contract as part of the trust discussion from the start. If the patient has not made a final decision about, or has not obtained, the medication, this step can be added to the contract at a later session (as described later in this chapter). You can suggest 12-step meetings and start urine drug screens in this session, but generally you do not add these to the contract initially to avoid confusion. These other supports for abstinence can be added to the written contract and calendar a little later.

TABLE 3.3. Therapist Checklist for Introducing Trust Discussion and Recovery Contract

_____ Introduce trust discussion concept.

_____ Explain and discuss trust discussion format.

_____ Couple practices trust discussion with coaching from therapist.

_____ Explain and discuss Recovery Contract, including possible recovery medication.

_____ Have each person verbally commit to Recovery Contract.

_____ Hand out Recovery Contract and Calendar Forms C.1 and C.2 from Appendix C.

_____ Assign home practice: trust discussion and completion of contract.

EXPLAIN AND DISCUSS THE RATIONALE FOR THE CONTRACT

When you first present it to the couple, describe the contract as a way a couple can address problems they face now that the substance-abusing patient has started to abstain. For relationships in which trust has been damaged, at least in part by alcoholism or drug abuse, partners often find it difficult to regain trust in each other.

The non-substance-abusing partner has been lied to on many occasions about the patient's alcohol and drug use and related behaviors. The non-substance-abusing partner often resents past substance abuse and fears future relapse. These feelings are intensified by the spouse's mistrust of the patient's promises to abstain. The patient helps to gradually bring peace of mind to the spouse by engaging in the trust discussion each day and doing other behaviors supportive of sobriety (e.g., attending AA meetings, having drug-free urine screens).

Substance-abusing patients need to earn back the trust and respect and allay the fears and misgivings of the spouse and other family members. They also need encouragement to deal with temptations and stressors without relapsing, especially in the first few months of abstinence, when they are most vulnerable to relapse from ambivalence about sobriety, protracted withdrawal symptoms, and triggers to use. Yet, many patients report that the spouse is very critical even when they have been sober for extended periods. Not surprisingly, patients' reaction is commonly one of "I can't get credit for trying, so why bother?" Explain that these problems and feelings are normal and typical for couples trying to make a new beginning after substance abuse. The contract tries to address the problems typically faced by the patient and the spouse. Based on the spirit of taking one day at a time, the contract can help the couple rebuild lost trust, support rather than unwittingly sabotage efforts to stay abstinent, and reduce arguments and tension about substance abuse.

EXPLAIN THE SPECIFICS OF THE TRUST DISCUSSION

After covering the rationale for the contract, review the following specifics of the trust discussion—the first part of the contract—with the couple.

1. The couple gets together privately at a specified time and place where they can talk without interruption for a few minutes. It is best to pick a time when this discussion will happen each day, so that it becomes part of the daily routine. Having the patient initiate the discussion works best (e.g., "Honey, it's time for our trust discussion. Is now OK for you?"). This initiative shows that the patient is taking responsibility for his or her own recovery and prevents spouse's having to remind or nag.

2. The patient makes a statement about his or her sobriety over the last 24 hours and his or her intentions over the next 24 hours. The spouse expresses appreciation for this reassurance. Although couples are encouraged to develop their own wording, giving them a template can be helpful at first.

> PATIENT: I have been sober for the last 24 hours and plan to stay sober for the next 24 hours. Thank you for listening and being supportive of my effort to be drug and alcohol free.
>
> SPOUSE: Thank you for staying sober for the last 24 hours. I appreciate the effort you are

making to stay clean and sober. (*Marks on the calendar that they had the trust discussion.*)

Figure 3.2 (a copy of which is Poster B.4 in Appendix B) displays this trust discussion formula. Reviewing this formula, displayed as a poster, helps familiarize them with the idea. If the patient is taking a recovery-related medication, he or she takes it while the spouse witnesses and thanks the patient as part of the trust discussion. (See section on medications below.)

3. Emphasize that the trust discussion is a way for the non-substance-abusing spouse to positively reinforce sobriety in the patient. Provide an example of introducing a negative into the discussion (e.g., "Thank you for staying sober, but I know this is only the calm before the storm because I have seen this before") and note that this should be avoided.

4. If the patient has not been sober for the past 24 hours or is not sure if he or she will stay sober in the next 24 hours, he or she should state that *and not lie*. If this occurs, the couple should contact the counselor by telephone.

5. Patient and spouse thank each other because each is receiving something from the other, and because they are finally doing something positive together about the substance use, which, in the past, has been a part of a very negative interaction between them.

6. Arguments and feelings about past or feared future episodes of substance use can lead to relapse. In the spirit of taking one day at a time, both the husband and the wife agree not to discuss past substance use or fears about future substance use outside of sessions. This restriction helps the couple avoid conflict and allows time to build a more positive relationship together without substance use.

Daily Trust Discussion Formula

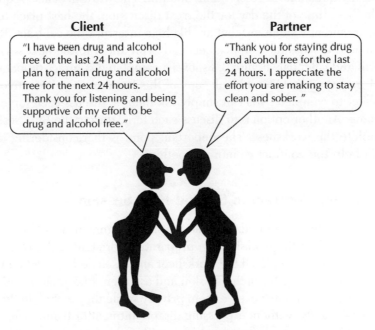

FIGURE 3.2. Daily trust discussion formula.

REHEARSE TRUST DISCUSSION IN THE SESSION

After reviewing the trust discussion, tell the couple that you would like them to try it for the coming week at home, after first doing it in the session. Have them fill in their names on the Recovery Contract form, then ask them to role-play the trust discussion. Keep it simple at first. As the sessions progress, some couples will personalize the contract and make it more involved. For example, couples have told us that they decided to read from AA's "Big Book" together, say a prayer together, or give each other a hug as part of their daily trust discussion. However, this first time most couples need to keep it simple and repeat the role play at least once to include all essential components (e.g., statement of intent to stay sober, both expressing thanks). If medication is part of the contract, include this as part of the trust discussion rehearsal. Provide corrective feedback liberally in a tolerant, cheerful manner. Join with the partners' initial awkwardness by stating that many couples feel uncomfortable with the contract at first, but that practice and repetition almost always make it easier. Rehearse all aspects of what they will be doing at home in the coming week, including when and where they plan to hold their daily trust discussions. Finally, on the calendar provided on the back of the contract form, have the spouse check off that they completed the discussion that day in session.

ASSIGN TRUST DISCUSSION FOR THE COMING WEEK

After discussing and rehearsing the contract, ask the couple to do the trust discussion at home, on a daily basis, and refrain from discussing past or future substance use in the coming week. In addition, ask them to consider signing a Recovery Contract, at least for the duration of BCT, in your next counseling session. To help in their decision making, each partner is asked to complete a contract preparation worksheet at home, describing potential benefits of doing the contract and raising any questions or reservations about it. The worksheet also requires the couple to determine the best time of the day for the trust discussion, the best place to keep the contract and calendar, and any situations that are likely to interrupt the contract. Request that the couple complete and discuss their worksheets and bring them to the next session, along with the contract form and calendar. Figure 3.3 shows a completed contract preparation worksheet (see Form C.31 in Appendix C for a blank copy of this form). As an alternative to giving partners the worksheet to complete, you can simply ask them to discuss each topic covered in the worksheet at home. Another option is to discuss each topic during the BCT session as you, the counselor, complete the worksheet. The important point is that considering these aspects of the contract can help the contract go more smoothly.

Establish Recovery Contract in Second BCT Session

After exchanging greetings, remind the couple that the assignment was to do the trust discussion daily and to complete the worksheet in preparation for signing the recovery contract in today's session. Ask if they completed the worksheet and discussed it, as agreed. If not, explain that you need the worksheet later in the session and ask them to complete and discuss it now. Leave the office for a few minutes to give them privacy while they complete the assignment. If you do this matter-of-factly, without expressing disappointment or blame, you will have sent a powerful message about the need for compliance with agreed-to assignments.

PREPARATION FOR THE RECOVERY CONTRACT

1. Write down any positive reasons for the two of you to be involved in a Recovery Contract together.

Patient	Partner
The trust discussion each day could help me stay focused on sobriety.	*Hearing him say he wants to stay sober could make me worry less.*
A little encouragement and no nagging would be nice.	*Appreciation for me sticking with him and helping him would be nice.*

2. Write down any questions or concerns you have about the contract:

Patient	Partner
Why does it have to be every day?	*I don't want to feel responsible for him staying sober. That's up to him.*
I'm not so sure about medication.	*What if he lies about using?*

3. Discuss the following together and write your decisions in the space provided:

   a. Best time of day to do the daily trust discussion

      Either in the morning before we leave for work or after supper when we're watching TV

   b. Best place to keep the calendar (hint—near where you will do the trust discussion so that you won't forget to mark it)

      In the kitchen cabinet

   c. Situations likely to interrupt the daily trust discussion (such as times apart, being angry)

      Our routine is different on Sundays when we don't go to work

      When Janice has to be gone overnight for work

FIGURE 3.3. Recovery Contract preparation worksheet.

Next, review and discuss the calendar and compliance with the contract in the past week. Praise the days when the contract was kept. Explore reasons for noncompliance on days when the contract was not kept. Ask about uncomfortable feelings when doing the contract. This is also the time to review the worksheets on pros and cons and procedural aspects of the contract.

When discussing the worksheets and any compliance problems, it helps to consider suggestions for both how to *do* the contract and how to *view* the contract. Most compliance difficulties relate to one or both of these aspects. In terms of *doing* the contract, the time for doing the trust discussion should be linked to a well-established habit when the patient and spouse are together each day, such as mealtime or bedtime. The couple should keep the contract with the calendar near the usual location of the trust discussion to make it easy for the spouse to mark the calendar each day. Couples also need to plan ahead to maintain the contract at times when the trust discussion routine most often gets broken, such as weekends, vacations, and times of marital crises. *Viewing* the contract constructively includes focusing on its individual and couple benefits and being very clear about who has what responsibility. The spouse is not responsible for keeping the patient sober. That is why the patient initiates the discussion: it signifies the patient is taking responsibility for his or her own recovery. The contract is not a weapon to force the patient to abstain or to bully the spouse into not nagging. It is extremely important that both partners view the agreement as a *cooperative method for rebuilding trust and feeling safe from substance abuse* and not as a coercive surveillance operation.

Finally, have the couple perform the trust discussion, as they did in the preceding session. Now it is time for you and each member of the couple to sign the contract. If the partners have been basically compliant with the contract in their first week (i.e., did contract at least 5 of 7 days without major problems or discomfort), then proceed with signing. If there were significant compliance problems in the first week, then postpone signing the contract until the following session. In such cases, compliance usually improves in response to the troubleshooting done in the second BCT session. Before signing the contract, add the length of time it will be in effect. The first installment of the contract typically lasts until the end of weekly BCT sessions, when it is often renewed for another period as part of the Continuing Recovery Plan (see chapter 8). Emphasize that, if the contract is skipped for 2 days in a row, they need to contact you. Add to the contract other components that have been agreed upon (e.g., medication, self-help meetings, urine drug screens) or defer these until the next session, if necessary. The couple takes the signed contract and calendar home to complete for the coming week.

Keep a copy of the signed contract and calendar for yourself. Each week, when you review the couple's calendar, update your copy so that both you and the couple have an ongoing record of progress. You can also mark days when strong urges or drinking or drug use occur on your copy of the calendar. By noting the circumstances surrounding these events, you gain information about triggers for substance use. Overall, the calendar gives you a detailed record for judging progress that does not rely on memory.

Maintain Recovery Contract in Third BCT Session and Beyond

Maintenance of the Recovery Contract, once it has been negotiated, is facilitated by monitoring compliance with the procedure at the beginning of each therapy session. The couple brings the calendar to each session, and the counselor probes for, and discusses, any lapses in compliance. Considering the distinction between doing and viewing the contract noted above may help the counselor understand the basis for the noncompliance. The couple can be asked to role-play the situations that interrupted the performance of the agreed-on behavior and to propose alternative strategies for dealing with such situations in the future.

Have the couple perform the trust discussion (with medication, if applicable) in each BCT session. This repetition highlights the importance of the contract. Phone calls from the counselor between sessions to monitor the contract also can be very useful in getting the procedure firmly established. Monitoring compliance with the Recovery Contract is especially important in the first month of the agreement, because most couples have some difficulty with the procedure during this period. (Frequently encountered difficulties are discussed in detail at the end of this chapter.) The first month is also the time period when other aspects of the contract (e.g., number, location, and type of self-help meetings) are finalized and fine-tuned. In later therapy sessions, briefly reviewing the calendar and performing the trust discussion (with medication, if applicable) in session usually suffice. Finally, a few weeks before the expiration of the agreement, the counselor should discuss whether or not the couple wants to renew the contract.

INCLUDING SELF-HELP MEETINGS AND DRUG SCREENS IN THE CONTRACT

Self-Help Meetings

BCT tries to increase and reward behaviors that support abstinence and long-term recovery. Participation in AA and NA are actions that support abstinence and a changed lifestyle conducive to long-term recovery. Therefore, participation in AA or NA for patients is frequently part of the Recovery Contract. Al-Anon or Nar-Anon for spouses can also be part of the contract, although in our experience this is somewhat less frequent than patient 12-step involvement. Occasionally another self-help group, such as Smart Recovery, will be part of the contract. BCT uses the contract and the patient's relationship with the spouse and the counselor to support activities that are associated with abstinence. BCT is only 1 hour a week; the contract supports behavior change the rest of the week.

Patient and spouse record specific commitments to self-help group meeting attendance on the contract and mark on the calendar the meetings that they attend each week. You review these commitments at each BCT session. Reinforce attendance at meetings and review circumstances surrounding planned meetings that were missed. When the couple completes a Continuing Recovery Plan toward the end of weekly BCT sessions, you can encourage continued participation in self-help groups to help prevent relapse.

Add self-help meetings to the contract early in the course of BCT sessions. Patients are most receptive when they are still feeling vulnerable from their most recent episode of substance abuse. After a few weeks of abstinence they may become less open to such suggestions and feel that they are doing fine without more help. Patients who have had extended abstinence in the past while actively taking part in a 12-step program are particularly good candidates.

The choice of number and type of meetings evolves over time as what is helpful and realistic becomes clearer. Keeping a schedule of local 12-step meetings to give to couples can help them plan the best times and locations to choose. Put in the contract only the number of meetings the person is truly committed to attend. A commitment that is kept to attend at least two meetings a week is better than a well-intentioned but unfulfilled promise to go to five meetings (only two are actually attended). Sometimes you will need to help the patient balance his or her commitment to 12-step with their commitment to spouse and family. This problem can arise when the patient feels pressure to do "90 meetings in 90 days" or something similar. For some, this daily attendance may be too much. For others it may be just what they need. You can help the couple find a number that is acceptable to both. This may mean suggesting that the patient focus on quality of meetings rather than quantity to allow for time to spend with the spouse and family. It can also mean encouraging the spouse to be understanding of the patient's time away, and helping the couple make the best use of the time they do have together. Getting the spouse involved in Al-Anon or Nar-Anon also can help. Much depends on the severity of the patient's addiction problem (the greater the severity, the greater the need for more meetings). We often recommend that a person consider three meetings per week for the first 90 days, and go to more if it is possible.

Meeting attendance is recorded on the contract and the calendar. We also discuss and encourage other key markers of participation, such as getting a sponsor, joining a group, going on commitments, attending smaller discussion group meetings, socializing with recovering individuals, and calling someone when help is needed. However, an in-depth introduction to the 12-step philosophy, similar to what is done in formal 12-step facilitation therapy,[1] is beyond the scope of BCT.

Urine Drug Screens

PROCEDURES FOR USING DRUG SCREENS IN BCT

We take urine drug screens at each BCT session for all patients with problematic drug use in the past year. Patients with a less recent drug history also may have drug screens if it seems clinically indicated (e.g., because they may be prone to return to a previous drug when abstaining from the current substance of choice). Results of urine drug screens are marked on the calendar and reviewed with the couple. We use the following codes on the calendar:

1. D+ = positive screen;
2. D– = negative screen; or
3. D0 = scheduled urine not taken due to missed appointment or other reason.

We also write the specific drug(s) that tested positive on the calendar. If a scheduled urine drug screen is not taken, we consider that abstinence on that occasion was not verified.

Based on the clinical history obtained in the first session, the patient is told if weekly drug screens will be part of the treatment plan, so this does not come as a surprise when he or she returns to sign up for BCT in the second session. Urine drug screens are initiated in the second session when the couple commits to starting BCT. Explain that urine drug screens provide objective data about recent drug use that serve two purposes. First, they corroborate the patient's reports of abstinence and are another way the patient can demonstrate changed behavior and win back the trust of the spouse. This is the most important reason. Second, the data tell you (as the counselor) if the patient is having difficulty staying abstinent and may give an early warning of problems before substance use gets too far out of control.

Some patients resent having to undergo drug testing and may complain that these procedures are overly coercive. It is important to listen and show that you understand their concerns, that it does not feel good to know that their word is not trusted fully. You can stress that even the most honest individuals, when they develop a substance abuse problem, will lie to conceal their use to avoid the wrath of those around them and protect their continued use. In short, nearly all substance abuse patients face a credibility crisis when they sober up. Now that they have started recovery, the drug screens can help them win back trust over a period of time.

Generally, we have had urine specimens tested by a laboratory on-site or contracted the testing to the clinics where we run BCT programs. Under routine procedures, a delay of at least a day is needed to get the test results, so the results from the current week's test is not reviewed and put on the calendar until the following week's session. At some locations we have started to use the newer disposable test cups that consist of a self-contained collection and testing device that provides results in a few minutes. A temperature strip also is provided on each cup so that temperature measurement can be used to verify that the specimen is freshly voided. The biggest advantage to the test cups is that you do not have to wait a week to review results with the couple and put them on the calendar. You can identify substance use earlier and intervene more quickly to prevent deterioration.[2]

LIMITATIONS TO DRUG SCREENS

Weekly drug screens are not foolproof. Patients can time their drug use to occur right after a session so that it will be out of their system by the time of the next urine screen; they can cancel sessions when they have used to prevent being detected; they can adulterate the sample (but this often can be prevented or detected). Labs can test specific gravity and temperature of specimens for signs of tampering, and test cups have a temperature indicator. Observing the specimen being given can prevent tampering, but many settings do not have staffing to accommodate same-sex screening of urination. Despite these limitations, if the patient regularly attends BCT sessions and submits to drug screens, it is unlikely he or she will get involved in very serious use without detection. The patient may be able to avoid detection on one or two occasions but not on a consistent basis. Even more importantly for the purpose of BCT, consistently negative drug screens contribute to rebuilding trust within the couple's relationship.

CASE EXAMPLES OF USING DRUG SCREEN RESULTS IN BCT

Two brief case examples illustrate different ways in which drug screen results can be helpful in BCT. *The first case of Mary and Jack*, in which Mary had both an alcoholism problem and daily marijuana use, was described earlier in this chapter. Drug screens were positive for marijuana in the first few weeks of BCT due to residual marijuana in her system. After a few weeks, the drug screens were negative for marijuana, and they stayed that way. In this case the drug screens verified Mary's reports that she had stopped marijuana use. This verification increased Jack's trust and helped their relationship.

In the second case of Ed and Belinda, the drug screens revealed drug use the patient was denying and forced him to choose between continued use and a stable home life. Ed was a 39-year-old self-employed roofer married for 11 years to Belinda, a stay-at-home mother. The couple had two children, both in elementary school. Belinda complained that for the past 8 years Ed had spent considerable time drinking in bars and using cocaine extensively on weekends. With some bitterness she stated that Ed had been "choosing drinking over his family." Ed acknowledged that his drinking had increased but felt that Belinda was exaggerating. Ed also admitted to using cocaine often on weekends but didn't think it was a problem. In the past year, the couple's arguments about the drinking and cocaine use had intensified. On more than one occasion, Belinda had threatened to separate if Ed did not change. A few weeks before the couple sought help, a neighbor called the police one evening when Ed returned home intoxicated and was pounding on the door and yelling at Belinda to let him in. Belinda insisted that Ed get some help. He called the BCT program based on a newspaper story he had seen about the program.

In the first session, the counselor told Ed he would be given a drug screen at the next session if they decided to start BCT. At the second session, Ed provided the urine specimen for testing. He also agreed to see the program physician about a possible disulfiram (Antabuse) prescription. Belinda suspected that he had been drinking on one occasion, but he denied it. She accepted Ed's denial, appearing relieved that he had agreed to continue BCT. They started the Recovery Contract with the daily trust discussion. For the next three sessions, Ed's urine screens came back positive for cocaine, which he denied using. He said he was taking nonprescription pain medication that contained codeine. The counselor explained that codeine would not produce a positive urine screen for cocaine. Then Ed said that the lab must have made an error. When asked for a urine specimen at that session, he gave a very small amount, saying it was all he could produce.

At the fourth session, the couple reported arguing frequently during the week because Ed had consumed alcohol on three occasions—twice before and once after saying that he had started taking Antabuse. In this session the counselor reported that urine screen results had been positive for cocaine again. Belinda was quite upset. She was fed up with Ed's continued cocaine use, drinking, and lying. Belinda told Ed he had to choose between his substance use and his family: He could not have both. The counselor asked Ed if he wanted to start again to stay clean and sober and be honest. Ed agreed that he did and admitted that he had been lying about the cocaine. Belinda agreed to try a few more weeks of BCT, although with some hesitation and skepticism.

At the following session they reported full compliance with the daily trust discussion and daily observation of Ed taking Antabuse. This compliance marked a turning point in the BCT sessions. From then on, Ed's urine screens were negative, and he did not drink. The couple made good use of the positive activities and communication skills training provided by BCT. At the end of the first year of sobriety, both Ed and Belinda were happy they had done the hard work needed to deal with their problems. In this case, the drug screens helped Ed confront and resolve his ambivalence about abstinence in favor of keeping his marriage and family together.

RECOVERY-RELATED MEDICATIONS AS PART OF THE CONTRACT

General Considerations to Using Medications in BCT

Including daily observation of the patient taking a recovery-related medication as part of the BCT recovery contract (1) helps the relationship because taking the medication in front of the spouse is another way for the patient to demonstrate that he or she is serious about abstinence, and (2) helps the patient by increasing compliance with medications that promote recovery. Currently the medications most frequently used to aid recovery are disulfiram (Antabuse) and naltrexone (ReVia) for alcoholic patients and naltrexone (Trexan) for opioid-dependent patients. Psychotropic medication for a comorbid psychiatric problem also can be considered a recovery-related medication and included as part of the BCT Recovery Contract. Such medications may include antidepressants for a comorbid mood disorder, antianxiety medications (with a low potential for abuse) for a comorbid anxiety disorder, and others. To be included in the contract, both patient and spouse need to view the medication as potentially helping the patient stay abstinent. Given the substantial efforts underway to develop and test medications to promote recovery from substance abuse, the number of medications that could be combined with BCT is likely to grow.[3]

It is important to note that having a medication witnessed by the spouse is not the same as having the spouse *dispense* the medication to the patient. Physicians will sometimes think of it this way and set up such an arrangement, with the goal of ensuring the patient's compliance with the medication. Such an arrangement may work for a while. However, unless relationship dynamics are addressed, the patient may come to resent the spouse, and the spouse may rebel at having to watch over the patient. Such feelings usually spell the end of the arrangement. In contrast, BCT emphasizes a noncoercive approach; the BCT counselor negotiates the daily contract between patient and family member as a positive, mutually beneficial arrangement—not as a watchdog approach and not as a way of putting the spouse in charge of keeping the patient sober. You need to be alert to how the patient and spouse view the medication taking, just as you monitor their view of the trust discussion. When medication is involved, such concerns may need greater attention than when it is not.

Next we describe the two medications for which there is the strongest evidence for effectiveness in combination with BCT. These are disulfiram for alcoholic patients and naltrexone for opioid-dependent and for alcoholic patients.[4]

Disulfiram (Antabuse) with Alcoholic Patients

The BCT Recovery Contract developed from behavioral contracts used to maintain disulfiram (Antabuse) ingestion among alcoholic patients, as described in Chapter 1. Originally we just had the spouse observe the patient take the disulfiram and then each thanked the other. Currently we combine the disulfiram observation with the other aspects of the Recovery Contract (i.e., the trust discussion, mutual thanking, agreement to refrain from discussing past or future substance use at home, attendance at 12-step meetings, and urine screens). Making the disulfiram observation part of this broader Recovery Contract solves two problems. First, the Recovery Contract provides ongoing behaviors that support abstinence and that can be continued by the patient and reinforced by the spouse after the patient stops taking Antabuse. This makes the transition off Antabuse much less anxiety-filled for the spouse, because the daily Recovery Contract can continue, albeit without Antabuse. Second, it also ensures that Antabuse is not used in isolation, as the only support for abstinence, but rather as part of a broader recovery program—a practice that reduces the risk of relapse when Antabuse is stopped.

Before making Antabuse part of the Recovery Contract, make sure that the drinker is willing and medically cleared to take the drug and that both the drinker and spouse have been fully informed about its effects. The prescribing physician should provide this information, but you should double-check both partners' level of understanding about it. If at the end of the first couple session the patient has expressed an interest in Antabuse, you can refer him or her to a prescribing physician at that time. Another way to include Antabuse from the start is to arrange to have willing patients started on Antabuse when they leave the detox or rehab program that is referring them to you for BCT. These patients should bring the medication to the second session, and you can include it with the trust discussion from the start. Antabuse can also be added after the second session—and it often is, for logistical reasons. Of course, the sooner the better, because patient receptivity decreases as time from the last substance-related crisis increases. Taking the Antabuse is immediately incorporated into the trust discussion. The dialogue between partners might go something like this.

PATIENT: Honey, it's time for our trust discussion and for me to take my Antabuse. Is now OK for you?

SPOUSE: Sure. Let me get the contract so I can mark the calendar.

PATIENT: I have been sober for the last 24 hours and plan to stay sober for the next 24 hours. I'm going to take my Antabuse (*shows spouse the pill so she can see it is Antabuse and then swallows it*). Thank you for listening and being supportive of my effort to be drug and alcohol free.

SPOUSE: Thank you for staying sober for the last 24 hours and for taking Antabuse to help with your recovery. I appreciate the effort you are making to stay clean and sober. (*Marks on the calendar that they had the trust discussion and that she observed the patient take Antabuse.*)

Couples bring the Antabuse to each BCT session and enact this brief ritual while the counselor observes. The counselor coaches the couple to help them find a comfortable, convincing way to perform this ritual, as already described above under the trust discussion. One additional element is added to the contract when a medication is involved: refilling the prescription before it runs out. This element is important because the contract often gets interrupted if the prescription runs out.

CASE ILLUSTRATION OF A RECOVERY CONTRACT WITH ANTABUSE

Figure 3.4 presents the Recovery Contract and calendar for Bill Jones, a 42-year-old postal worker with a chronic alcoholism problem, and his wife Nancy, who drank only occasionally. (Forms for the Recovery Contract and calendar are in Appendix C; see Form C.1 for contract and Form C.2 for calendar.) They entered our BCT program following Bill's completion of a 2-week residential rehabilitation program at a local treatment center. Daily ingestion of Antabuse, observed and reinforced by the wife, was part of their contract in addition to the daily trust discussion. They illustrate a somewhat less cooperative, less compliant case than Mary and Jack (earlier in this chapter), who did most of what was asked of them right from the start of BCT.

Bill's drinking had been a problem for many years. Three prior treatment programs had been followed by a few weeks, to a few months, of abstinence. The couple seemed distant and estranged with an air of tension and discomfort in the session. They did not report extensive overt hostility or emotion or threats to separate. Nancy said that they had "gone through all that" earlier. Now they both seemed resigned to a stable but unhappy relationship in which Bill had short periods of sobriety and long periods of daily addictive drinking. Bill's reaction to his most recent treatment was the only indication that change might be possible. He had been quite sick physically in the week before he checked into the treatment center. This illness had scared him because his father had died from medical complications of alcoholism. He also had made a strong connection with one of the counselors and liked a few of the patients in the rehab program.

During the first 2 weeks of trying out the trust discussion and Antabuse observation, Bill and Nancy were inconsistent in their performance. Their noncompliance was due partly to logistical problems but mainly to their continued underlying anger and distrust with each other—a common problem. The counselor worked with the couple to overcome these prob-

RECOVERY CONTRACT CALENDAR

☐ ✓ = Trust Discussion Done ☐ N = Al-Anon or Nar-Anon

☒ ⊘ = Trust Discussion with

Medication (_Antabuse_) ☐ D = Drug Urine + or –

☐ O = Other

☐ A = AA or NA Meeting (_____)

Mo & Yr: _September, 20XX_

S	M	T	W	T	F	S
				5	6	7
2	3	4	5	6	7	8
9	10	11	12	13	14	15
16	17	18	19	20	21	22
23	24	25	26	27	28	29
30						

Mo & Yr: _October, 20XX_

S	M	T	W	T	F	S
		1	2	3	4	5	6
7	8	9	10	11	12	13
14	15	16	17	18	19	20
21	22	23	24	25	26	27
28	29	30	31			

Mo & Yr: _November, 20XX_

S	M	T	W	T	F	S
				1	2	3
4	5	6	7	8	9	10
11	12	13	14	15	16	17
18	19	20	21	22	23	24
25	26	27	28	29	30	

Mo & Yr: _December, 20XX_

S	M	T	W	T	F	S
1	2	3	4	5	6	7	8
9	10	11	12	13	14	15
16	17	18	19	20	21	22
23	24	25	26	27	28	29
30	31					

RECOVERY CONTRACT

In order to help (patient) _Bill_ _____ with his/her recovery and to bring peace of mind to
(partner) _Nancy_ _____, we commit to the following.

Patient's Responsibilities	Partner's Responsibilities
☒ DAILY TRUST DISCUSSION	
(with medication _Antabuse_ _____ if taking it)	
• States his or her intention to stay substance free that day (and takes medication, if applicable).	• Records that the intention was shared (and medication taken, if applicable) on calendar.
• Thanks partner for supporting his or her recovery.	• Thanks patient for his or her recovery efforts.
☒ FOCUS ON PRESENT AND FUTURE, NOT PAST	
• If necessary, requests that partner not mention past or possible future substance abuse outside of counseling sessions.	• Agrees not to mention past substance abuse or fears of future substance abuse outside of counseling sessions.
☐ WEEKLY SELF-HELP MEETINGS	
• Commitment to 12-step meetings: _____	• Commitment to 12-step meetings: _____
☐ URINE DRUG SCREENS	
• Urine Drug Screens: _____	
☐ OTHER RECOVERY SUPPORT	
• _____	• _____

EARLY WARNING SYSTEM
If, at any time, the trust discussion (with medication, if taking it) does not take place for 2 days in a row,
we will contact (therapist/phone #: _Dr. Tim O'Farrell 123-456-7899_ _____) immediately.

LENGTH OF CONTRACT
This agreement covers the time from today until the end of weekly therapy sessions, when it can be
renewed. It cannot be changed unless all of those signing below discuss the changes together.

Bill Jones _____   _Nancy Jones_ _____
Patient   Partner

Tim O'Farrell PhD. _____   _9 / 13 / xx_ _____
Therapist   Date

FIGURE 3.4. Contract and calendar for Bill.

63

lems. Logistical problems were overcome by discussing the best time to have the trust discussion. The original plan was to do the trust discussion first thing in the morning. However, this did not work on Wednesdays or Sundays, when Nancy got up before Bill to attend an aerobics class. The time was changed to just before Bill went to bed in the evening. Bill's bedtime varied, but he and Nancy were always together at that time, and she generally retired when he did or stayed up a bit later.

The biggest interference with the contract was the couple's continuing discomfort with each other. At home they did not talk a lot other than what was required for practical reasons. They were living separate lives. The counselor empathized with them about how the contract and the BCT sessions represented a big change for them. It meant being vulnerable to reconnecting with each other, raising hopes for change, and risking possible failure in these attempts. The counselor also had Bill and Nancy repeatedly rehearse the contract in session, until they did it with some positive feeling and comfort. The couple eventually did the trust discussion consistently, each day, and felt that they benefited from it.

Urine drug screens were not part of the contract because Bill did not have a problem with any substance other than alcohol. The counselor thought that both Bill and Nancy were good candidates to benefit from 12-step meetings, but Bill steadfastly refused AA. He had gone to AA previously and suspected that an AA member had told a coworker that he had seen Bill at a meeting. He no longer trusted that his anonymity and his story would be safe in AA. Nancy was reluctant to attend Al-Anon because she felt drinking was Bill's problem and she was already doing enough by attending BCT sessions. Thus, 12-step meetings were not part of their contract.

The counselor stressed how important other supports for abstinence were, that it was not wise to rely solely on the BCT sessions, particularly given the severity of Bill's alcoholism. The possibility of individual substance abuse counseling at the treatment center was considered, but Bill refused this too. The counselor was about to give up when Bill mentioned that he had enjoyed the alumni group meeting last week for patients who had completed the treatment center's rehab program. The counselor Bill liked had led the group, and Bill saw some people who had been in rehab with him. Bill did agree to go to weekly meetings of the alumni group. However, he was not willing to make this part of his contract and write it on the calendar. He did not want to be bound by a commitment to go to alumni group meetings, only to go if he "felt like it."

After 6 months Bill stopped taking Antabuse but continued the daily trust discussions for an additional 12 months. This routine proved to be a satisfactory arrangement for both Bill and Nancy. Bill went weekly to the alumni meetings for about 6 months and then two to three times per month after that. The alumni group had a cake for him when he reached his 1-year anniversary of sobriety. Nancy attended the celebration. Eventually they started to socialize with one of the couples from the alumni group.

Naltrexone with Opioid-Dependent and Alcoholic Patients

Naltrexone is an opioid antagonist drug with proven ability to block the subjective reinforcing effects of opioid-based drugs.[5] Naltrexone prevents addicts from getting high when they take heroin or some other opioid drug. Without the high, the motivation to seek and use the drug decreases. However, naltrexone has not been widely used in drug abuse treatment, largely because of poor patient compliance.[6] Daily observation of naltrexone ingestion as part of the

Recovery Contract improves medication compliance and overall clinical outcomes. In a study of male opioid patients taking naltrexone, BCT patients, compared with their individually treated counterparts, had better naltrexone compliance, which led to greater abstinence and fewer substance-related problems.[7]

Among alcoholic patients, results for naltrexone are similar to those for opioid patients. Naltrexone reduces craving to drink and relapse to heavy drinking.[8] However, patient compliance must occur to get maximum benefit from this medication.[9] For alcoholic patients, BCT with daily observation of medication ingestion as part of the Recovery Contract also has improved compliance with naltrexone and overall clinical outcomes.[10]

COMMON PROBLEMS WITH THE RECOVERY CONTRACT

Many couples have some initial discomfort with the Recovery Contract procedure and some difficulty carrying it out. When first starting to use BCT, the counselor may be surprised and discouraged by these problems. Our view is that you have to expect such difficulties. Your job as a BCT counselor is to discover the nature of the difficulty and help the couple resolve it so that they can use the Recovery Contract successfully. Difficulties with the contract are a chance for you to repeat the reasons behind the contract and the specific actions needed by each person. In our experience, nearly every couple will have some problems establishing and maintaining the contract, but you can overcome these difficulties in most cases. The more experience you gain in BCT, the easier it is to recognize and deal with the many common resistances and problems encountered.

Counselor Failure to Prioritize the Contract

Many problems can be traced to the counselor's failure to give adequate attention to the contract. Counselors often fail to explain sufficiently the purpose and actions required in the contract. Without such detailed and repeated explanation, both members of the couple may not understand exactly what to do and why. Failure to be sufficiently careful and specific in monitoring compliance with the contract is another common error. An example may help you visualize how it should be done. When checking the calendar for the case of Bill and Nancy, above, an experienced BCT counselor would have held the calendar, looking at it, and said something like this:

> "So let me be sure I understand your calendar. Every day that has a checkmark means that Bill, you told Nancy that you were going to stay sober that day. And every day that has a circle around the checkmark means that Bill took the Antabuse while you, Nancy, watched. And you thanked each other. Is that right?"

Failure to elicit the couple's reactions and thoughts about the contract, especially negative feelings or concerns, prevents discussing and neutralizing the reactions that may interfere with compliance. Failure to perform the procedures of the contract in session, or doing it in a perfunctory manner, is another error. Finally, when the counselor addresses the contract late in the session and devotes little time to it, it should come as no surprise when the couple does not abide by the contract faithfully.

Spouse Complaints about the Contract

The spouse may object that the contract gives him or her responsibility for keeping the patient sober. The spouse may have learned through long and bitter experience, or through Al-Anon participation, that he or she cannot control the patient's substance use. Based on this belief, the spouse may feel that the contract is a step backward and dangerous to his or her mental health. You must stress that the spouse is not responsible for the patient's sobriety, or for the contract, or for any medication that is part of the contract. Rather the spouse is responsible *only* for doing his or her part, as specified in the contract. The spouse must be present at the agreed-upon time to witness and appreciate the patient's stated intention to stay abstinent (and take medication, if applicable) and record that he or she witnessed this on the calendar. The patient must do the rest.

What happens if the patient needs to be reminded to do the contract? The spouse may interpret this as the patient's resentment toward the contract or the spouse, or as a sign of general irresponsibility, or as failure to make recovery a priority ("He doesn't forget Monday night football"). Generally, we recommend having the patient be the one who initiates the contract. This provision is particularly important if the spouse is very concerned about being saddled with responsibility for the patient's recovery or if the patient fears that the spouse will try to force the agreement on him or her. In such cases, if the patient is forgetting to initiate the contract, you can help the patient find ways to remember (e.g., putting the contract where it is easily seen, linking the contract closely with some behavior the patient already does). In other cases, the spouse's reminding the patient occasionally is perceived by both as a sign of mutual caring. For still others, who initiates the contract is not an issue of concern. Having the couple perform the contract in each session is a good way to establish exactly how the couple will enact the contract at home, and it also allows you to elicit and discuss reactions and feelings the couple has to the contract during the session.

Negative Substance-Related Conversations

A common problem early in therapy is the spouse who, despite the agreement, continues to talk about past or possible future substance-related events. Often during such conversations, the patient passively listens and says as little as possible, while inwardly becoming quite angry. Interpreting the spouse's behavior as an attempt to punish the patient or sabotage the patient's recovery, or overtly disapproving of the spouse's behavior in other ways, usually is not helpful. Instead, you need to empathize with the spouse. Often you can do this by reframing the spouse's behavior as trying to protect the couple from further problems due to substance abuse. From this perspective, the spouse's conversations about the past are intended to ensure that the patient (1) knows fully the negative impact of the substance abuse (and this is a plausible reason, given that often the patient does not remember all that happened) and (2) is aware of the full extent of the problem so that his or her motivation to maintain sobriety will be fortified. Similarly, talk about "possible" future drinking is intended to fortify the patient against lapses in motivation and all-out relapse. If you sympathetically interpret the spouse's intent for the repeated substance-related conversations as just described, most often the spouse agrees that he or she has been correctly understood. Frequently the spouse then becomes more receptive to your statement that he or she has been "doing the wrong thing for the right reason" and to suggestions about more constructive methods to achieve the same goal. The spouse's compliance with the contract often improves greatly after such a discussion.

Substance-related conversations are infrequent for many couples who have signed a contract. Nevertheless, it is still important to monitor compliance with this part of the contract at each session. Failure to do so can lead to the patient's feeling that the agreement is one-sided. In addition, such substance-related discussions, although infrequent, can be quite revealing. Situations that stimulate the spouse's anger or fear about drinking are likely to lead to negative feelings and comments by the spouse. Situations that remind the spouse of the past negative effects of substance abuse (e.g., receiving an overdue bill that resulted from the patient's most recent drinking binge) often precipitate feelings of anger. Recurrence of situations that formerly signaled that the patient was drinking or using drugs often produces fear. For example, the patient is late getting home from work on Friday evening because of a traffic jam or car trouble, whereas in the past arriving home late meant the patient had been out drinking with companions from work. Similarly, upcoming situations (e.g., family gatherings or the holiday season) that were associated with embarrassing substance-related incidents in the past often stimulate fear and anger in the spouse.

When there have been no overt discussions about substance use, you can ask if the spouse has been tempted to engage in such talk. This question allows you to reinforce the spouse for resisting such temptations and to show the patient that the spouse indeed is making positive efforts. It also permits you to explain that such feelings are quite normal and that the contract requires only that the spouse does not discuss the feelings with the patient outside of BCT sessions.

Problems with Contracts Involving Medication

As you review a couple's performance of the Recovery Contract since the last BCT session, you frequently will discover that on one or more days the patient took the medication but the spouse did not observe it. Sometimes the patient does not fully see the point of the contract: "What's the difference, I took the medication anyway?" In other cases, the couple initially reports that medication ingestion was observed daily, but your probing reveals that the spouse did *not* actually observe it. For example, the patient called to the spouse from the next room, saying that he or she was taking the medication. In such cases, reiterate how the contract specifies something more than just the patient taking medication. Emphasize that the contract involves *the spouse observing the patient take the medication*. Remind the couple that the contract has advantages for both of them (peace of mind for the spouse, help to stay on the medication for the patient, as detailed above) that just taking of the medication by the patient does not. The couple also may need to adjust the time and location for performing the contract to make it work successfully.

Sometimes a couple's earlier experiences with a medication make them reluctant to include it in the contract. We have observed this reluctance most often with Antabuse. Some couples report having failed when they tried to include spouse observation of Antabuse taking without a counselor's assistance. Frequently, the Antabuse observation was initiated in a coercive manner by the spouse, and the patient had resented it and deceived the spouse by not actually swallowing the tablet or by substituting another pill (e.g., aspirin in the Antabuse bottle). Alternatively, the spouse had stopped observing the Antabuse ingestion after a brief period, once his or her fear and anger had subsided.

To overcome such reluctance, differentiate the counselor-assisted BCT contract from the previous failed attempt. First, in BCT you will help them with any problems they encounter. Second, insist that the couple not sign the contract if either partner feels coerced by the other to enter into the agreement. In this regard, reviewing the patient's current motivation toward sobriety can be useful. Often, partly because of past failed treatment attempts, the patient verbalizes that his or her current motivation is stronger than in the past, indicating a willingness to enter into the contract freely. The fact that the spouse has to refrain from substance-related conversation often makes the agreement seem less one-sided to the patient. Third, the fact that the contract is for a set time period with periodic counselor monitoring is an important difference that makes it more likely to succeed. Finally, when there has been deception about Antabuse taking in the past, you must deal with this issue directly. Have the patient show the spouse the pill prior to taking it and crush it in liquid (e.g., coffee or juice) to eliminate possible deception.

OVERCOMING PROBLEMS WITH THE RECOVERY CONTRACT: A CASE EXAMPLE

The previous section covered common problems with the Recovery Contract that are fairly easy to resolve. The following case example illustrates more serious problems with setting up the Recovery Contract that, although not typical, do occur periodically. In this case these problems included high levels of distrust in the couple and a substance-abusing patient who was mandated to treatment, denied the problem, lied about substance use, and falsified urine samples. As this example shows, the combination of a patient, persistent BCT counselor, a willing couple, and external pressure to encourage abstinence can often overcome these difficulties.

James was a 27-year-old married white male referred to outpatient substance abuse treatment by his probation officer for treatment of suspected cocaine dependence. James had been arrested recently for resisting arrest in an altercation during a police raid on a local crack house. James initially denied any problem with cocaine or other drugs, but urine testing by the probation officer revealed consistent cocaine use, which James ultimately admitted. James was informed by his probation officer that continued use of illegal drugs would constitute a violation of his probation conditions and would likely result in incarceration. James subsequently admitted that he had a cocaine problem and agreed to outpatient treatment.

During his intake interview at the outpatient treatment program, James described a 5-year history of problematic cocaine and alcohol use. He and his wife Cindy were living with his parents, largely because of financial problems resulting from his poor employment history. He and his wife had been married 3 years at the time of his admission to treatment; he noted that they married after Cindy got pregnant. He emphasized how much he loved his wife and daughter, Emma, as well as his guilt over his difficulties in supporting them.

James was admitted to the intensive outpatient program, which consisted of two group sessions and one individual session each week. He was required to submit urine samples at all appointments. Vocational training was also an important part of his treatment plan. Finally, he and his wife were referred to the couples therapy program for initial evaluation and assessment to determine eligibility.

When James and Cindy arrived for their interview at the couples therapy program, it was evident that Cindy was more interested in participating than was James. Cindy, who was 25 years old and working part-time as a cashier in a local discount store, said she was strongly considering leaving James, taking their daughter, and moving in with her parents. She had already consulted an attorney, who advised her that there was little doubt she would get custody of Emma. Cindy convinced James to take part in BCT, saying "this is our last chance to be a family." James, fearing the breakup of his marriage and loss of his daughter, agreed to participate.

Initial couples therapy sessions revealed significant distrust between them. Cindy openly stated her suspicions that James was using cocaine, despite his assertions to the contrary and urine screening results showing no drug use. James denied any use but repeatedly expressed concerns that some issues needed to be kept "private" and that he needed to finish treatment with no problems to "get my life back." Cindy and James engaged in the daily trust discussion and James attended twice-weekly AA meetings as part of his Recovery Contract (and as part of his general outpatient treatment plan). All of his urine assays were negative for cocaine and other drugs, which was reported by the counselor during the regular couples therapy sessions. Yet, Cindy remained unconvinced and held onto her suspicions that "something is wrong" because "James keeps hanging out with all the bad actors he always hangs out with." Many of the initial BCT sessions were spent discussing compliance with the Recovery Contract, Cindy's suspicions about James's continued use, and James's indignation about being accused of lying, despite the results of the urine assays.

About a month after starting BCT, James's individual therapist informed the BCT counselor that the probation department recently discovered that James had been submitting someone else's urine for analysis. More specifically, James had a friend who supplied urine to him, which he put in a concealed bottle and then squirted it into the urine cup when asked to provide a sample. This deception was discovered by the probation officer when he was supervising James as he provided a urine sample. Subsequent urine samples were found to be positive for cocaine. Although the probation officer allowed James to continue in outpatient treatment, he told James that any other positive urine samples would lead to a probation violation and a recommendation for incarceration. In addition, the probation department would be conducting regular and random urine screenings in addition to the ones performed in the outpatient program.

In the BCT sessions, James admitted to Cindy and the therapist that she was, in fact, correct. He had been regularly using cocaine since starting the program. Cindy said she would "give this another month," but only under the condition that they move in with her parents, so that "if he screws up again, it's him who gets kicked out, not me and Emma." James agreed to this new arrangement. The Recovery Contract was revised to provide more structured support for abstinence (see Figure 3.5; blank forms for the Recovery Contract and calendar are in Appendix C [see Form C.1 for contract and Form C.2 for calendar]). James agreed (1) to increase attendance at AA meetings from twice weekly to daily, at least for the next 2 months; (2) to get an AA sponsor and contact him at least twice weekly; and (3) to attend vocational training faithfully (he had been missing some classes) until he graduated. The couple also continued to do the daily trust discussion. Finally, the BCT counselor began calling each member of the couple between the weekly BCT sessions to check on compliance with the Recovery Contract.

Although Cindy remained understandably suspicious, after another month of BCT treatment, she noted that James was not seeing his old friends and was very involved with AA, his sponsor, and trade school. James said that the move out of his parents' house to a new (and better) neighborhood helped, and that Cindy's parents were "great with Emma and liked hav-

RECOVERY CONTRACT CALENDAR

☒ ✓ = Trust Discussion Done ☐ N = Al-Anon or Nar-Anon
☐ ⊘ = Trust Discussion with ☒ D = Drug Urine + or −
Medication (_____) ☒ O = Other
☒ A = AA or NA Meeting (used + lied)

Mo & Yr: September, 20XX

S	M	T	W	T	F	S
						✓O 1
✓O⁻ 2	✓OD⁻ 3	✓OA 4	✓D⁻ 5	A 6	✓D⁻ 7	✓O 8
✓ 9	✓D⁻ 10	✓A 11	✓OD⁻ 12	A 13	✓D⁻ 14	✓O 15
16	✓D⁻ 17	✓A 18	✓OD⁻ 19	OA 20	✓OD⁻ 21	22
✓ 23	D⁻ 24	OA 25	✓OD⁻ 26	OA 27	✓OD⁻ 28	29
✓O 30						

Mo & Yr: October, 20XX

S	M	T	W	T	F	S
	D+ 1	✓A 2	D+ 3	A 4	✓AD⁻ 5	✓ 6
✓ 7	✓AD⁻ 8	A 9	✓AD⁻ 10	✓A 11	✓AD⁻ 12	✓ 13
14	AD⁻ 15	✓A 16	A 17	A 18	✓D⁻ 19	20
21	✓AD⁻ 22	A 23	✓D⁻ 24	✓A 25	✓D⁻ 26	✓ 27
28	29	30	✓AD⁻ 31			

Mo & Yr: November, 20XX

S	M	T	W	T	F	S
				A 1	✓AD⁻ 2	✓ 3
4	✓AD⁻ 5	A 6	✓AD⁻ 7	✓A 8	✓AD⁻ 9	10
11	AD⁻ 12	✓A 13	AD⁻ 14	✓A 15	AD⁻ 16	✓A 17
✓ 18	AD⁻ 19	✓A 20	✓AD⁻ 21	✓A 22	AD⁻ 23	A 24
✓ 25	✓D⁻ 26	✓A 27	✓AD⁻ 28	✓ 29	AD⁻ 30	

Mo & Yr: December, 20XX

S	M	T	W	T	F	S
						✓A 1
2	✓AD⁻ 3	✓A 4	AD⁻ 5	A 6	✓AD⁻ 7	A 8
✓ 9	D⁻ 10	✓A 11	AD⁻ 12	✓A 13	✓AD⁻ 14	✓ 15
16	D⁻ 17	✓A 18	AD⁻ 19	✓A 20	✓AD⁻ 21	A 22
23	AD⁻ 24	✓A 25	AD⁻ 26	✓A 27	✓AD⁻ 28	A 29
30	✓AD⁻ 31					

RECOVERY CONTRACT

In order to help (patient) _James_ with his/her recovery and to bring peace of mind to (partner) _Cindy_, we commit to the following.

Patient's Responsibilities	Partner's Responsibilities

☒ **DAILY TRUST DISCUSSION**
(with medication _NA_ / if taking it)

- States his or her intention to stay substance free that day (and takes medication, if applicable).
- Thanks partner for supporting his or her recovery.

- Records that the intention was shared (and medication taken, if applicable) on calendar.
- Thanks patient for his or her recovery efforts.

☒ **FOCUS ON PRESENT AND FUTURE, NOT PAST**

- If necessary, requests that partner not mention past or possible future substance abuse outside of counseling sessions.

- Agrees not to mention past substance abuse or fears of future substance abuse outside of counseling sessions.

☒ **WEEKLY SELF-HELP MEETINGS**

- Commitment to 12-step meetings: _AA mtgs Tues & Thurs—changed to at least 5 days per week_

- Commitment to 12-step meetings:

☒ **URINE DRUG SCREENS**

- Urine Drug Screens: _3x/wk at Tx center random by p.o._

☒ **OTHER RECOVERY SUPPORT**

- _vocational training classes & p.o. mtgs._

EARLY WARNING SYSTEM
If, at any time, the trust discussion (with medication, if taking it) does not take place for 2 days in a row, we will contact (therapist/phone #: _Dr. Bill Fals-Stewart 123-456-7899_) immediately.

LENGTH OF CONTRACT
This agreement covers the time from today until the end of weekly therapy sessions, when it can be renewed. It cannot be changed unless all of those signing below discuss the changes together.

James Cox Patient   _Cindy Cox_ Partner
William Fals-Stewart Therapist   _9 / 7 / xx_ Date

FIGURE 3.5. Contract and calendar for James and Cindy.

ing us there." Although initial emphasis was placed largely on compliance with the Recovery Contract, the BCT sessions eventually moved toward increasing positive activities, including weekly "dates" and other regularly shared rewarding activities. James completed job training and got a full-time job as an auto mechanic, and Cindy also moved to a full-time position at the discount store. By James's report and from results of the urine assays (which were collected multiple times during the week by both the outpatient program and the probation department), he had remained abstinent from cocaine and alcohol.

James successfully completed weekly BCT, outpatient treatment, and probation. As part of the couple's Continuing Recovery Plan, negotiated near the end of weekly BCT sessions (see Chapter 8 for more details), they agreed to continue the daily trust discussion for 6 more months, and James agreed to attend at least two AA meetings weekly. Cindy also started attending Al-Anon weekly to obtain additional support, which she found very helpful.

During quarterly checkup visits for the year after the end of weekly BCT sessions, James and Cindy reported they were saving money to move into their own apartment, and Emma was getting ready to enter kindergarten. Cindy acknowledged that James was doing much better and was very involved with AA and some newer friends from work. She said she remained concerned that he would relapse, but that he was doing "all of the right things." Her parents described being "very impressed" with the changes they saw in James and considered him to be a good father and husband.

This case example shows how a patient, persistent BCT counselor helped a couple decide to use the Recovery Contract to help themselves, despite some serious problems in their first attempt with it. (The increased external pressure from probation no doubt also was quite important.) When it was discovered that James had lied about his drug use and falsified his urine samples, the BCT counselor did not give up, or stop couples sessions, or recommend divorce; instead, the counselor let Cindy and James make their own decision about what to do. The BCT counselor did say that she was willing to restart BCT sessions to see if things could improve, but only if both members of the couple were willing. She said it would be understandable if Cindy wanted to call it quits. Once the couple agreed to try again for another month under changed conditions, the counselor suggested some changes in the Recovery Contract to increase structure in support of abstinence. These changes included midweek phone calls to prompt compliance, increased attendance of AA meetings and contact with sponsor, and the addition of job training.

FREQUENTLY ASKED QUESTIONS

The following FAQs voice concerns raised by patients and spouses receiving BCT.

- *Question 1*: I have a disease over which I am powerless. How can I promise to stay sober? I can't guarantee I won't drink or use drugs. I do not see how I can do the trust discussion each day.
- *Answer*: The trust discussion asks you to tell your spouse that it is your *intention* not to drink or use drugs in the next 24 hours, that you *plan* to stay clean and sober for the next 24 hours, that you will *do your best* to stay sober for the next 24 hours. It does not ask you for a guarantee. That would be unreasonable and unrealistic. Admitting that you have a disease of alcoholism or chemical dependency over which you are powerless is an important step in your

recovery. The trust discussion can be a helpful reminder to make sobriety your first priority one day at a time. It also can reassure your spouse that you admit you have a serious alcohol or drug problem and are making a sincere effort to stay sober. Gradually your spouse may begin to trust you more, to forgive your for the past problems, and to look forward to a future together.

• *Question 2*: I am not sure I like this Recovery Contract. I'm supposed to watch him take Antabuse everyday and listen to him say he'll stay sober. It seems like you're making me responsible for his sobriety. I learned in Al-Anon that taking care of him isn't my responsibility. I need to detach from worrying about him and take care of myself.

• *Answer*: Yes, I absolutely agree you are not responsible for his sobriety. That is not the purpose of the contract. Making you responsible for his sobriety would be bad for you and for him. You could worry yourself sick trying to control something (his drinking) over which you are powerless, and he could become less likely to take responsibility for his own drinking. In the trust discussion part of the contract, your job is to be a daily witness to your husband while he takes Antabuse and promises to stay sober. It may help him when you do this, but it doesn't mean you are *responsible* for his recovery. It is not your job to keep him sober. That is his job. In the Recovery Contract, your husband has the primary role of initiating the trust discussion and the Antabuse taking. You have a secondary role as a witness and a supportive person, but you are not responsible for his sobriety.

I also agree that it is better for you *not* to worry about him and to take care of yourself. In an odd sort of way, the contract actually may help you with this. Knowing he has taken the Antabuse and hearing him promise to stay sober may make it easier for you not to worry about what he is doing the rest of the time. The part of the contract in which you agree not to bring up past drinking or possible future drinking, except at the couple sessions, also may help you focus less on him. It's a bit of a paradox—focusing on him a few minutes each day when he takes Antabuse and promises sobriety may help you "let go" of your worry and desire to control him for the rest of the day. We see the contract as a small way in which you can take care of yourself by letting yourself receive some peace of mind by witnessing his words and actions regarding his intended sobriety.

• *Question 3*: I don't see why I have to take Antabuse. It seems like you think I need it to stay sober, that I'm going to drink at any moment. I don't need it, and I would prefer not to take it.

• *Answer*: Whether or not you take Antabuse is your decision. Certainly you don't have to take it if you don't want to. But let me clarify a few things. I don't think you need Antabuse to stay sober now. You just got out of detox. The problems that led up to the detox are fresh in your mind, and you are very motivated not to drink. I'm thinking more of the immediate bene-fits of Antabuse to your wife. When she sees you take Antabuse, she doesn't have to worry whether you are going to drink that day. Taking the Antabuse while she observes sends a safety signal to your wife. It is a way you can give her the gift of peace of mind. It shows her you are really serious about your recovery, that you are willing to take an extra step to earn back her trust. Even though you don't need the Antabuse now to stay sober, taking it now and agreeing to stay on it for at least the next few months while you are attending couple sessions may turn out to be an insurance policy for the future. A number of weeks from now you may have some unexpected stress in your life, or the memory of your last detox may have started to fade, or you may find yourself strongly tempted to drink for other reasons. At that time, the Antabuse may help you by preventing an impulsive choice to drink.

SUMMARY

- The Recovery Contract starts with the trust discussion, in which the patient states his or her intent not to drink or use drugs that day, the spouse expresses support for the patient's efforts to stay abstinent, and the patient thanks the spouse for the encouragement and support. The spouse records performance of the discussion and other recovery supports (self-help meetings, drug screens, medication) on a calendar that is provided. The couple agrees not to discuss substance-related conflicts that can trigger relapse, reserving these discussions for the counseling sessions.

- Although the Recovery Contract seems simple enough, generally it takes three or more BCT sessions before the couple performs the contract smoothly. In the first BCT session the couple rehearses the trust discussion part of the contract and agrees to try it each day for the coming week at home. In the next BCT session, if they performed the trust discussion faithfully at home, the couple signs the contract for a specific time period. In each subsequent BCT session, the counselor reviews the contract performance in the past week, and the couple does the contract in session to highlight its importance.

- Self-help meetings, urine drug screens, and recovery-related medication are part of the contract for many patients because each helps the patient stay abstinent and demonstrates to the spouse the patient's commitment to abstinence and a changed lifestyle.

- It is important for couples to realize that the Recovery Contract does not conflict with 12-step beliefs. For patients, stating that they do not intend or plan to drink or use drugs in the next 24 hours does not constitute a guarantee or conflict with the view of having a disease over which they are powerless. For spouses, being part of the trust discussion or observing the patient take recovery medication in no way makes them responsible for the patient's recovery.

- For patients who object to Antabuse because they don't feel they need it to stay abstinent, it can help to stress the peace of mind that Antabuse brings to the spouse. This perspective puts the patient in a position of strength (giving a safety signal to the spouse), rather than a position of weakness (needing a medication to stay abstinent).

- Many couples' problems with the contract can be traced to counselors' failure to give adequate attention to the contract's components. Other common problems involve the spouse feeling responsible for the patient's recovery, continuing negative substance-related conversations, and issues related to medication.

- This chapter covered the daily Recovery Contract, a major support for abstinence in BCT. The next chapter considers other procedures used in BCT to promote abstinence.

NOTES

1. For details on 12-step facilitation therapy, see Nowinski, Baker, and Carroll (1992).
2. For information on procedures for urine drug screens, see Verebey and Turner (1991) for laboratory

testing, and see the Instant Technologies, Inc. website (www.tryi.com) for use of a self-contained collection and testing device.

3. For reviews of the psychopharmacology of addiction, see the chapters on pharmacological interventions in *Principles of Addiction Medicine* (Graham, Schultz, Mayo-Smith, Ries, & Wilford, 2003), published by the American Society of Addiction Medicine.

4. For a review of BCT to increase compliance with disulfiram, see O'Farrell, Allen, and Litten (1995). For studies of BCT to increase compliance with naltrexone, see Fals-Stewart and O'Farrell (2003; results with opioid-dependent patients) and Fals-Stewart and O'Farrell (2002; results with alcoholic patients).

5. Kleber and Kosten (1984).

6. Kosten and Kleber (1984).

7. Fals-Stewart and O'Farrell (2003).

8. Kranzler and Van Kirk (2001).

9. Chick et al. (2000); Volpicelli et al. (1997).

10. Fals-Stewart and O'Farrell (2002).

4

Other Support for Abstinence

The previous chapter covered the daily Recovery Contract, a major support for abstinence in BCT. This chapter considers four other methods used in BCT to promote abstinence. These include (1) reviewing substance use or urges to use at each session, (2) decreasing exposure to alcohol and drugs, (3) addressing stressful life problems, and (4) decreasing spouse behaviors that trigger or reward substance use. Whereas each BCT session reviews urges and use, time spent on each of the other supports for abstinence depends on the needs of the couple. As described in Table 1.7 in Chapter 1, if needed by the couple, other components (i.e., decreasing substance exposure, stressful problems, and enabling) are initially addressed in the first four BCT sessions. Most couples need to give some attention to stressful problems and substance exposure. Whether these other components are continued in subsequent sessions is based on the particular needs of the couple.

REVIEW SUBSTANCE USE OR URGES TO USE SINCE LAST SESSION

A typical BCT session begins with an inquiry about any drinking or drug use, or urges to drink or use drugs, that has occurred since the last session. The counselor's question might go something like this: "Could you tell me about times since we last met when you drank or used drugs or had an urge or temptation to do so?" If the patient and spouse report that no drinking or drug use has occurred since the last BCT session, then review urges to drink or use drugs that occurred. If the patient drank or used drugs, make dealing with this your top priority. Address the substance use right away and defer other issues, as described in the next section.

Reviewing Urges to Drink or Use Drugs

Reviewing urges to drink or use drugs experienced in the past week is part of each BCT session. Thoughts and temptations that are less intense than an urge or a craving are included. At first, many spouses fear that having an urge means the patient still wants to drink or use drugs or that a relapse is imminent. Similarly, the patient may be reluctant to discuss urges for fear it will upset the spouse. Therefore, the first time you discuss urges, you need to normalize them as an expected part of recovery.

Discussing situations, thoughts, and feelings associated with urges helps identify potential triggers for alcohol or drug use and often leads to consideration of ways to deal with such triggers without using. The patient's report can alert you to the possible risk of a relapse depending on the intensity of the urges described and how close the patient came to using. Such discussions should include successful coping strategies (e.g., distraction, calling a sponsor) that the patient used to resist an urge. Celebrating the patient's success in resisting urges and temptations gives credit for important steps in maintaining abstinence and builds self-confidence that future obstacles can be overcome. Finally, discussing urges in session prepares the couple for discussing them at home—a practice that many patients report helps them considerably.

The case of Eric and Jon, a gay male couple in their late 20s, illustrates these points about reviewing urges to drink or use drugs. Both were heavy drinking regulars in the local gay bar scene when they met 5 years ago. They had lived together as roommates and lovers since then. During this time Eric's drinking had increased and he continued to frequent the bars, but Jon had decreased his drinking and no longer enjoyed the bar scene. Their arguments increased about Eric's drinking and Jon's suspicions that Eric was having casual encounters with other men at the bars. Then Eric lost his job as a graphic designer because he missed too much work and showed up late too frequently after drinking the night before. At Jon's insistence, Eric sought help at the substance abuse program of a health center serving the gay and lesbian community in a large Eastern U.S. city. Over the course of four BCT sessions, they started a Recovery Contract that included daily Antabuse and regular AA meetings for Eric. Then they agreed to attend eight more weekly BCT sessions. They missed doing the daily trust discussion with Antabuse on only four occasions during the 12 weeks of BCT, when Jon was gone or had to work late and Eric had already gone to bed before he returned home. Eric also said that his regular attendance at AA meetings helped him cope with the frustration of trying to find work and stay sober in spite of this frustration.

At the start of each BCT session, Eric reviewed a form on which he had recorded any urges or thoughts of drinking or drug use from the previous week. He recorded the day, time, and circumstances surrounding the urge to drink and how strong the urge had been on a 1 ("weak") to 10 ("very strong") scale. Through many of the early BCT sessions, Eric reported moderate to intense thoughts of drinking. Two types of situations triggered Eric's thoughts of drinking: (1) incidents in which Jon commented about his being unemployed and their serious financial problems, and (2) times when he was alone and his mood became depressed after thinking about unresolved problems in his life. Eric benefited from discussing these thoughts of drinking in the BCT session. Learning that others had similar experiences also helped, as did the counselor's pointing out that he had successfully coped with the urges. The counselor suggested that he try to distract himself with other thoughts and activities when confronted by the thought of drinking. This tactic appealed to Eric, who liked the prospect of actively controlling his urges to drink. As time went on Eric's urges and thoughts about drinking became less frequent and less intense. Figure 4.1 (a copy of which is Form C.30 in Appendix C) shows a sample record of urges completed by Eric. Although this written record of urges was used in Eric's case, it is more typical in BCT to verbally review urges and use without the written form.

THOUGHTS OF HAVING A DRINK OR DRUG
(IF NONE, WRITE "NONE")

Time & Day	Situation (where, with whom, doing what, your mood)	How Strong (1–10)
Wed 11/20	Jon asked when was I going to give him my half of the rent. I felt like hitting him. He knows I am looking for a job. Thought getting drunk would teach him not to be so mean.	6
Sat 11/23	At home alone on Saturday night. Jon visiting his family. Felt lonely and depressed. Thought about going to bar where friends hang out. Called my sponsor instead.	9

FIGURE 4.1. Sample record of urges to use.

Crisis Intervention for Drinking or Drug Use

GENERAL APPROACH

Crisis intervention for substance use is an important part of BCT. Drinking or drug use episodes occur during BCT, as they do with any other treatment. BCT works best if you intervene before the substance use goes on for too long a period. In an early BCT session, negotiate an agreement that either member of the couple should call you if substance use occurs or seems imminent. You can link this strategy to the early warning system of the Recovery Contract in which they agree to call you if the daily trust discussion does not occur for 2 days in a row. Once substance use has occurred, try to get it stopped and to see the couple as soon as possible to use the relapse as a learning experience.

At the couple session, you must be extremely active in defusing hostile or depressive reactions to the substance use. Stress that drinking or drug use does not constitute total failure, that inconsistent progress is the rule rather than the exception. Help the couple decide what they need to do to feel sure that the substance use is over and will not continue in the coming week (e.g., restarting recovery medication, going to AA and Al-Anon together, reinstituting a daily trust discussion, entering a detox unit). Finally, try to help the couple identify what trigger led up to the relapse and generate alternative solutions other than substance use for similar future situations. Table 4.1 summarizes the general approach to dealing with urges and substance use in BCT.

TABLE 4.1. Dealing with Urges and Use

- Reviewing urges to drink or use drugs:
  - Helps identify substance use triggers.
  - Builds confidence in resisting urges.
- Crisis intervention for substance use:
  - Get substance use stopped quickly.
  - Use relapse as a learning experience.
  - Repeated episodes need special focus.
  - Shifting of blame and couple issues may be involved in repeated use.

REPEATED SUBSTANCE USE BASED ON INDIVIDUAL, NOT RELATIONSHIP, FACTORS

Repeated substance use can present a particularly difficult challenge. Use each episode as a learning experience. Depending on what is discovered, different strategies may be helpful. Sometimes a careful analysis shows that the substance use is being triggered by factors outside the couple relationship, such as work pressures or job-related drinking situations. In such cases, help the patient devise methods to deal with the nonrelationship triggers. Another nonrelationship factor that can lead to repeated episodes of substance use is the patient's ambivalence about whether to embrace abstinence or try to drink "socially" or use drugs "recreationally." Often an individual session with the patient will help you establish that this ambivalence is the basis for the repeated substance use. Then you can use a motivational interviewing[1] approach to help the patient consider costs and benefits of different choices about his or her drinking or drug use.

WHEN REPEATED SUBSTANCE USE HAS COUPLE BENEFITS

At times, repeated episodes of substance use are related, at least in part, to couple relationship issues. The substance use has relationship benefits for some couples. For example, it may facilitate sexual interaction or emotional communication for one or both spouses. In such cases, your first task is to help the patient strengthen controls against substance use. You can do this by coaching the patient to do things that will make him or her less likely to drink or use drugs, such as increasing 12-step involvement (e.g., attending more meetings, joining a group, getting a sponsor), taking recovery medication formerly refused, or getting alcohol completely out of the house. Then you can help the couple learn, through a process of problem solving and communication (see Chapters 6 and 7), to get the same relationship benefits without the aid of substances.

REPEATED SUBSTANCE USE BASED ON COUPLE CONFLICTS AND SHIFTING OF BLAME

For other couples, repeated episodes of substance use are a response to recurring, intense relationship conflicts. Often these conflicts involve complex couple dynamics that circle around blame and responsibility. The patient blames the spouse for their drinking, saying they cannot stay sober unless spouses change how they act. Spouses insist that patients have to stay sober, that their own actions are justified, and that they do not have to change.

The case of Janet and Ken illustrates this all too familiar pattern. Janet was a stay-at-home mother of two preschool children. She started to drink heavily during a period of depression after the birth of her first child. When they both started BCT, Janet was attending an intensive outpatient program. Social services had referred her for treatment because a neighbor reported that Janet looked intoxicated while caring for her two kids. Ken drove a delivery truck and took medication prescribed by the local mental health center for bipolar disorder.

During the first four BCT sessions, they reported complete abstinence and total compliance with the daily trust discussion, the only part of the Recovery Contract to which they agreed. Janet refused AA because there was no one to care for the children during the day, and Ken did not want her going out at night. At the fifth BCT session, Ken looked agitated. He said he could not keep on lying. Janet had cut down her drinking. She no longer drank during the day when at home with the kids. However, in the evening while Ken watched the kids, she would go out to buy a half-pint to a pint of liquor, bring it home, drink it in the basement recreation room, and fall asleep on the couch. At first he had agreed not to tell the therapist about her evening drinking for fear it would be reported to social services and they would lose their children. Now Ken was afraid Janet would get out of control, go back to daytime drinking, and they would lose their kids anyway. He insisted she had to stop drinking totally.

Janet said the main reason she drank was to escape Ken's yelling and criticizing, and also to relax after caring for the children all day. She said Ken would return home many evenings and start complaining that the house was a mess, dinner wasn't ready, or it didn't meet with his approval. When she tried to explain she was tired from caring for the kids, Ken would raise his voice and loudly tell her his mother had raised four kids, kept a spotless house, and always had a home-made meal ready on time. Why couldn't she? What was wrong with her? Janet reported that she would get quiet, finish dinner, and then head out to the liquor store. She said it was his fault she kept drinking. Unless Ken stopped yelling and started treating her better, there was no way she could stop drinking.

The best approach for couples such as this one is to (1) clarify that each person has responsibility for his or her own behavior; (2) devise specific methods that both partners can use to contain conflict and that the patient can use to avoid substance use; (3) strengthen individual coping mechanisms; and (4) teach alternative communication and problem-solving skills. These principles were applied to Janet and Ken, as follows.

First, the BCT therapist empathized with Janet's feeling criticized and devalued by Ken's frequent put-downs and negative comparisons with his own mother. The therapist then stated that Janet was responsible for whether or not she drank. Clearly it was more difficult to stay sober in the face of Ken's criticism, but he could not make her drink or make her stay sober. That was up to her. If she wanted to stay sober, she would have to find a way to cope with Ken's criticism without drinking over it. Similarly, the therapist empathized with Ken's frustration over Janet's continued drinking and her level of homemaking. Still, Ken had a choice about whether to vent his anger by yelling or to find a less hostile way to express his concerns. Clearly his current approach was not helping. The therapist delivered this message of individual responsibility in a quiet, deliberate manner, and asked each person to comment. Both Janet and Ken agreed they could see the wisdom in this message, even if it might be hard to put into action.

Second, to restructure the high-risk early evening hours, they agreed to try to make the first 15 minutes after Ken returned home a "conflict-free zone." Ken would eat a snack bar on the way home so that he wasn't so hungry, tired, and on edge. Even if they had argued, Janet would relax and watch TV after dinner rather than go out to the liquor store.

Third, to strengthen individual coping mechanisms, the therapist referred Janet to a twice-weekly morning therapy group for substance-abusing mothers at a clinic that provided child care. The therapist also encouraged Ken to rejoin a biweekly therapy group at the mental health center where he got his medication. Fourth, as the BCT sessions progressed, the couple worked on problem solving and communication to address their conflicting expectations and the many stressors in their lives.

ACTUAL OR SUSPECTED SUBSTANCE USE AT TIME OF BCT SESSION

On occasion, a patient will appear to be under the influence of alcohol or drugs when the couple comes to a BCT session. This is a good time to speak with each member of the couple alone for 5–10 minutes while the other sits in the waiting area. Speak with the patient first. Give the patient the opportunity to admit having used. If the patient denies use, suggest a breathalyzer or urine screen to determine his or her current state. Results will provide evidence of the patient's denial if results are negative. If results are positive, discuss how the patient is going to share the truth with the spouse when you go back to the couple session. Then see the spouse alone to convey information about the results of the breathalyzer or urine screen. Allow the spouse to express anger and disappointment if the results were positive. Listen to the spouse's opinions about factors that led to the use and what should happen now to prevent a recurrence. Finally, bring the couple back together to decide the best course of action, much of which you will have already determined in your separate interviews with each person alone. Usually you will have to wait until the next session to process the episode of substance use in more detail because this is not feasible when the patient is under the influence.

When deciding how to deal with a patient who is under the influence, safety issues should be paramount, including preventing an intoxicated patient from driving. Most substance abuse clinics have written procedures for dealing with intoxicated patients. Generally if the patient's blood alcohol level (BAL) is greater than or equal to the legal limit for driving, or if the patient refuses a breathalyzer and shows signs of impairment, the therapist tries to prevent the patient from driving. Frequently the spouse can drive the patient home if there are no contraindications to this arrangement (e.g., patient showing erratic behavior, or any doubt by therapist or spouse that doing so will be safe). Alternatively, you can arrange other transportation or you can ask the patient to surrender his or her keys and wait at the clinic until the BAL drops below the legal limit. Written procedures are intended to ensure that you will be prepared when faced with such a problem, and they should include options for dealing with a patient who refuses to follow your recommendations, especially when you are concerned that the patient, upon leaving, may harm him- or herself or others. Such options can range from documenting that you advised the patient that it was not safe to drive to contacting emergency response personnel for assistance. Options used will depend on your judgment of the seriousness of the risk presented by the patient's intoxication.

WHEN THE COUPLE DISAGREES ABOUT WHETHER THE PATIENT DRANK OR USED DRUGS

It is not uncommon for the spouse to report suspicions that the patient drank or used drugs during the week, whereas the patient strongly denies this. You can try to determine which is most likely true by listening to each person's story. Sometimes the patient eventually admits drinking or drug use. Other times the patient continues to deny this behavior even when it seems clear to you that the patient most likely did use. This stalemate can be a frustrating situation for the therapist and the couple. When partners remain at odds, it is better not to add to their conflict by getting upset yourself. (Sometimes this is easier said than done; most people, including counselors, do not like thinking they are being lied to.) In response to this type of situation, we tell the couple that in our experience, a spouse who suspects that the patient has used is usually correct—not always, but most of the time. We also admit that we do not really know the truth, and in the long run it may not matter too much. Most cases will clarify themselves over time. "Time will tell." If a person with a serious alcohol or drug problem is using, that behavior will gradually increase to a point that it becomes unmistakable. On the other hand, if the person is not using or if using occurred only once or twice and the person remains abstinent in the future, then this behavior will become evident.

DECREASE EXPOSURE TO ALCOHOL AND DRUGS

Exposure to situations where alcohol or drugs are available or others are using such substances is a high-risk situation for relapse among individuals in treatment for substance abuse. BCT sessions can reduce the risk of relapse by discussing how the patient and spouse will deal with such situations. The safest plan is for the patient to avoid all contact with situations where alcohol or drugs are available, especially in the early months of abstinence. However, many people are not willing or able to follow this suggestion. You should help each couple develop their own plan for dealing with common exposure situations.

Alcohol at Home and Spouse's Substance Use

Start by helping the couple decide if the spouse will drink in the patient's presence and whether alcoholic beverages will be kept and served at home. For example, Jane and Ed were a couple in their early 40s. Ed had a serious alcohol problem that had caused many problems in their lives. Jane had been a moderate drinker but, after discussing the dangers of Ed's exposure to alcohol at an early BCT session, she decided to stop drinking except for an occasional glass of wine when she was out with one of her female friends, unaccompanied by Ed. Jane also wanted to stop keeping alcohol in their home. But Ed wanted to keep liquor, beer, and wine on hand to serve to friends or family members who might visit them. He felt it was unfair to penalize others because he could not drink. The couple's discussion became more intense as the Thanksgiving and Christmas holidays approached. Past holiday gatherings had often been marred by Ed's excessive drinking, but he insisted on having alcohol on hand to serve family and friends even though he had been abstinent for only 2 months.

The therapist helped Ed and Jane reach a compromise. They would not keep any alcohol in their home on an ongoing basis. Jane would purchase wine specifically for each holiday and then remove any that was not consumed that day. It turned out that most guests did not want the wine at the holiday gatherings. Most were so happy that Ed was sober that not having alcohol was not a problem. Ed continued his AA meetings and became more committed to ongoing abstinence. Eventually he decided it was better to declare his home an "alcohol-free zone" altogether.

Complications can arise when you are helping couples decide whether the spouse will drink in the patient's presence. Couples in which spouses are unwilling to change their own drinking or drug use to support patients' abstinence may not be good candidates for BCT. Sometimes such reluctant spouses change their minds after carefully considering the cost and benefits of their own substance use and that of the patient's abstinence. In other cases, when spouses remain unwilling, it may be better to pursue individual counseling for the patient than BCT. We consider this problem further in Chapter 9, when we discuss special considerations for couples in which both members have a substance problem.

Social Gatherings Involving Alcohol or Drugs

You also need to help the couple decide whether to attend social gatherings that include alcohol or drugs and, if they do attend, how to deal with these situations. Help them identify particular persons, gatherings, or circumstances that are likely to be stressful. This decision can be particularly difficult to reach when exposure situations involve members of the patient's or spouse's extended family who are heavy drinkers or drug users and do not fully support the patient's abstinence. For a couple deciding whether or not to go to an event, encourage the patient to confide in the spouse how uncomfortable they feel about the event. A patient often does not want to inconvenience the spouse or admit vulnerability. If a couple decides to attend such social gatherings, you can help them rehearse how to refuse offers of alcohol or drugs, what alternate beverages to drink, and how the spouse can help if the patient feels awkward or tempted to drink. You also can help by discussing how the patient will signal the spouse if he or she gets uncomfortable and wants to leave. The important point is to help couples talk about these situations so that they can anticipate problems rather than be caught off guard.

The case of Joe and Sue, a couple in their early 30s, illustrates these points about social gatherings. Joe and Sue started BCT after Joe's discharge from a residential treatment program for alcohol and cocaine dependence. At their fourth BCT session, Joe reported that they had gone to a Halloween party where he almost drank. Someone at the party whom they didn't know unexpectedly handed Joe a can of beer. Joe held it for a minute (unopened), felt nervous and edgy, and had a strong urge to drink. Then he made eye contact with his wife and put the beer back in the refrigerator without getting any comments from anyone. This "close call" convinced the couple that they needed to plan ahead for other social gatherings. They decided not to go to the wife's work-related Christmas party because it was too alcohol focused. They discussed at length whether to attend family holiday gatherings, because cousins and siblings were heavy drinkers and one brother-in-law had smoked crack with Joe. Eventually they decided to attend these gatherings with the following plan. Joe and Sue would stay together in the house rather than join the heavy drinking group on the enclosed porch. Joe would not have contact with the crack-smoking brother-in-law except at the party. Finally, they would leave if Joe's discomfort became too great.

Other Exposure Situations

Other exposure situations also require careful attention in BCT. For many individuals, work-related situations present a high risk because coworkers drink or use drugs often on the job during work hours, during breaks, or after work. For others, old habits associated with prior use (e.g., buying lottery tickets in a bar where one formerly drank) have to change to avoid risky exposure situations. The spouse often knows details about the exposure situations and can support the patient's efforts to find alternative solutions. To achieve long-term abstinence, some individuals may have to change jobs, find new friends, and avoid or limit contact with certain family members. Others may need to cautiously limit exposure to substance-related sit-

---

TABLE 4.2. Exposure to Alcohol and Drugs

- Will alcohol be kept and served at home?
- Will the spouse drink in front of the patient?
- Will they attend social gatherings involving alcohol?
- Identify other exposure situations (work, friends, family).
- Extent that exposure must be restricted will vary.
  - Some can use partial avoidance.
  - Others need total avoidance and major life changes.

---

uations for the first 6–12 months of abstinence, and then be less restrictive as their confidence increases in their ability to handle such situations. As a BCT therapist, you help the patient and spouse weigh the risks involved and make decisions that fit them. Table 4.2 summarizes key points about reducing the patient's exposure to alcohol and drugs.

ADDRESS STRESSFUL LIFE PROBLEMS

Rationale for Addressing Stressful Life Problems

Stress caused by unresolved life problems can be a trigger for relapse. Common problems experienced by substance abuse patients and their spouses include (1) medical problems, (2) job problems, (3) legal concerns, (4) financial difficulties, (5) psychiatric distress, and (6) social or family-related stressors, including concerns about children and parenting.[2] Research shows that helping patients deal with these life problems increases their chances of staying abstinent.[3]

Resolving or working on life problems reduces relapse risk in a number of ways. First, it reduces stress with which the patient may be tempted to cope by drinking or drugging, and it makes abstinence more rewarding. Second, taking an active role to help couples deal with life problems strengthens the therapeutic relationship. They see you as someone who cares about their broader life concerns, not just the patient's recovery from alcohol/drug abuse. A strong therapeutic relationship increases the chances that they will keep coming to BCT sessions, which in turn is linked to greater recovery success. Finally, getting help for some problems can create links to other community providers who have a vested interest in the patient's abstinence and the couple's well-being. These providers usually will encourage BCT, and you can support the patient's involvement with them.

How to Address Stressful Life Problems in BCT

Start by identifying life problems during the initial assessment in the first or second BCT session. Then, in the early BCT sessions, address these problems directly or by referral to another source of help. Help the patient and spouse discuss alternative solutions and resolve disagreements about the best course of action. Invite the couple to take some step to resolve a problem and report back at the next session on their progress. Actions that address life problems can become individualized elements of the Recovery Contract, which is reviewed at each BCT session. For example, medications for medical or psychiatric problems can be taken together during the daily trust discussion time. Including such elements strengthens the contract as a sign of a couple's joint commitment to improve their lives together.

Not all problems should be addressed in early BCT sessions, however. You want to start with problems where some improvement can be made fairly quickly. However, some problems are not amenable to quick action or solution because they are part of entrenched couple conflicts and disagreements or may have become chronic life patterns. Delay addressing such problems until the patient has stayed abstinent for a while, the couple is getting along a little better, and you have taught them communication and problem-solving skills (see Chapters 6 and 7).

When they start BCT, many couples will already have one or more community providers for help with various life problems. You also may refer them to new providers. Such community providers can include physicians or other health care workers, vocational rehabilitation personnel, probation officers, mental health therapists, and child protective and other social service workers. Your job is to identify these other providers during the initial assessment for BCT. Then, after getting signed releases,[4] you can arrange periodic contacts with these other providers to keep them informed about, and to coordinate efforts supporting, the patient's and the couple's progress.

For many couples who take part in BCT sessions, the patient or spouse will also be seeing an individual counselor or therapist. Communicating with these providers presents some special issues. When you contact the individual therapist, in addition to mutual sharing of information to coordinate treatment efforts, you want to set some boundaries between BCT and individual sessions, if possible. Ideally BCT sessions will focus on couple issues and individual sessions will focus on individual (not relationship) issues. Often a counselor will not agree to this artificial division of therapy material. However, most therapists will agree that if their client shares couple issues in individual sessions, then they will encourage the person to also discuss these issues in BCT. This compromise avoids the situation where a person describes negative feelings about his or her partner in individual sessions but does not share these feelings in BCT, where they could be addressed. Table 4.3 summarizes key points about how BCT helps the couple deal with stressful life problems.

Case Example of Addressing Stressful Life Problems

The case of Bob and Penny, a couple in their mid-30s with a 3-year-old daughter, illustrates these points about addressing stressful life problems. They started BCT after Bob's discharge from a residential treatment program for alcohol and cocaine dependence. This was Bob's second professional treatment episode. He had only stayed abstinent for a month after his first treatment program. Penny entered BCT to give their marriage "one last chance." They had many stressful life problems, mostly a result of Bob's substance abuse. The therapist began addressing these problems in the first month of BCT, usually in the second half of the session after reviewing standing agenda items (e.g., urges, Recovery Contract).

Medical problems of elevated blood pressure and abnormal liver function tests had been identified during Bob's residential program. At the first session, the BCT counselor made sure that Bob had an appointment to see the clinic physician. Liver function tests returned to normal quickly, so Bob could take Antabuse (which the physician prescribed). Daily observation of

---

TABLE 4.3. Addressing Stressful Life Problems

- Resolving life problems reduces relapse risk.
- Identify such problems in first or second session.
- Address these problems in early sessions.
  - Work with couple on solutions.
  - Refer to other providers, as needed.
  - Communicate with other providers to encourage patient's problem solving and abstinence.
- Start with problems that may show quick progress.
- Defer complex, contentious problems until gains in abstinence and communication have been made.

---

his Antabuse taking was made part of the couple's Recovery Contract, starting after the second BCT session. Bob's blood pressure stayed high after 2 months of abstinence, so the physician prescribed blood pressure medication, which also became part of the Recovery Contract. The BCT counselor contacted the physician to discuss Bob's progress in the BCT sessions and to learn about Bob's attendance at his medical appointments and the progress on his medical problems.

Job problems were a major concern. Bob had lost his job due to drinking, and the couple had serious financial problems. After the first session, the BCT counselor referred Bob to vocational services at the hospital where the BCT program was located. Bob got temporary part-time employment at minimum wage and would receive help to secure a full-time position in the community. To receive these vocational services, Bob had to attend his part-time job faithfully, in a sober state, and attend BCT sessions. The BCT therapist spoke with the vocational counselor every few weeks to report on Bob's abstinence and attendance at BCT sessions and to learn about his job performance. Progress on the job problems was discussed briefly at each BCT session. After a few months Bob eventually got a full-time job.

Financial difficulties were a major source of stress for both Bob and Penny. They owed over $20,000 in credit card and other debts. Frequent phone calls from creditors were quite stressful because the couple was living with Penny's family who often answered these calls. They were considering filing for bankruptcy. At the third BCT session, the counselor suggested referral to a nonprofit credit counseling agency[5] to evaluate their financial options. Penny and Bob agreed to organize and list all their debts before the next session. At the next BCT session, the couple brought their list of debts, the therapist gave them specific referral information, and they agreed to contact the credit agency before their next BCT session. They followed through and got an appointment quickly because they already had the needed information organized. The credit agency worked out a repayment plan that would stop interest payments and creditor calls, withdraw a set amount from their bank account each month, and pay off the entire debt in 4 years. They set up the payment plan with the agency when Bob got full-time work. The BCT counselor periodically asked about their progress on the payment plan and their efforts to avoid a recurrence of the problem. Despite some difficulties, especially in the first few months of the plan, Bob and Penny reported, with some pride, that they did keep up their payments.

Legal problems were a major reason Bob sought help. He had been arrested and put on probation for a year after being charged with domestic violence. The arrest had occurred when a neighbor heard them arguing and called the police. Bob was not court-mandated for treatment, but his arrest had led to his detox and rehab admission. The BCT therapist contacted Bob's probation officer, who agreed to set up regular communication about Bob's attendance, abstinence, and other aspect's of his progress. Bob's contacts with the probation officer were reviewed at ongoing BCT sessions. Standard BCT methods were used to prevent partner violence (see Chapters 7 and 10). However, this was not a big concern to the couple because during the incident that led to his arrest, Bob had not hit Penny, and she had not been afraid he was going to hurt her. They both saw it as an argument that got out of control because Bob was intoxicated. As long as he stayed abstinent, neither feared a recurrence.

Psychiatric distress was a significant problem for Penny. She was emotionally overwhelmed. She was working full time as the couple's sole support after Bob was fired. She felt humiliated by the embarrassment of the police coming to the house and arresting Bob. She feared that the couple's frequent arguments were starting to affect their daughter. She was thinking seriously about ending the marriage. Because of this emotional stress, she had been seeing a therapist and taking antidepressant medication for a number of months before starting BCT. The BCT therapist contacted Penny's individual therapist, who said she shared Penny's misgivings about Bob and the viability of the marriage. The individual therapist did agree to encourage Penny to discuss her concerns about the relationship in BCT sessions. The BCT and individual therapist had periodic contact to share information and monitor progress. Penny added her antidepressant medication and counseling appointments to the couple's Recovery Contract.

Social and family-related stressors also troubled the couple. They had lost their apartment because they could not afford the rent after Bob got fired. They were sharing cramped quarters with Penny's mother and older brother, who were very critical of Bob. Her mother was also paying for some of their food, letting them live rent free, and babysitting for the couple's daughter while Penny worked. The couple argued whenever they tried to discuss this problem at home or in a BCT session. The BCT therapist decided that this emotionally charged set of problems did not have a ready solution. Therefore, this problem was deferred until the couple had made progress on other issues and had been taught problem-solving and communication skills. Only then did the therapist try to help couple deal with it. Bob wanted to move out as soon as he got a full-time job. Penny felt more secure staying with her mother awhile longer. She wanted Bob to have at least a year of abstinence and 6 months full-time work before they got their own place again. The therapist helped each understand the other's viewpoint and gradually work out a compromise solution.

Resolution of life problems occurred slowly for Bob and Penny over a period of 3 years. After 24 weekly BCT sessions, they continued periodic relapse prevention sessions for the next year, and then quarterly checkup visits for the next 18 months (see Chapter 8). Bob used cocaine once to celebrate getting full-time work, but otherwise remained abstinent. When asked at his 3-year checkup why he thought he had done well this time when he had relapsed quickly after his earlier treatment, Bob offered the following reasons. First, Penny's credible threat to end the marriage and being on probation had created an initial strong motivation for change that made him willing to use recovery tools he had not tried before. Second, the structured BCT program with Antabuse for the first 18 months, regular AA attendance, and Penny's daily support gave him the consistent help he needed to stay abstinent. Finally, life got better with abstinence because he and Penny were also resolving some of their other problems.

DECREASE SPOUSE BEHAVIORS
THAT TRIGGER OR REWARD USE

Partners and spouses try many ways to cope with their loved one's substance abuse. Unfortunately, some frequently used coping behaviors by spouses unintentionally trigger or reward substance use. Common examples are buying, or giving the user money to buy, alcohol or drugs and making excuses or lying to others to protect the user. Often such coping behaviors have a short-term benefit, such as avoiding conflict with the substance abuser or protecting the family from negative economic and social consequences. However, such actions may increase the chances of current and future use.

A recent study of couples starting BCT[6] showed that such behaviors, often called *enabling behaviors*, occur quite frequently. In this study, alcoholic patients and their spouses completed a questionnaire to determine the extent of spouse behaviors that might reasonably be thought to reinforce drinking or hinder recovery. These included behaviors that would likely reinforce drinking directly as well as making it easier for the drinker to minimize the negative consequences of his or her actions. Most patients *and* spouses reported that the spouses engaged in such behaviors. For example, many spouses (1) took over the patient's neglected chores or duties when the patient was drinking; (2) drank or used drugs with the patient; and (3) lied or made excuses to others to cover for the drinker. Other frequently endorsed behaviors were buying alcohol for the drinker or giving the drinker money to buy alcohol, helping nurse the patient through a hangover and cleaning up (vomit, urine, etc.) after the patient became sick from drinking.

To reduce spouse behaviors that trigger or reward substance use, BCT helps the couple identify such behaviors that have occurred in the past or may still be occurring if abstinence has not yet been established. Start by reviewing the definition and examples of enabling, as shown in Figure 4.2 (a copy of which is Poster B.27 in Appendix B). Reviewing this poster helps familiarize the couple with the idea. It is important to help both members of the couple see the potential harm of such actions. Finally, BCT helps the couple plan to stop such actions in the future by identifying specific alternative behaviors to do in situations that might have elicited enabling behavior in the past.

Noel and McCrady[7] described implementing procedures as part of BCT to decrease spouse behaviors that trigger or reward abusive drinking. They presented an illustrative case study of a female alcohol abuser, Charlotte, and her husband Tom. The couple identified behaviors by Tom that triggered drinking by Charlotte (e.g., drinking together after work, trying to stop her from drinking, arguing with her about drinking). Charlotte reacted by criticizing Tom until he left her alone, whereupon she would drink still more. Moreover, Tom unwittingly reinforced Charlotte's drinking by protecting her from the consequences of her drinking (e.g., by helping her to bed when she was drunk, cleaning up after her when she got sick).

Noel and McCrady helped the couple find mutually comfortable and agreeable methods to reverse Tom's behaviors that inadvertently had promoted Charlotte's drinking. Tom decided to give up drinking so that his drinking after work or at a restaurant would not be a trigger for Charlotte to drink. Tom indicated that drinking was not that important to him, and he wanted to do something to help his wife. He worked hard to change his feelings that he must protect Charlotte from the negative consequences of her drinking. In the past, when she would drink until late at night, he would argue with her to stop drinking, but she would continue. Then, often he would help her to bed and clean up the area where she had been drinking—but she usually did not remember this the next morning. The couple agreed that if Charlotte was drinking by herself in the kitchen in the evening, he would check on her occasionally to be sure she was not in a dangerous state. However, he would not put her to bed. "If she is downstairs on the floor, then that's where she'll stay." Both agreed it was better to let Charlotte "face the music" by herself. Interestingly, after the couple agreed to this plan, Charlotte remained abstinent—so the plan was not actually implemented. The therapist also taught Tom to provide positive reinforcers (e.g., verbal acknowledgment, going to movies and other events together) only when Charlotte had not been drinking.

Enabling

- Spouses try many ways to cope with their partner's substance abuse. Some coping behaviors unintentionally trigger or reward substance use.

- Enabling by spouse
  - Rewards partner's drinking or drug use directly.
  - Protects partner from the consequences of his or her drinking or drug use.

- Enabling often has short-term benefit.
  - It may avoid conflict or protect family from legal or economic problems.
  - *But* enabling increases chance of future substance use.

Examples of spouse's enabling of substance-abusing partner:
- Bought alcohol or drugs for partner.
- Gave partner money to buy alcohol or drugs.
- Drank or used drugs with partner.
- Took over partner's neglected duties when partner was drinking or drugging.
- Lied or made excuses to family, friends, or others to cover for partner.
- Helped nurse partner through a hangover or helped partner to bed when drunk.
- Borrowed money to pay bills caused by partner's drinking or drug use.
- Cancelled family plans or social activities because partner was impaired.
- Paid lawyer or court fees or bailed partner out of jail due to substance use.
- Cleaned up (vomit, urine, etc.) after partner got sick.
- Asked family members to be silent about partner's drinking or drug use.
- Helped conceal partner's drinking or drug use from employers or coworkers. (e.g., called in sick for partner; lied to supervisors or customers).
- Reassured partner that his or her drinking or drug use wasn't that bad.
- Lied or told a half-truth to a physician, counselor, probation officer, judge, or police officer about partner's substance drug use or about partner's participation (or nonparticipation) in treatment/recovery programs.

FIGURE 4.2. Enabling. These examples of enabling behaviors are from "Enabling Behavior in a Clinical Sample of Alcohol Dependent Clients and Their Partners," by R. J. Rotunda, L. West, and T. J. O'Farrell, 2004, *Journal of Substance Abuse Treatment*, 26, p. 272. Copyright 2004 by Elsevier Inc. Adapted with permission.

FREQUENTLY ASKED QUESTIONS

- *Question 1*: In the case of the woman who said she drank in response to her husband yelling at and criticizing her, you emphasized her responsibility to stay abstinent despite the husband's outrageous behavior. This seems unfair.
- *Answer*: You are referring to the case of Janet and Ken described earlier in this chapter. Janet said that the main reason she drank was to escape Ken's yelling and criticizing. She said it was his fault that she kept drinking. Unless Ken stopped yelling and started treating her better, she felt there was no way she could stop drinking. The BCT therapist told Janet that she was responsible for whether or not she drank. Clearly it was more difficult to stay sober in the face of Ken's criticism, but he could not make her drink or make her stay sober. That was up to

her. If she wanted to stay sober, she would have to find a way to cope with Ken's criticism without drinking over it. Similarly, Ken had a choice about whether to vent his anger by yelling or to find a less hostile way to express his concerns.

At times this approach does seem unfair to the patient or spouse. That is why it is important that you empathize with the person who is complaining before giving the message of individual responsibility for one's feelings and actions. In this case, the BCT therapist empathized with Janet's feeling criticized and devalued by Ken's frequent put-downs before clarifying that she was responsible for her reaction to Ken's criticism. It also is important that you deliver this message of individual responsibility in a quiet, deliberate manner, and that you ask the person for his or her reaction. Such a careful, respectful dialogue often helps the person see the wisdom in this message.

Most counselors and self-help groups subscribe to a similar philosophy of individual responsibility. However, when they first start seeing couples, many counselors find that issues of blame and responsibility are complex and confusing. As discussed in Chapter 1, BCT encourages a good-faith–individual-responsibility approach in which each member of the couple freely chooses to make needed changes in his or her behavior, independent of whether or not the partner makes corresponding changes in behavior. Thus, we ask each person to voluntarily make the changes needed to help the patient stay abstinent and to improve the couple's relationship. In BCT, we emphasize abstinence as a primary goal that must be achieved before lasting change in couple and other problems is possible.

- *Question 2*: What impact does repeated use of alcohol or drugs have on the validity and usefulness of the daily trust discussion, in which the patient states his or her intent to stay abstinent? How is this problem addressed in BCT?
- *Answer*: It seems like such experiences would make the daily trust discussion useless and ineffective. However, often this is not the case. Spouses and patients often are willing to restart using the trust discussion even after there have been multiple occasions of use. Frankly, this willingness surprised us when we first noticed it. After all, the patient had pledged not to use but had done so anyway, suggesting that the patient may have lied or, at best, been unable to keep his or her pledge. However, if the spouse perceives that the patient is making a sincere effort to abstain, then the spouse is more likely to be willing to continue the trust discussion after the patient "slips." Also, if it seems that the patient planned the episode of use, then it can make a difference if the patient refused or avoided doing the trust discussion on the days when he or she used. A spouse may respond that at least the patient didn't lie by saying he or she was going to stay abstinent on days when he or she knew that using was likely. Many couples seem to view the trust discussion like they view other tools for recovery (e.g., self-help meetings). Even though the person may not have used the tool when he or she drank, or the person used the tool but drank or drugged anyway, this is no reason not to return to using the tool when he or she recommits to abstinence after a slip. As a BCT counselor, you will have to check with each couple to see if the partners would find it meaningful to restart the trust discussion after multiple slips. But do not assume, as we mistakenly did, that most or all such couples will not want to resume the trust discussion.

- *Question 3*: You advocate starting to address stressful life problems in early BCT sessions. Many problems, such as job losses and legal charges, were caused by the patient's drinking and drug use. These problems can motivate the patient to stay abstinent. Dealing with these problems too early can distract the patient from the number one priority of staying abstinent. Many counselors have written a letter to a judge, probation officer, or employer on behalf of a patient, who then discontinued counseling because the immediate substance-related problem (e.g., impending incarceration or job loss) had been avoided. It seems like this boomerang effect could be a risk of the approach you advocate.

   • *Answer*: First, we agree that if you help the patient resolve immediate substance-related problems without making the efforts needed to develop an ongoing abstinent lifestyle, then the patient will keep developing new substance-related problems until the root cause has been addressed. The patient's motivation for change at the start of counseling may come more from external events than from a strong internal commitment to abstinence. So you do not want to undercut, but rather to build on, this motivation for change. The primary focus in early BCT sessions is the Recovery Contract and actions to promote abstinence. Problem-solving efforts are always secondary to the Recovery Contract and abstinence efforts in early BCT.

   Second, we also agree that it is better not to intervene to help the patient avoid the natural negative consequences of a substance-abusing lifestyle unless you can build in increased support for ongoing counseling and abstinence. Frequently, in exchange for your initial letter indicating that the patient is seeing you for counseling, you can arrange to have the judge or employer require the patient to continue in counseling, with ongoing reports from you on attendance and progress. You also can provide such letters or other interventions on the patient's behalf only after you have seen some faithful attendance at BCT and some clear commitment to abstinence.

   Finally, despite these cautions, which most substance abuse counselors understand, studies show that addressing patients' life problems actually increases abstinence and reduces dropout from counseling.[8]

SUMMARY

• Start each BCT session with a question about drinking or drug use since the last session. If substance use has occurred, make dealing with this your top priority. If not, review urges to drink or use drugs that occurred.

• When the patient blames substance use on the spouse's criticism or other negative actions, empathize with each person and clarify each person's role in the problem. The patient is responsible for how he or she reacts to the spouse's criticism, including the substance use. Because the spouse's behavior makes it harder for the patient to stay sober, the spouse is responsible for changing this behavior.

• Do not assume that repeated use episodes make the trust discussion no longer effective. Instead, check with the couple to see if they would find it meaningful to restart the trust discussion after multiple slips.

• Patients' exposure to situations where alcohol or drugs are available or others are using such substances is a high risk situation for relapse. Help the couple decide if the spouse will drink in the patient's presence, whether alcohol will be kept and served at home, if the couple will attend social gatherings involving alcohol, and how to deal with other exposure situations.

• Stress caused by unresolved life problems (e.g., medical, job, financial problems) can be a trigger for relapse. Identify such problems during the first or second BCT session. Then, in the early BCT sessions, address these problems directly or by referral to another source of help. Start with problems where some improvement can be made fairly quickly.

- Problems from substance use can motivate patients to change, so take care not to undercut this motivation when intervening with external legal or job problems. Intervene only after the patient has made a strong commitment to change or you can arrange leverage for change in exchange for the problem solving.

- Some spouse-coping behaviors can unintentionally trigger or reward substance use. Common examples are giving the user money to buy alcohol or drugs and lying to others to protect the user. BCT helps the couple identify and stop such behaviors.

NOTES

1. Miller and Rollnick (2002).
2. McLellan et al. (1985).
3. McLellan et al. (1997); McLellan, Hagan, Levine, Gould, et al. (1998); McLellan, Hagan, Levine, Meyers, et al. (1998).
4. In the United States, federal confidentiality regulations are stricter for substance-abuse-related information than for general health-related information. Special release forms are required when sharing substance abuse information about a patient. Readers who work in substance abuse settings will be familiar with these regulations. Others will need to learn about and follow the correct procedures. For more information, see the Legal Action Center's (2003) guidebook or contact your state substance abuse agency.
5. We referred this couple to the local office of a nationally accredited, nonprofit credit counseling agency that had been operating in our area for many years. As with all referrals, it is important to know the quality of help they provide. Particular care should be taken with debt management services, which have proliferated in the United States in recent years.
6. Rotunda, West, and O'Farrell (2004).
7. This case example is from "Alcohol-Focused Spouse Involvement with Behavioral Marital Therapy," by N. E. Noel and B. S. McCrady in T. J. O'Farrell (Ed.), *Treating Alcohol Problems: Marital and Family Interventions* (pp. 230–232), 1993. New York: Guilford Press. Copyright 1993 by The Guilford Press. Adapted with permission.
8. McLellan et al. (1997); McLellan, Hagan, Levine, Gould, et al. (1998); McLellan, Hagan, Levine, Meyers, et al. (1998).

5

Increasing Positive Couple
and Family Activities

Previous chapters introduced you to substance-focused interventions used in BCT to support the patient's abstinence. Now we turn to relationship-focused interventions used to improve the couple's relationship functioning.

BCT aims to increase positive couple and family activities in order to enhance positive feelings, goodwill, and commitment to the relationship. This chapter describes how BCT increases such positive activities by using methods such as "Catch Your Partner Doing Something Nice," participating in shared rewarding activities, and scheduling caring days.

As described in Table 1.7 in Chapter 1, Catch Your Partner Doing Something Nice may start as early as the first BCT session. Shared rewarding activities and caring days are phased in during the early BCT sessions. Starting with the middle BCT sessions (i.e., session 5 of a 12-session format) and continuing to the end of BCT, the couple picks at least one of the three assignments to carry out each week.

CATCH YOUR PARTNER DOING SOMETHING NICE

Catch Your Partner makes both members of the couple more aware of the benefits they are already getting from the relationship. It increases how often the man and woman notice, acknowledge, and initiate pleasing or caring behaviors on a daily basis.

Introducing the Catch Your Partner Assignment

Table 5.1 provides the therapist checklist for introducing the exercise Catch Your Partner Doing Something Nice (from the checklist for session 1 of the 12-session BCT manual contained in Appendix A). Next we describe how the counselor completes each of these steps.

92

TABLE 5.1. Therapist Checklist for Introducing "Catch Your Partner Doing Something Nice"

_____ Show *Sample Caring Behaviors Poster B.6* from Appendix B.

_____ Discuss rationale for this exercise.

_____ Ask each person to name one caring behavior the partner did in past week.

_____ Show *Sample Catch Your Partner Poster B.7* from Appendix B.

_____ Solicit questions or concerns about this exercise.

_____ Hand out *Catch Your Partner Form C.3* from Appendix C.

_____ Assign home practice: Write down one nice thing partner does each day.

Couples struggling with substance abuse often complain that love and caring have gone out of their relationship. You can help them start to change this. You might begin this way:

"When a couple faces serious problems such as substance abuse, both partners can get so wrapped up in their unhappiness that they ignore positive aspects of the relationship. Even couples without problems tend to take each other for granted over time. No wonder couples entering recovery often complain they have lost touch with their loving feelings.

"The first step to more caring feelings is to notice nice behaviors your partner does already, instead of taking them for granted or letting problems blind you to positive behaviors. The 'Catch Your Partner Doing Something Nice' game will help."

The Catch Your Partner game requires each person to notice one caring behavior performed by his or her partner each day. Explain that caring or pleasing behaviors can be compliments, words of appreciation, or gestures of affection such as a hug. Caring behaviors also can be actions that make life easier, such as doing errands, caring for children, or working to earn money for the family. Figure 5.1 shows a list of sample caring behaviors (a copy of which is Poster B.6 in Appendix B). Reviewing this list displayed as a poster helps familiarize the couple with the idea.

After explaining what a caring behavior is, ask each person to give an example of one or two caring things his or her partner did or said in the previous week. Depending on the functioning of the relationship, it may be difficult for the partners to recall one another's caring behaviors. You may need to probe areas of the relationship to get them thinking. For example, "You mentioned that a strength of your relationship is in how you raise your children. Can you think of something your partner did to help you take care of your children in the past week?"

Once you are sure that they understand the caring behavior concept, assign the Catch Your Partner exercise for the coming week. Indicate that the purpose is "to notice the little things your partner does for you rather than take them for granted." Instruct them to notice one nice thing their partner does each day and write it on the Catch Your Partner form (a copy of which is Form C.3 in Appendix C). What they should look for are ordinary, "everyday" actions that express caring and affection or make life together easier and more pleasant. Tell them to bring the completed form to the next session, but not to share their lists with each other at home (to avoid arguments about the accuracy of recordings).

Emphasize that it is always possible to notice at least one caring behavior, even if they have an argument or don't see each other that day. On such days, the caring behavior noticed might be something fairly mundane like "went to work to earn money" or "made the bed." This

Sample Caring Behaviors

Paid the bills
Went to work to earn money
Helped with shopping
Packed a lunch for me
Cooked dinner
Did the dishes
Straightened up the house
Set the table
Did the yard work
Played with the children
Changed the baby's diaper
Gave the kids a bath
Helped kids with homework
Let me sleep in
Hugged or kissed me
Cuddled close to me in bed
Brought me a cup of coffee, tea, etc.
Complimented me on my appearance
Thanked me for doing something
Called to tell me where he or she was

FIGURE 5.1. Sample caring behaviors.

exercise may seem strange or unnatural to the couple in the beginning, but it becomes easier with practice.

Reviewing the Assignment to Notice Caring Behaviors

At the next BCT session, after going over the Recovery Contract and other substance-focused assignments, review the Catch Your Partner assignment. First, restate the rationale and specifics of the assignment. Then have each person take turns reading the caring behaviors recorded in the previous week. We usually start with the woman because she is more likely to have done it completely. Ask her to read what she wrote for the day after the last session. Then ask the man to read what he wrote for that same day. Proceed in this manner through the week, day by day, alternating partner reports for each day.

After each person reads a behavior, you can empathize with the intent behind what the person is saying. Amplify the underlying meaning a little. Don't nitpick about negative aspects (e.g., " She made a great dinner Tuesday—first time she cooked in a month"). Save this until after you talk with them about how to acknowledge the good stuff. Your dialogue might go something like this.

JAKE: On Friday, Ginny made a special trip to pay the cable bill at the office because I forgot to pay it earlier.

THERAPIST: So you really appreciated that Ginny was thinking about you and went out of her way to pay the cable bill.

JAKE: Yeah, that was really thoughtful of her. She knew I didn't want to miss the big game Sunday. So she did this for me.

Often reading and listening to noticed caring behaviors, especially with your amplification of the meanings underlying the stated appreciation, will create a pleasant, positive warmth that may have been lacking or infrequently voiced. An example of a Catch Your Partner sheet completed by a couple in BCT is shown in Figure 5.2 (a copy of which is Poster B.7 in Appendix B). A copy of the form for couples to use in BCT is Form C.3 in Appendix C.

"Catch and Tell": Adding Acknowledging to Noticing

Table 5.2 provides the therapist checklist for introducing the Catch Your Partner Doing Something Nice and Tell Him or Her exercise (from the checklist for session 2 of the 12-session BCT manual contained in Appendix A). Next we describe how the counselor completes each of these steps.

After reviewing the couple's efforts at noticing caring behaviors, introduce the concept of acknowledging the caring behaviors that were noticed. This step expands Catch Your Partner to Catch Your Partner Doing Something Nice *and Tell Him or Her*, or "Catch and Tell" for short. Catch and Tell involves asking each person to notice and acknowledge one nice thing each day that their partner did. By acknowledging caring behaviors, a couple can increase posi-

Catch Your Partner Doing Something Nice

Each day, notice at least one nice thing that your partner does and note it on the following chart. It is ALWAYS POSSIBLE to notice at least one CARING BEHAVIOR—even if you do not see your partner for an entire day. Don't share your list with your partner yet!

Day	Date	Caring Behavior
Mon.	4/6	Waited to have dinner with me because I had to stay late at work. Made me feel good.
Tues.	4/7	Told me she loved me.
Wed.	4/8	Cooked a delicious Italian dinner and afterwards we had a very romantic evening.
Thurs.	4/9	Was patient with me when I came home tired and moody from work.
Fri.	4/10	Enjoyed a walk together around the neighborhood.
Sat.	4/11	Woke me gently and rubbed my back.
Sun.	4/12	She asked me how my day was and listened to me talk.

FIGURE 5.2. Sample "Catch Your Partner" sheet.

TABLE 5.2. Therapist Checklist for Introducing Catch Your Partner Doing Something Nice and Tell Him or Her

_____ Show *Acknowledging Caring Behaviors Poster B.8* from Appendix B.

_____ Explain importance of telling partner about (acknowledging) caring behaviors.

_____ Therapist models how to acknowledge caring behaviors.

_____ Couple practices acknowledging caring behaviors, with therapist coaching.

_____ Hand out *Catch and Tell Form C.5* from Appendix C.

_____ Assign home practice: Acknowledge one nice thing partner does each day.

tive feelings, reward acts they would like to see more often, and start opening their hearts to each other. Catch and Tell begins the work of improving communication skills, starting with communicating positive feelings. Table 5.3 summarizes steps used in BCT to teach a variety of relationship skills. You can follow these steps in teaching Catch and Tell.

THERAPIST INSTRUCTS COUPLE ON HOW TO ACKNOWLEDGE CARING BEHAVIORS

Indicate that learning about Catch and Tell will follow the same steps used in all BCT work on improving communication skills. First you will explain the skill and show them right and wrong ways to do it. Then they will practice with you before they try it at home. Start by reviewing "what to say" and "how to say it" when acknowledging caring behaviors, as shown in Figure 5.3 (a copy of which is Poster B.8 in Appendix B). Reviewing this poster helps familiarize them with the idea.

THERAPIST MODELS ACKNOWLEDGING CARING BEHAVIORS

Then you can show them how to acknowledge caring behaviors correctly. As you do so, you can use an example from your own day. You might say to the couple: "Thank you for coming on time to the session. It shows that you have a real commitment to your relationship and to your recovery." In making this statement, be sure to incorporate positive nonverbal components (e.g., pleasant tone of voice, smile). Ask them to point out which of the elements listed on the chart were included in your demonstration. Point out elements that they miss and be sure they understand.

TABLE 5.3. Steps in Teaching Relationship Skills

- Instruction—therapist tells couple how to do it.
- Modeling—therapist shows couple how to do it.
- Rehearsal—couple practices skill while therapist coaches.
- Home Practice—couple tries skill at home.
- Review—therapist reviews how home practice went and coaches further practice in session.

Acknowledging Caring Behaviors

What you say:
- "I liked it when you . . . ."
- "It made me feel . . ."
- *(Leave out the negative)*

How to say it:
- Look at the other person
- Use pleasant tone of voice
- Smile
- Be sincere

FIGURE 5.3. Acknowledging caring behaviors.

Next, model an ineffective example so that the couple can see the difference between correct and incorrect ways of acknowledging caring behaviors. For example, you might say to one of the partners chosen to help you in your role play: "I liked it when you did the laundry yesterday, but you should try doing it every day. Besides, you don't thank me when I do *your* laundry." Making this statement in a low tone of voice, without smiling or looking at the partner, will also show incorrect nonverbal communication. Solicit feedback on your modeling in relation to the elements on the chart. First ask them to say what aspects you did well (e.g., the statement started off positive) and what needed improvement (e.g., had a lot of negative content and nonverbal aspects were all wrong). Then reenact the scenario correctly, incorporating the feedback provided by the couple.

COUPLE PRACTICES ACKNOWLEDGING CARING BEHAVIORS WITH THERAPIST COACHING

Each person takes a turn acknowledging caring behaviors, using the most pleasing example from the Catch Your Partner form, completed about the previous week. Ask them to try to follow the guidelines on the chart (i.e., Figure 5.3). Indicate that you will give them feedback, the way they did with you. After the first person has stated his or her acknowledgment, identify positive aspects first and then move on to any constructive suggestions. You can model, if necessary, to demonstrate improvements. The person tries the acknowledgment again. Give positive feedback, noting even small improvements made. Usually one, or at most two, "replays" are needed for the person to get it right. The process might go something like this:

THERAPIST: OK, Ben. It's your turn. Pick the thing you liked the most that Katie did in the past week. Tell Katie what you liked and how it made you feel. Try to get across to her your appreciation. You could start with "I liked it when you . . . "

BEN: (*looking at the therapist*) OK. I liked it when Katie went to my mother's birthday party on Saturday.

THERAPIST: That was good, Ben. You said specifically what she did that you appreciated. Could you do an "instant replay"? This time talk to, and look directly at, Katie, telling her why you liked this the most, and maybe smile a little.

BEN: (*looking at Katie with a shy smile*) Katie, I really appreciated that you made my mom's party a success. I know how pressed for time you are right now, but you went out of your way to help plan the party and make it a special time for my mom. Thanks.

THERAPIST: Thanks, Ben. That was much better. Katie, what did you think?

KATIE: Yeah, the second time it really came through loud and clear.

Practice, not perfection, is the goal, especially when doing this exercise for the first time. Try to elicit a convincing, sincere statement of appreciation within the current limits of the couple's relationship and each partner's background and skill level. Men often have more trouble with this exercise and other communication skills at first. It is important to make a start. You will continue to work on these skills throughout the remaining BCT sessions.

ASSIGN CATCH AND TELL FOR HOME PRACTICE

After both members of the couple have practiced, it is time to assign Catch and Tell for home practice in the upcoming week. Each person is to notice and acknowledge one nice thing that his or her partner does each day. Ask them to write down the behavior and have a 2- to 5-minute daily communication session in which each person acknowledges one pleasing behavior noticed that day. (The Catch and Tell form, a copy of which is Form C.5 in Appendix C), is the same as the Catch Your Partner form, with the addition of a place to check whether the person acknowledged the caring behavior.) It takes special effort to help each couple find a realistic time for this communication session. Many couples do these daily brief acknowledgments at the same time as the trust discussion that is part of the Recovery Contract. Others make this a time to chat about their day, have a cup of tea, and start on a positive note by writing down and then sharing the most pleasing thing they have noticed in their partner's behavior in the last 24 hours.

REVIEW HOME PRACTICE OF CATCH AND TELL AT NEXT BCT SESSION

At the next session, ask the couple if they completed the Catch and Tell assignment and how they felt noticing and acknowledging their partner's behaviors as well as giving caring behaviors. Table 5.4 summarizes the steps involved in checking home practice assignments in BCT. In the session have them practice acknowledging the caring behaviors they noticed in the past week. With prompting and feedback, help them improve the specificity and explicitness of their descriptions of the caring behaviors they noticed. Use the same format for practicing the acknowledgment of caring behaviors that you used in the prior session, when you introduced

---

TABLE 5.4. Checking Home Practice Assignments in BCT

- Restate assignment to be sure it was clear.
- Restate rationale for assignment to be sure reason behind assignment was clear.
- Ask each person to what extent they did assignment and what they got out of it.
- Conduct in-session practice of skill assigned.

---

it. Catch and Tell continues as part of most remaining BCT sessions, although the extent of emphasis may decrease over time. After a few weeks in which the assignment goes well, you may no longer require them to write down caring behaviors daily. However, encourage them to continue the daily acknowledgment at the time of the trust discussion. Also in each session have them practice acknowledging their partner's most pleasing behavior in the prior week.

As couples begin to notice and acknowledge daily caring behaviors, you may find that each partner begins initiating more caring behaviors. Often the weekly reports of daily caring behaviors show that one or both partners are fulfilling requests for desired change voiced before the therapy. In addition, many couples report that the 2- to 5-minute communication sessions result in more extensive conversations. You can tell couples about the importance of timing caring behaviors they initiate at key points in the day when they have a greater impact (e.g., upon awakening, bringing a cup of coffee to partner or simply giving a hug or kiss; before leaving for the day, saying goodbye, expressing affection; upon greeting after work, giving a hug or kiss or inquiring about day's events). Conversely, these are times of the day to avoid negative interactions that can color the mood for hours to come. Introduction of shared rewarding activities, described next, is another way you can help the couple initiate positive activities together.

SHARED REWARDING ACTIVITIES

The upset and unhappiness that comes with a substance abuse problem can cause a couple to stop doing enjoyable things together. Often a pattern develops wherein the couple spends less time together, becoming more distant from each other, and the patient spends more time isolating or using substances. They no longer do activities they once enjoyed. The spouse often fears that the substance-abusing member will get intoxicated and embarrass the family. Furthermore, they may not enjoy each other's company anymore. Hobbies, sports, and other interests often take a back seat to trying to keep the family together, the bills paid, and the substance abuser out of trouble. As a result, it is not surprising that many couples have not done anything "fun" together or with the family in a long time. The goal of participating in shared rewarding activities is to reverse this pattern and to begin to put fun back in the relationship.

Increasing shared fun activities helps both the couple's relationship and the patient's recovery. Joint fun activities can bring the couple closer together. Moreover, patients who do enjoyable, non-substance-using activities with their spouse and children have better recovery rates after substance abuse treatment.[1]

Assign List of Possible Shared Activities for Home Practice

Start work on increasing shared activities by discussing the rationale for such activities given above. Most couples readily identify with this description and see why increasing shared activities could be important. Indicate that as part of BCT, you will ask them to plan and engage in fun activities together each week. Remind the couple that they don't need to feel that everything about their relationship is perfect in order to have a good time together. Usually, change in behavior comes first and then feelings will change. In other words, they may not be enthusiastic about doing a shared rewarding activity, but if they plan and do the activity, they may see their feelings change about the situation. The bottom line: They need to try to improve their relationship through positive activities.

The first step is to identify activities they would like to do. Figure 5.4 provides a list of possible shared activities (a copy of which is Poster B.9 in Appendix B). Review this list of possible activities, displayed as a poster to familiarize them with the idea. As home practice ask each person to list possible shared fun activities on the form provided and to bring the completed form to the next session. The form (a copy of which is Form C.7 in Appendix C) asks each person to identify three types of activities to do with their partner:

1. Activities by themselves as a couple;
2. Activities with other couples and friends, without the children;
3. Activities with the children, as a family alone or with other families.

The goal is for the couple to have some alone time as well as spending quality time with children, friends, and relatives. Activities can take place at home (e.g., family games or "a date at

Possible Shared Activities

As a couple:
• Pop popcorn and rent a movie
• Go out to our favorite restaurant
• Go out to the movies
• Go bowling
• Do a project at home together

With other couples:
• Have a cookout for our families
• Hike with my sister and her boyfriend
• Invite sponsor and his wife for dinner
• Go to church supper with neighbors
• Invite couples to our house after high school concert

With the kids:
• Have a picnic by the river
• Go to Jimmy's T-ball game
• Play board games—no TV
• Go camping
• Play miniature golf as a family

FIGURE 5.4. Possible shared activities.

home") or out (e.g., restaurant or movie theater). Activities can be simple and inexpensive (e.g., taking a walk, using free passes to the zoo) or more extensive, with considerable planning required (e.g., a weekend away, a dream vacation). However, encourage the couple to include mostly things that are easy and inexpensive and that they can do without a great deal of advance planning. This approach will make it easier to meet the goal of planning an activity each week.

Couples can get ideas for fun activities from a listing of sample activities for couple and family fun. You may wish to develop your own list of low- or no-cost local recreational activities in your area. Your list could include any social groups or settings that have a substance-free policy.

Help the Couple Plan a Fun Activity Together for the Following Week

The goal for the next session is to have the couple plan a fun activity together for the following week. Three steps achieve this goal. First, review the list of possible shared activities that they completed for homework. If either partner failed to complete the list of activities, wait while they complete it in session. Then ask each person to share their list. If one member of the couple has been reluctant to do activities together, start with this person; doing so may reverse a pattern in which the more enthusiastic partner initiates an idea that gets rejected. The nonspeaking partner is to listen attentively, without interrupting, to the other person's ideas for fun. After both have shared their lists, return to the first partner and ask which of the spouse's ideas he or she liked and might want to do. Do the same thing with the second partner. Be careful to cut off comments about what is not liked or about obstacles. The best rule to follow is: Give positive feedback first. Your goal is to find one or more activities that both partners want to do. Usually this is not difficult because, even when a couple has serious conflicts about recreation, a number of the same activities appear on both partners' lists.

Second, discuss and model an effective way for the couple to plan a fun activity together for the following week. Start by suggesting the following guidelines for planning a fun activity:

1. Each partner should state an activity he or she wants to do—not what he or she doesn't want to do.
2. Start with something that both partners want. If the couple cannot agree on one activity they both want to do, they can alternate activities week to week.
3. Make specific plans for the day and time of the activity, as well as the activity itself.
4. Make sure the chosen activity is feasible, meaning they can afford it, have the time to do it, and have a reasonable idea of how to do it. The activity does not need to be elaborate or expensive. The important point is that they both think it might be fun, and they are willing to give it a try.
5. Try to think of any obstacles (e.g., weather, babysitter, money) that may arise when engaging in the activity and ways to handle those obstacles.
6. Do the activity this week and plan on talking about it at the next BCT session.

Next, model how to plan a shared rewarding activity. Your overview might go something like this.

"I will plan an activity using the guidelines we just talked about to show you how it works. I want to be specific when choosing my activity. Therefore, I might say to my partner, 'I would like to rent a movie this Saturday night.' I stated what I want to do, not what I wouldn't want to do.

"Next, I would check to see if my partner would want to do the same thing. Let's say that the movie idea is appealing to my partner.

"But then we realize that Saturday can't work because the kids will be home. Brainstorming on what we could do, we realize that it is high time the kids had a 'sleepover' at Grandma's house. I will call my mom and make the arrangements for the kids, so that we can watch a movie and spend some time alone.

"Now that solution worked out, but what if there was no babysitter for Saturday night? Maybe we would consider a different night or decide that the activity could still be on Saturday but it will be a family night."

Third, now that you have given them some guidelines, the couple practices planning an activity for the coming week. Suggest that partners start with ideas they both liked from their list of possible activities to see if any of these would be feasible in the coming week. Guide them through the discussion, if necessary. Help keep them focused on the task and using the guidelines just presented when planning the activity: (1) the plan needs to specify a day and time; (2) they should be sure the plan is feasible; and (3) they should consider any obstacles to completing their plan and be prepared to deal with them. For example, if they are planning an outdoor activity, what will they do if it rains: do it anyway, reschedule to the next day, or have a backup activity to do instead? Your questions and comments can help them form a specific, feasible plan that has some options built in to deal with likely obstacles and problems.

Once the plan is formulated, their home practice assignment is to do the planned activity in the coming week. Instruct the couple to refrain from discussing problems or conflicts during the planned activity. It is a time for lighthearted fun, not heavy communication or problem solving. Finally, ask them to plan an activity for the following week and write it down on their home practice assignment sheet to bring to the next session.

Continue Planning a Fun Activity Together Each Week

When the couple returns for the following session, review the success of the planned activity. Consider any difficulties and help them figure out how they might have overcome the problems they encountered. Also review the new activity they planned for the next week. Help them make or finalize this plan, if they did not do so for homework, as assigned. Most couples continue to do a shared fun activity each week and plan an activity for the following week for remaining BCT sessions. Table 5.5 summarizes key points about shared rewarding activities in BCT.

CARING DAY

Table 5.6 provides the therapist checklist for introducing the caring day exercise (from the checklist for session 3 of the 12-session BCT manual contained in Appendix A). Next we describe how the counselor completes each of these steps.

TABLE 5.5. Shared Rewarding Activities

- Each partner lists possible activities.
- Therapist models planning an activity.
- Couple plans one activity each week.
- Activity can take place at home or out, be simple or large.
- Three types of activities are planned:
  - As a couple
  - With the kids
  - With other couples
- Such activities are linked with recovery.

Start by commending the couple on the progress they have made so far with Catch and Tell and shared rewarding activities. They have done a good job noticing and acknowledging caring behaviors that currently exist in their relationship and planning fun together. Now you have something new to help them *put more caring into their relationship*. Giving each other a *caring day* is next.

Explain that in the caring day assignment, each person plans ahead to surprise his or her partner with a day when the person does some special things to show their caring. A caring day can involve doing a number of little things throughout the day or a bigger, special gesture of caring. Give examples of what other couples have done for a caring day, such as those shown in Figure 5.5 (a copy of which is Poster B.10 in Appendix B). Reviewing this information about the caring day exercise, displayed as a poster, helps familiarize them with the idea.

This exercise is important because caring actions and feelings often decrease as people get busy and forget to take the time to show their partners that they care. It is even worse when the stress and unhappiness of substance abuse cause partners to hold back such caring behaviors out of anger and disappointment. Therefore, active efforts are needed to increase caring and to help partners repair the damage done to the relationship by the substance abuse and other problems.

After answering questions and discussing any comments, assign the caring day home practice for the coming week. Ask each person if they are willing to commit to giving their partner a caring day in the coming week. Encourage each person to take risks and to act lovingly toward the other rather than wait for the other to make the first move. Remind them that at the start of therapy they agreed to *act* differently (e.g., more lovingly) and then assess changes in feelings,

---

TABLE 5.6. Therapist Checklist for Introducing the Caring Day Exercise

_____ Show *Caring Day Poster B.10* from Appendix B.

_____ Explain importance of doing special things to show caring to your partner.

_____ A caring day is when you plan ahead to do special things for your partner.

_____ Couple gives examples of possible caring day actions.

_____ Assign home practice: Give your partner a caring day this week.

Caring Day!

♥ A day when you plan ahead to do some
special things to show you care for your
partner. Make it a surprise.

♥ You can do a number of little things
throughout the day or a bigger, special
gesture of caring.

Examples:

♥ *"I left work early to cook a lasagna dinner
with strawberry shortcake for dessert. Also
gave him a card to let him know I love him."*

♥ *"I picked up a new bike for my wife. Picked up
her medication. Cut the lawn and cleaned the
shed. Took her for an ice cream."*

FIGURE 5.5. Caring days.

rather than wait to feel more positively toward their partner before instituting changes in their own behavior. Finally, ask them, in the coming week, to write on the bottom of their Catch and Tell form what they did for their partner on the caring day so that they can discuss it at the next session.

At the next session, review the caring day assignment using the same format used for checking other assignments in BCT. First, restate the assignment to be sure it was clear. In this case, each partner was to pick one day on which to do some special things for the other. Second, state the rationale for the assignment: to encourage the partners to increase the level of caring in the relationship. Finally, ask if they completed the assignment and have each person describe what they did for a caring day. It is interesting to see if the receiving partner realized which day it was!

You can continue the caring day assignment each week in subsequent BCT sessions. As another option, partners can alternate the weeks on which each one does a caring day. Alternatively, you can give them a choice to pick which two out of three assignments designed to increase positive feelings and activities they want to do: Catch and Tell, caring day, or shared rewarding activities.

When you start, the caring day assignment will vary with the couple. Whether you introduce caring days after Catch and Tell depends on how estranged the couple is. You may want to delay the caring day assignment for very distressed, disengaged couples, in which one or both partners are unwilling to take the risk involved in showing such obvious caring to the partner. In such cases, do Catch and Tell and shared rewarding activities first and delay caring days until the partners have started to open up to each other and reengage a little.

CASE EXAMPLE

Background

The following case example describes a couple that was very estranged when they started BCT. Most couples seeking BCT are not this estranged and do not require such a cautious, painstaking approach to increase positive activities and feelings. The case is presented here to show that the persistent, creative counselor can use BCT to increase positive couple activities even with very distressed couples.

The case of Jackson and Marie, an African American couple in their early 30s, illustrates the potential benefit, as well as the substantial challenges, in increasing positive couple and family activities for couples in early recovery. Jackson and Marie had known each other in high school, when both drank heavily and smoked marijuana regularly. Both had grown up without a father in the home. Their fathers had been substance abusers who left their families before either started elementary school.

After high school Marie went to secretarial school, took a job in a law office, cut down on her drinking, and stopped drug use. Jackson moved to a larger city, worked as a mover, increased his drinking, and started using crack cocaine regularly. When he lost his job due to substance abuse, he returned to his hometown. After a family friend hired him, he and Marie started "hanging out" together. They drank heavily and smoked pot together, as they had done in high school. Jackson introduced Marie to crack cocaine. When Marie got pregnant, they got married. Marie stopped alcohol and drug use when she was pregnant and intended to stay abstinent. However, a few months after the baby was born, she was back drinking heavily both alone and with Jackson. Marie was very upset about this; she felt guilty that she was not being a good mother to her son, and she knew she needed to be stable for his welfare. She went back to church, joined an AA group at the church, and stopped drinking and drug use. She had been abstinent 4 years when the couple was seen by the BCT counselor.

Jackson, on the other hand, had increased his substance use. He was arrested and sent to jail for 90 days for crack cocaine possession. He came out and went right back to drinking and drugging. Within a month he had lost the job that the friend had held for him, hoping that jail would have straightened him out. Marie said he could no longer live with her. By this time Marie was working as an office manager in a busy law firm, with care for her son split between day care and her mother. After the couple separated, Marie took an additional job transcribing depositions from her home at night after she put her son to bed. A few months later, after a random urine screen came back positive for cocaine and marijuana, Jackson's probation officer said he had to get help and stay abstinent or go back to jail.

Jackson admitted himself to the county detox program, from which he was referred to a 30-day residential treatment program. The BCT counselor met with Jackson and Marie to plan the next steps in Jackson's treatment and to discuss whether they wanted to try BCT. Jackson wanted to return to live with Marie and their son. Marie said no. She needed to see at least 90 days abstinence, his faithful adherence to a recovery program, and a full-time job before she would consider taking him back. She did not want to see him, except when he visited their son, until these conditions had been met. Jackson went to a sober house to live and went to 90 AA meetings in 90 days. He tried to get a full-time job but had to settle for temporary day labor work.

The couple met with the BCT counselor for a second time about 3½ months after the first meeting to discuss treatment options. The couple had not seen each other very often while separated for the past 9 months. Jackson had met Marie's conditions, except that he didn't have a job. Marie seemed anxious, depressed, and overwhelmed from the stress of her daily grind and from being uncertain about the future of her marriage. She often thought it would be easier just to get divorced. However, she did not want her 5-year-old son to grow up without a father the way she and Jackson had. Marie decided to reconcile and give it one last try with BCT, despite being fearful of taking another chance on Jackson, especially since he did not yet have a job. Jackson knew Marie's reservations about the marriage. He also wanted to see his son have a father, but he was not willing to live in a loveless marriage for the rest of his life. The couple started BCT. After the daily Recovery Contract was going smoothly, they began work on the difficult task of increasing positive feelings and activities.

Increasing Positive Couple and Family Activities

The therapist noted that Jackson and Marie were quite distant and estranged from each other. The outcome for their relationship seemed uncertain even if Jackson stayed abstinent. Marie, in particular, feared that reconnecting with Jackson would only lead to more heartache if Jackson relapsed. The therapist decided to start with shared fun activities because this generally is less threatening than the Catch Your Partner or caring days exercise for couples in which one or both partners have a high degree of anxiety about getting closer.

SHARED REWARDING ACTIVITIES

Jackson and Marie had stopped doing fun activities together because in the past, Jackson had frequently sought enjoyment only in alcohol-involved situations, where he invariably embarrassed his wife when he drank too much. Further, as their relationship deteriorated over the years, Jackson and Marie had spent less and less time doing activities together. The first activity they planned—having pizza together at a local pizza parlor—did not work out too well. Marie started to discuss their financial problems, and Jackson, who felt guilty about the lack of money, became angry at Marie for wanting to discuss the problem. He walked out of the pizza parlor and waited in the car while Marie finished eating. When they discussed this incident at the next BCT session, the therapist suggested that they both avoid combining problem discussions with fun-together time because it tended to ruin the fun.

The second activity involved going to a movie together. Marie reported that this went better than the pizza date, but Jackson said he did not enjoy himself. When he tried to hold Marie's hand during the movie, she withdrew it and moved away from him in her seat. Although he did not say anything at the time, he had felt rejected. He wondered if she would ever warm up to him again. The therapist suggested that at least for the next few weeks, Marie should be the one to initiate any physical displays of affection. The therapist also concluded that this couple was even more seriously estranged and fearful of reconnecting with each other than she had realized.

Hoping to build on their mutual bond with their son, the therapist asked if they might like to do something as a family with their son for their next activity. They decided to go for a walk and then have a picnic with their son at a park by the river where they used to go in happier times. They both enjoyed this activity. Marie reported that she had felt good watching Jackson play with their son. She held his hand as they walked together. It seemed a little bit like old times together. For the next few weeks, the fun activity involved special time together with their son.

Now that they had gotten more comfortable spending time together, Marie and Jackson returned to couple activities just for the two of them. As they progressed during BCT sessions, they gradually tried longer and more meaningful activities together: For example, they went out to dinner to a nice restaurant, and they invited another couple Jackson had met in AA to their home to play cards. These activities seemed to bring them closer together.

CATCH YOUR PARTNER DOING SOMETHING NICE

The therapist waited until the fifth session to make this assignment, which usually would have been given after the second session. Still there were problems. Jackson brought in a blank Catch Your Partner form and Marie had filled in a pleasing behavior she had noticed for only 1 day of the past week. The therapist asked what had kept them from noticing something nice their partner had done each day. Jackson's response was "She didn't do anything special, so how could I notice it?" The therapist suggested that Jackson was looking for expressions of affection or special, out-of-the-ordinary behaviors but overlooking small, daily behaviors (e.g., his wife going to work or preparing meals). Marie's response was "I started out noticing some minor things he did. But then I got angry. He still doesn't have a job. I am carrying the total load at work and at home with no help from him at all. It wouldn't be this way if he hadn't been a drunk and a crackhead." Responding to Marie required considerable sensitivity. The therapist empathized with her feelings of anger and of being overwhelmed with shouldering most of the family responsibilities for a very long time. The therapist said she could understand if Marie did not want to try to make the relationship better and asked if she had had a change of heart from when she agreed to start BCT. Marie indicated she still wanted to work on the relationship, but it was harder than she expected. She was tired from carrying the load for so long, depressed at how long it was taking for Jackson to find a job, and frightened about the prospect of a relapse. But she wanted to continue with BCT and recommitted herself to doing the recommended assignments.

The therapist asked each of them to think back over the past week and pick out the two things their partner had done that pleased them the most. This is a typical response to noncompliance with a home practice assignment in BCT: Ask the partners to do in session at least part of what they did not do at home. Marie said she liked that Jackson had been putting their son to bed many evenings and that he had been very faithful to his AA commitments. Jackson appreciated that Marie continued working in her stressful job to support them and that she seemed genuinely supportive of his sobriety when they did their daily trust discussion. Then the therapist modeled, and had them practice, acknowledging these two pleasing behaviors. After considerable coaching, they did a reasonable job acknowledging and agreed to Catch and Tell for home practice in the coming week.

When they returned for the seventh session, both had recorded a pleasing behavior for most of the days but had only acknowledged what they had noticed on the 2 days following their last BCT session. Jackson said they "forgot" after that, and Marie said she had felt awkward telling Jackson something she appreciated. The therapist praised them for their efforts and coached them to practice acknowledging in the session the two best things their partner had done last week. The therapist suggested that for the coming week, they try acknowledging one another's pleasing behaviors right after they did their trust discussion. The therapist also scheduled a phone check-in with them midweek to see how the assignment was going—another common way to increase compliance with home assignments in BCT.

At session 8, they reported nearly complete compliance with Catch and Tell. Marie still felt awkward on some days, especially when she had only fairly mundane things to acknowledge. The therapist asked Jackson how he felt about being acknowledged for mundane things, and he said he liked it; it was better than having his efforts go unnoticed. The therapist also suggested to Marie that it probably would feel less awkward with more practice. Although Jackson and Marie continued to struggle with Catch and Tell, repeated practice with coaching and modeling by the therapist succeeded in getting them to acknowledge one another genuinely both in the session and at home.

CARING DAYS

The caring day assignment, which involved planning ahead to do something special for the partner, was saved until last. Given how estranged they were at the start of BCT, the therapist waited until Jackson and Marie had started to open up to each other a little. The caring day exercise was introduced at the eighth BCT session and went surprisingly well, considering the earlier difficulties with fun activities and Catch and Tell. On one occasion Jackson cleaned the house, did the laundry, and had dinner waiting when Marie came home from work, and a few weeks later he brought her flowers. Marie gave Jackson a card acknowledging his efforts in his recovery program. On another occasion, she made his favorite meal to celebrate his 6 months of sobriety.

THE COUPLE'S OPINION ABOUT WHAT HELPED THEM

When asked which aspects of the BCT sessions had been most helpful, both Jackson and Marie identified the Recovery Contract and Jackson staying abstinent as the most important because their relationship had no chance of success without abstinence. Increasing positive activities and opening up their hearts (especially Marie) to each other was the second most important element. Their communication was adequate when Jackson wasn't drinking or using, but the big question was whether they wanted to be together after all the past hurt even if Jackson stayed abstinent. Both felt the fun activities with their son were very important. At the start, when they were both uncertain about their future together, sharing activities with their son helped them focus on a major reason to keep working to see if their relationship could be saved. It wasn't easy, but it was what they really wanted to do. Both indicated that Catch Your Partner Doing Something Nice (especially daily acknowledgment of pleasing behaviors at home) and caring days contributed a great deal to a more positive relationship. Marie noted that these assignments helped decrease her resentment about Jackson's past transgressions by helping her see the positive things he was doing now. Finally, they were grateful that their therapist had been patient and persistent in helping them get closer, even when they didn't follow through on what they said they would do.

FREQUENTLY ASKED QUESTIONS

• *Question 1*: What is the difference between the shared rewarding activity and caring day assignments? They both seem like positive couple activities. Don't couples in BCT get these two confused?

- *Answer*: Yes, sometimes couples do get confused about the difference between these two assignments. A shared rewarding activity is an activity that partners plan together and may do with others, including their kids, other couples, and other families or relatives. With the caring day assignment the emphasis is on each person taking the initiative to plan to surprise the partner with a special day on which the initiator shows his or her caring for the partner. Caring day is focused just on the two of them. A caring day could include a fun activity together, planned by one of the partners as a surprise for the other, but very often it does not. More frequently a caring day involves one person doing a number of little things to show caring and concern for the partner or a bigger, special gesture of caring. Caring day involves a greater degree of personal vulnerability than a shared fun activity because the person has to go out of his or her way to do something to actively show caring. Often this effort involves opening his or her heart to the partner or letting go of anger and resentment over past hurts. Doing a fun activity together often does not require the same level of personal risk. This is the reason that caring day is often delayed until other positive activities have been accomplished.

- *Question 2*: Is it acceptable for these positive activity exercises to be verbal and not written down? Many couples don't like writing down anything. Some couples do not write or read very well, and they are embarrassed by that.
    - *Answer*: That is a good point. As we described methods in this chapter to increase positive activities, they all involved writing down something. For Catch Your Partner, each person writes down one thing he or she appreciates each day, and both bring their sheets to the BCT session for review. The shared rewarding activities exercise involves each person making a list of possible fun activities to do together, and then using this written list each week to plan an activity. For the caring day exercise, the counselor asks partners to write down what they did for the other so that they can discuss it at the next session.

    However, you can change each exercise in small ways so that couples can do them verbally, with little or no writing. For Catch Your Partner, eliminate the form. Simply ask each partner to start by remembering two or three things from the previous week that the partner did that was appreciated. Then have each person practice acknowledging these pleasing behaviors in session. Ask them to do the Catch and Tell assignment at the same time they do the trust discussion, but they do not have to write down what pleasing behavior they noticed. You may want to ask them to mark on the Recovery Contract calendar when each gives the other this "daily compliment." For the discussion of possible shared rewarding activities, you can make the list of possible activities yourself by interviewing them in session. Then you can coach them each week in session to plan an activity for the coming week. For caring days, the important point is that they increase caring for each other, not that they write down what they did. Most people remember what they did, so you can discuss it in session without their writing it down.

- *Question 3*: When you ask couples to increase positive couple and family activities, what kinds of problems do you encounter frequently and what do you do about them?
    - *Answer*: Common problems and solutions for the three exercises presented in this chapter are listed below. Most of these problems were discussed in the case example in this chapter.

Problem	_Solution(s)_

Catch Your Partner

1. One or both partners failed to notice any pleasing behaviors for most or all days in prior week.	1.1. Clarify why: Often partners are looking for "special," not typical, things. 1.2. Ask them to pick out the two most pleasing things their partner did in past week and share it now. 1.3. If the reason is anger and resentment, empathize with these feelings. Then ask if person will do exercise any way. If refused, revisit later.
2. When acknowledging a caring behavior in Catch and Tell, the speaker ends with a negative comment.	2. Restate guideline of no negative comments in Catch and Tell and ask person to do "instant replay," leaving out the negative.
3. Couple does not want to write down pleasing behaviors noticed.	3. Do the exercise without written record (see Question 2, p. 109).

Shared Rewarding Activities

1. The couple argues or discusses problems during planned fun time.	1. Suggest couple agree to make fun time separate from time for problem discussions; both are needed, but not together.
2. The couple does not complete planned activity due to changed conditions (e.g., weather, movie not playing, babysitter cancels).	2.1. Suggest they have a backup plan if first plan does not work. 2.2. Stress that fun together is more important than specific activity. So need to improvise if first plan does not work.
3. Couple has trouble agreeing on fun activity to do.	3.1. Alternate who chooses activity. 3.2. Help them find a compromise activity or an activity they both might like (e.g., things they used to do).

Caring Days

1. One or both persons feels threatened by doing nice things for the other.	1.1. Agree it makes you vulnerable but maybe the only way is to try. 1.2. If still resist, then defer until later.
2. One person follows through and the other does not.	2. Praise person who complied, noting individual responsibility ethic. Explore reason for other person's lower compliance.

SUMMARY

• Once abstinence has begun, most patients need help to improve their relationships. The first goal of relationship-focused interventions in BCT is to increase positive couple and family activities in order to enhance positive feelings, goodwill, and commitment to the relationship.

- Catch Your Partner Doing Something Nice asks each person to notice and acknowledge one nice thing each day that the partner did. Have them do the daily acknowledging when they do the trust discussion at home. Also have them practice, in session, acknowledging one another's most pleasing behavior in the prior week.

- Shared fun activities, either by themselves or with their children or other couples, can bring the couple closer together. Also, patients who do enjoyable substance-free activities with their spouse and children have better recovery rates.

- Giving each other a caring day helps the couple put more caring into their relationship. Each person plans ahead to surprise the partner with a special day involving caring behaviors.

- Although both are positive couple activities, the shared rewarding activity exercise (the couple plans together for fun) differs from the caring day exercise (each person plans to surprise the other with a special day involving caring behaviors).

- Methods described in this chapter to increase positive activities all included a writing component in which the couple is asked to write down something. However, we also described how you can change each exercise in small ways so that couples can do them verbally, with no writing, for those couples who do not write or read very well.

- We also described problems frequently encountered when you ask couples to increase positive couple and family activities, and what to do about them.

- A case example illustrated how it is possible to increase positive feelings and activities even in a very estranged couple. The therapist's patient determination in the face of the couple's many challenges was rewarded by slow, steady progress.

NOTE

1. Moos, Bromet, Tsu, and Moos (1979); Moos, Finney, and Cronkite (1990).

6

Improving Communication, Part I
Listener and Speaker Skills

The last chapter discussed how to increase positive feelings and activities to create a warmer, more cooperative atmosphere for dealing with relationship concerns. The next two chapters focus on teaching communication skills. Better communication helps the couple resolve conflicts, problems, and desires for change.

Inadequate communication is a major problem for patients with alcoholism and drug abuse and their spouses.[1] Once the patient is abstinent, inability to resolve conflicts and problems can cause substance abuse and relationship tensions to recur.[2] Teaching couples how to resolve conflicts and problems can reduce family stress and decrease risk of relapse. BCT teaches basic communication skills (described in this chapter) of effective listening and speaking as well as use of planned communication sessions. Couples also learn more advanced skills (described in Chapter 7) of negotiating agreements for desired changes, conflict resolution, and problem solving. Table 6.1 lists these communication skills.[3]

TABLE 6.1. Key Points about Teaching Communication Skills

Basic skills

- General guidelines
- Communication sessions
- Listening skills
- Expressing feelings directly

Advanced skills

- Negotiating for requests
- Conflict resolution
- Problem solving

As you begin helping the couple to improve their communication, keep in mind the emphasis on individual responsibility and self-control that are key principles of BCT. Each person is responsible for their own behavior, which includes how they communicate. If one partner does not follow through on using new communication behaviors, it does not relieve the other spouse of the responsibility to use the new communication skills learned in BCT. For example, one partner, when angry may yell, accuse, and refuse to listen to the other's viewpoint. This does not mean it is OK for the other spouse to respond in kind. If one person uses the other's bad behavior as a reason to act the same way, then all too often communication only worsens. On the other hand, one person's use of the BCT skills when the partner is not using them often defuses the situation and both return to better communication. In short, one's own change should not be dependent upon seeing the other person change.

As noted Table 1.7 in Chapter 1, basic skills of effective listening and speaking and use of planned communication sessions are introduced at the end of the early BCT sessions (i.e., session 4 of a 12-session format). These basic skills are part of all subsequent BCT sessions because they are used in all the more advanced communication skills (negotiating requests, resolving conflicts, problem solving). Each of these more advanced skills is introduced for two sessions, starting toward the end of the middle BCT sessions (i.e., session 7 of a 12-session format) and may be continued in later BCT sessions, depending on the particular needs of the couple.

INTRODUCTION TO COMMUNICATION SKILLS TRAINING

Communication training starts with nonproblematic areas that are positive or neutral and moves to problem areas and emotionally charged issues only after the couple has practiced each skill on easier topics. Chapter 5 described the general approach for teaching each skill. First the therapist tells and shows the couple how to do it. Then the couple practices the skill with therapist coaching and at home on their own. Finally, the therapist reviews how the homework went and coaches further practice.

Before teaching specific communication skills, you need to give the couple some general guidelines about key elements of effective communication. These guidelines, describing good and not-so-good communication, set the stage for the couple to learn how to improve their communication together.

Table 6.2 provides a therapist checklist for introducing communication skills training (from the checklist for session 4 of the 12-session BCT manual contained in Appendix A). Next we describe how the counselor completes each of these steps.

Overview of Good Communication

Couples with substance abuse problems often have major difficulties communicating with each other. You might begin to address the area of communication this way:

"Now we are going to talk about communication. Many things get in the way of effective communication. Busy lifestyles often make it difficult to talk regularly. Also, conflict and disagreement may make us reluctant to talk about certain topics.

"The communication of couples struggling with substance abuse is often marked by hostility and sarcasm. Some couples basically stop talking because they are tired of argu-

TABLE 6.2. Therapist Checklist for Introducing Communication Skills Training

____ Show *Message Intended = Message Received Poster B.11* from Appendix B.

____ Explain that good communication exists when speaker's intended message matches message received by listener.

____ Show *Nonverbal Communication Poster B.12* from Appendix B.

____ Explain nonverbal communication.

____ Show *Barriers to Communication Poster B.13* from Appendix B.

____ Explain barriers to communication.

____ Show *Direct and Indirect Communication Poster B.14* from Appendix B.

____ Explain direct and indirect communication.

____ Hand out *"Dos and Don'ts" Form C.9* from Appendix C.

____ Explain "Dos and Don'ts" of communication.

____ Elicit partners' reactions and examples of these aspects of communication.

ing. Regardless of the cause, a breakdown in communication is often at the root of many problems.

"To learn how to communicate better, you need to understand the ideas behind good communication. Let's start by defining good communication."

GOOD COMMUNICATION DEFINED

Good communication exists when the intended message of the speaker matches the message received by the listener. Use the chart shown in Figure 6.1 (a copy of which is Poster B.11 in Appendix B) to explain this definition to the couple. Emphasize that the chances of the message intended matching the message received increases dramatically when the speaker clearly states what he or she wants, thinks, or feels instead of assuming the listener already knows. In turn, the listener should make every effort to understand the message without filling in gaps with his or her own assumptions.

This definition helps the couple understand that both speaker and listener must work together to ensure that the message intended equals the message received. A clear understanding of what constitutes good communication sets the stage for learning both listening and speaking skills. Finally, coverage of this concept includes a discussion of the "filters" in each person (described on the next page) that can get in the way of good communication.

NONVERBAL COMMUNICATION

It is also important to introduce the concept of nonverbal communication. All messages have two components: the words themselves and the nonverbal aspects of the message. The same words may convey different meanings depending on the accompanying nonverbal behavior. The nonverbal communication often outweighs the words themselves. For example, if the speaker says "OK, let's go out to dinner tonight," but speaks loudly and sighs afterward, it may sound as if the speaker is not happy about going out to dinner. On the other hand, if the speaker says the same words with a smile and a pleasant tone of voice, just the opposite message is conveyed.

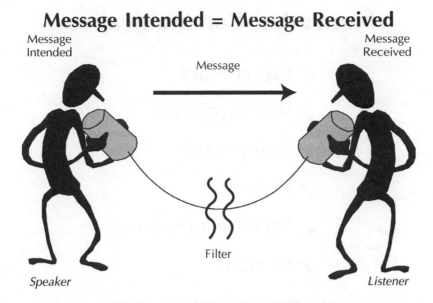

FIGURE 6.1. Good communication defined. From *A Couple's Guide to Communication* (p. 1), by J. Gottman, C. Notarius, J. Gonso, and H. Markman, 1976, Champaign, IL: Research Press. Copyright 1976 by Research Press. Adapted with permission.

Couples need to understand the impact of nonverbal communication so that the intended message will match the message received. Body language and tone of voice are key. Positive *body language* includes facing the person speaking, maintaining eye contact, and using nonverbal body cues such as nodding the head to indicate that the message is being heard. *Tone of voice* used when expressing a feeling or thought should be in line with the speaker's intended message and easy for the listener to receive. When a message is delivered in a loud, angry tone, the chance of the person actually listening drastically decreases because he or she is focusing on the negative. When the speaker uses a neutral or pleasant tone without raising his or her voice, the listener is more likely to really hear what the speaker is trying to say. Figure 6.2 (a copy of which is Poster B.12 in Appendix B) lists these aspects of nonverbal communication that you explain to the couple.

Barriers to Good Communication

Unfortunately, there are many ways communication can go wrong, and when it does, the message intended does not equal the message received. As part of introducing the couple to communication skills training, explain the following barriers to good communication.

FILTERS

There are factors in each person that function as filters and may block good communication. Filtering occurs when a person is tired, in a bad mood, under the influence of substances, or particularly sensitive about a certain subject. Each person's filters can prevent the speaker's intended message from being received correctly by the listener.

Nonverbal Communication

✓ Eye contact

✓ Voice volume

✓ Voice tone

✓ Posture

✓ Facial expression

✓ Gesture

FIGURE 6.2. Nonverbal communication.

Filters affect how the listener interprets messages. The listener may not hear the message the way it was sent because it was distorted by the listener's "filter." For example, if a wife is feeling depressed or moody, a compliment from her husband might sound insincere because of her negative mood, not because of the husband's actual message. However, if she were in a better mood, she might appreciate the compliment intended by the husband.

Filters also affect how the speaker sends a message. The message may pass through the speaker's filter and come out in a distorted way. For example, if a husband comes home in a bad mood, he may say something to his wife in a harsh tone when he is really angry at someone else. He may not even be aware of sounding cross.

The filters described so far tend to be temporary or situational. For example, if a speaker comes across as irritable because he or she is tired (a filter), then the speaker is likely to be more pleasant when well rested (and the filter is gone). A second type of filter tends to last longer, be more persistent, and affect communication attempts more frequently. These more enduring filters may consist of a person's sensitivities, beliefs, and expectations. For example, a person could be very sensitive to criticism and respond to perceived criticism with intense anger. Such a filter certainly distorts communication, especially when a couple discusses problems in their relationship. Effective communication requires that partners be aware of these two types of filters and work together to reduce or eliminate any distorting effects.

"ALL-TALK-AND-NO-LISTEN" SYNDROME

The "all-talk-and-no-listen" syndrome is a very common pattern that occurs when both partners think they are right and are unwilling to listen to what the other has to say. They each just state their points again and again, but neither is heard. Often, each partner is thinking of what to say while the other person is speaking, rather than listening to the message being sent. The result is that both partners feel frustrated, not listened to, not respected. An example of this syndrome might look like this for a typical husband and wife:

HUSBAND: Blah blah.

WIFE: Yak yak.

HUSBAND: What I said was "blah blah."

WIFE: What I said was "yak yak."

HUSBAND: Don't you see, I am saying "blah blah"?

WIFE: Yes, but I already said "yak yak."

You can fill in the "blah blah" or the "yak yak" with anything you like. The point is that each person continues restating his or her own position and does not listen. All talking and no listening prevents good communication and weakens the couple's ability to resolve disagreements and relationship issues. Couples experience many negative effects from this pattern of communication. Both partners believe that the other person doesn't see their point of view. Conversations drift to other problems and topics. The couple does not stay on one topic long enough to resolve a problem or disagreement. Conversations end with both partners feeling frustrated and not heard.

BLAMING AND SHAMING

Communications that include blaming and shaming are often filled with hostility and antagonism. Each partner is on the defensive, trying to protect their own point of view. Use of blame and shame communication allows a person to avoid responsibility for their own actions, distracts partners from the issue at hand, and prevents any discussion and resolution. Such behaviors are all too common in couples with substance abuse. Consider the example of Beth and Sam, who have financial problems because Beth spent a lot of money on alcohol and drugs and got fired from her job for missing work.

BETH: Sam, we got another call today from the bank. They threatened to foreclose on the mortgage. What are we going to do?

SAM: You're the one who caused these problems, not me. If you hadn't been drinking and doing coke, we wouldn't be in this mess. You're a worthless drunk, just like your father.

Sam has a right to be angry and upset, but this is not a healthy way to express it. Certainly this way of communicating will not help the couple deal with their very serious financial problems.

Additionally, in the face of Sam's shaming and blaming, Beth may be more likely to relapse. However, we are not suggesting that Sam's hostility would make him responsible if Beth relapsed. As we discussed in detail in Chapter 4, Beth would be responsible for whether or not she relapsed. However, it still is true that Beth might find it more difficult to stay abstinent in the face of Sam's withering criticism, particularly if it was a frequent occurrence. So blaming and shaming are a communication barrier that can damage the relationship and become a high-risk situation for relapse.

INDIVIDUAL COMMUNICATION STYLES

A final barrier to good communication that is important to explain to couples is a person's use of an overly aggressive or an overly passive communication style. An *aggressive* communicator makes demands and expects them to be followed, or makes nasty remarks in order to get his or her own way. A *passive* communicator does not stand up for him- or herself, often gives in to others, and may neglect his or her own needs. At times a person with a passive style may agree to do something, even when he or she doesn't want to, in order to avoid conflict. The preferred communication style emphasized in BCT is an assertive one. An *assertive* communicator can negotiate compromises without being taken advantage of or taking advantage of others, and can express his or her feelings or thoughts without resorting to attacks on the other person. The assertive communicator can typically get his or her point across without making others feel bad.[4]

Table 6.3 lists the specific barriers to good communication that are covered with couples in BCT. (Poster B.13 in Appendix B is a simpler version that can be used to guide discussions of communication barriers.)

Communication Dos and Don'ts

The final introductory comments about communication describe the differences between direct and indirect communication and other ideas about effective communication. Key differences between direct and indirect communication are displayed in Figure 6.3 (a copy of which is Poster B.14 in Appendix B). Reviewing this poster helps familiarize the couple with this idea.

Direct communication involves clear, direct expressions of thoughts, feelings, and ideas. The speaker expresses his or her own feelings and opinions in the spirit of communicating, not judging the other person. This attitude reduces the listener's defensiveness and makes it easier to receive the intended message. The listener pays attention to the content of the speaker's message instead of planning his or her response or feeling offended.

Indirect communication involves indirect expression of thoughts and feelings. The speaker uses barriers and defenses to try to avoid responsibility for actions and remove focus

---

TABLE 6.3. Barriers to Good Communication

- Filters
  - Distort message sent or received
  - May be a temporary mood or an ongoing attitude
- "All-talk-and-no-listen" syndrome
  - Each states their point again and again
  - No one listens
  - Nothing gets resolved
- Blaming and shaming
  - Linked with hostility and resentment
  - Common in substance abuse couples
- Individual communication styles
  - Overly aggressive style
  - Overly passive style
  - Assertive style just right

Direct and Indirect Communication

Direct Communication:

⇒ Taking responsibility for your feelings

⇒ Not waiting to share your feelings

⇒ Actively expressing yourself

⇒ Being assertive

Indirect Communication:

∅ Accusing and blaming the other person

∅ Delaying

∅ Passively withdrawing

∅ Sulking or aggressing

∅ Mind reading

FIGURE 6.3. Direct and indirect communication.

from the issue being discussed. When indirect communication predominates, partners report feeling hurt, not listened to, and that the other does not see their point of view. Conversations drift off topic before they reach a resolution. Partners have a tendency to "mind read" and fill in the blanks themselves.

The following statements are examples of direct and indirect communication.

Direct communication

1. I like you.
2. I feel uneasy in this kind of situation.

3. I'm mad at you for being late.
4. I really linked that dinner.
5. I feel uneasy when you drive this fast.

Indirect communication

1. You're a very likeable person.
2. This is the kind of situation that makes a person feel uneasy.
3. Why can't you be on time?
4. That was a nice dinner.
5. You shouldn't drive so fast—it's dangerous.

Additional examples of direct and indirect communication describe different situations in which such communication might occur.

Direct communication

1. Owning up to feeling hurt by your partner's forgetting anniversary.
2. Spontaneously and immediately telling partner that not helping with chores makes you feel overburdened.
3. Directly saying that you feel hurt or angry by something the other person said or did.

4. Pointing to some actions of the other person and saying how *you* feel about them.

Indirect communication

1. Beating around the bush and hinting indirectly that your feelings are hurt.
2. Storing up antagonisms and letting them come out later in a burst of pent-up rage.
3. Expressing hurt and angry feelings by inducing guilt (e.g., "I know you were so busy last week you forgot my birthday").
4. Reading into the other person's actions the idea that he or she feels something bad or negative.

DOS AND DON'TS

DO

- Use "I" statements.
- Take responsibility for your feelings.
- Tell how you feel in reaction to something your partner did: "I felt . . . when you . . . "
- Express negative feelings with words, not actions.
- Discuss one issue at a time.
- Show respect.
- Work together to solve problems.

DON'T

- Accuse: "You . . . "
- Blame partner for how you feel.
- Say "You never . . . " or "You always . . . "
- Yell, insult, or swear at partner.
- Use angry gestures or tone of voice.
- Threaten violence or separation/divorce.
- Bring up past or other issues.
- Try to "win" the discussion or "punish" partner.
- Call partner names.
- Passively withdraw.

FIGURE 6.4. Communication dos and don'ts.

Conclude the general guidelines about effective communication by giving the couple simple suggestions they can use to improve their communication. Review the handout on Communication Dos and Don'ts shown in Figure 6.4 (a copy of which is Form C.9 in Appendix C) with the couple to be sure they understand. Ask if they see any of these points in their relationship and indicate that all of the points will be covered in more detail in future BCT sessions on communication. Encourage them to keep these simple suggestions in mind in the meantime.

COMMUNICATION SESSIONS

After providing general guidelines about effective communication, your next step is to introduce and explain the concept of a communication session. Table 6.4 provides the therapist checklist for introducing communication sessions (from the checklist for session 4 of the 12-session BCT manual contained in Appendix A). Next we describe how the counselor completes each of these steps.

A communication session is a planned, structured discussion with the following ground rules. The couple talks privately, face-to-face, without distractions. Each spouse takes turns expressing his or her point of view without interruptions. Each gives the other full attention. They use communication skills learned in BCT so that the message intended by the speaker matches the message received by the listener.

TABLE 6.4. Therapist Checklist for Introducing Communication Sessions

_____ Show *Communication Session Poster B.15* from Appendix B.

_____ Explain concept of a communication session.

_____ Therapist models a communication session about a positive or neutral topic.

_____ Couple practices a communication session about a positive or neutral topic.

_____ Hand out *Communication Session Form C.10* from Appendix C.

_____ Assign home practice: Have a 10- to 15-minute communication session at home.

The couple uses communication sessions for in-session and at-home practice of communication skills. We first mention the term "communication session" when we assign a 2- to 5-minute daily communication session for couples to practice acknowledging caring behaviors in the Catch and Tell exercise described in Chapter 5. We expand on the communication session concept when we begin communication skills training in earnest. Communication sessions help the couple set aside time to practice good communication. Practice starts with positive or neutral topics, moves over time to relatively "safe" concerns (e.g., squeezing the toothpaste in the middle), and progresses to more sensitive topics (e.g., partner's perceived flirting) as their communication skills improve. Practice time increases from 2 to 5 minutes on positive topics up to 10- to 20-minute sessions three to four times a week in later BCT sessions, when the couple discusses current relationship problems or concerns.

Teaching the couple to set aside time for a communication session helps them develop and practice effective communication skills. These sessions provide a time for the couple to express thoughts, feelings, and opinions on day-to-day topics as well as more conflict-laden topics. Holding regular communication sessions reduces the likelihood of problems snowballing and partners holding onto grudges and fostering bitterness. Establishing a routine for discussing topics also prevents partners from blurting out thoughts when running out the door to work or, conversely, keeping silent about their thoughts or feelings. The communication session encourages open, clear discussion to help improve communication and facilitate problem solving.

The goal is that the couple will continue regular use of communication sessions after completing BCT. You should encourage partners to ask each other for a communication session when they want to discuss an issue or problem, keeping in mind the ground rules of behavior that characterize such a session. Asking for a communication session becomes a signal that this is a time when each person will listen carefully to the other and use the skills learned in BCT. Figure 6.5 (a copy of which is Poster B.15 in Appendix B) summarizes key points about communication sessions. (Form C.10 in Appendix C provides this same information on a handout, which can be given to couples for easy reference.)

The First In-Session Practice of a Communication Session

The goal of conducting the first communication session is to increase the partners' awareness of the benefits of practicing effective communication. For this exercise, the couple has a brief conversation, paying specific attention to the use of effective verbal and nonverbal communication skills. Partners can use the *dos and don'ts* sheet (Form C.9 in Appendix C) for helpful hints. This is

Communication Session

➤ Sit down face to face.

➤ Plan time and place ahead so that you will have privacy.

➤ Do not allow distractions, such as TV.

➤ Schedule 10–15 minutes.

➤ Use communication skills learned in couples therapy.

➤ Discuss concerns and problems.

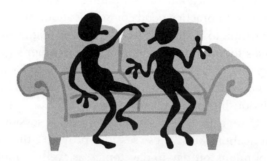

FIGURE 6.5. Communication sessions.

an opportunity for the partners to slow down their speech and learn how to communicate effectively with one another. You might introduce the exercise to the couple as follows:

"We have been talking about communication. We covered points about how to ensure that the intended message matches the message received, such as body language, tone of voice, paying attention to mood, and so forth. We also talked about things that can make communication more difficult, such as shaming and blaming, harsh voice tones, and accusations. Now I would like to introduce a helpful technique that we will use quite frequently throughout the rest of treatment.

"A communication session is a planned conversation. It is a brief, simple, and safe way to exchange thoughts, ideas, and feelings. It also is a time to practice good communication skills. These sessions will become more advanced as we build on communication skills and use more and more of the skills that we will talk about."

In-session practice begins with you, the therapist, modeling a communication session with one of the partners. Then have the couple do their own communication session, being sure each partner chooses a neutral or positive topic to discuss. You can suggest some examples of neutral or positive topics each partner may want to use for this practice session. Neutral topics might be:

1. "Where would your dream vacation be?"
2. "What would you do if you won a thousand dollars?"
3. "What is your favorite childhood memory?"

Positive topics might include:

1. "What is your fondest memory from your relationship with your partner?"
2. "What do you love the most about your partner?"
3. "Talk about when you first met each other."

Tell the couple that the goal of this first communication session is for both of them to pay attention to their body language, their tone of voice, and how they are feeling. Also ask them to *really* listen to each other. Suggest they sit face-to-face. Each person takes a turn as the speaker and then the listener. The speaker should use brief statements (two or three sentences) to describe his or her chosen topic. This brevity makes it easier for the listener to hear and remember what the speaker said. The listener should not respond to the speaker except to ask related questions to understand better what the speaker is saying. Explain that future sessions will involve a lively interchange between speaker and listener. However, the purpose of this first effort is to experience talking and listening to each other without interrupting or giving feedback. They will have about 5 minutes to talk. Let them know you may interrupt, if necessary, to help keep the conversation focused.

Observe the couple enacting their first communication session and interrupt if they go off topic. Provide corrective and supportive feedback to each partner after both complete the communication session. Ask how the conversation felt to them. Did they communicate differently or more positively than they typically have done with each other in the past? Ask if they would be willing to continue this communication practice at home in the coming week.

Home Practice and Ongoing Use of Communication Sessions

After this first in-session communication session is completed, assign a similar activity for home practice. Review the following guidelines for their communication sessions at home during the upcoming week:

1. Sit face-to-face.
2. Plan ahead a time and place where they will have privacy.
3. Do not allow distractions such as TV, radio, etc.
4. Work together, taking turns; decide who will go first as speaker.
5. Schedule about 5 minutes on 2 or 3 different days.
6. Choose a topic that is neutral or positive.
7. Speaker should be brief (two or three sentences).
8. Listener should not respond to the speaker except to ask related questions.
9. Pay specific attention to body language, tone of voice, filters, and avoid the all-talk-and-no-listen syndrome.
10. Use the dos and don'ts sheet (Form C.9 in Appendix C).

Discuss with the couple the time and place that they plan to have their communication practice sessions. At the next BCT session, assess the success of their plan and suggest any needed changes.

Once introduced, communication sessions are part of nearly all subsequent BCT sessions. A familiar rhythm develops. First, you review the communication home practice from the last week. Second, you have the couple practice during the session, using the communication skills learned up to that point. Third, teach a new skill (e.g., listening) by explaining and modeling it and having partners practice it in session, with coaching from you. Finally, assign more practice at home for the coming week. Guidelines 1–4 above, remain the same throughout BCT. However, the other guidelines change over time. Practice sessions get longer and cover harder topics, moving from everyday issues and problems to major emotionally charged issues. The couple practices and masters more communication skills, as we describe next. The core communication skills that are taught include structured listening techniques and direct expression of positive and negative feelings.

EFFECTIVE LISTENING SKILLS

Table 6.5 provides a therapist checklist for introducing the communication skills of listening and understanding (from the checklist for session 6 of the 12-session BCT manual contained in Appendix A). Next we describe how the counselor completes each of these steps.

Effective listening accomplishes three important goals: (1) It helps each member of the couple feel understood and supported; (2) it slows down couple discussions and prevents quick escalation of negative exchanges; and (3) it helps make the message intended by the speaker equal the message received by the listener. Teaching a partner to summarize the spouse's message and check the accuracy of the received message before stating his or her own position is often a major accomplishment that can only be achieved gradually. A partner's failure to separate *understanding* the spouse's position from *agreeing* with it often is an obstacle. Although often new to couples, the concept that they can understand each other's position without agreeing with it is stressed repeatedly.

TABLE 6.5. Therapist Checklist for Introducing Communication Skills of Listening and Understanding

_____ Show *Listening and Understanding Poster B.17* from Appendix B.

_____ Listening: Listener restates and checks accuracy of message received from speaker
("*What I heard you say was _____. Did I get that right?*").

    _____ Therapist explains and models listening.
    _____ Each person practices listening while therapist coaches.

_____ Understanding: Listener acknowledges that speaker's ideas make sense
("*It makes sense that you feel _____ because . . .*")
and shows empathy ("*That must make you feel . . .*").

    _____ Therapist explains and models listening with understanding.
    _____ Each person practices listening with understanding while therapist coaches.

_____ Assign home practice: Practice listening with understanding.

During communication, particularly emotionally charged communication, partners must learn to check that their perceptions of the message received match the speaker's intent. The short-term goal of listening effectively is for partners to slow down the communication process in an effort to decrease the potential for misunderstanding. In the long term, listening effectively, when used with other communication skills, can help decrease the number and intensity of arguments. BCT works first on basic listening skills and then helps couples add a deeper level of understanding to their communication.

Basic Listening Skills

EXPLAIN LISTENING RESPONSE TO THE COUPLE

Introduce listening skills to the couple by reminding them that good communication happens when the intended message of the speaker matches the message received by the listener. Refer back to Figure 6.1, which illustrates this definition. Tell the couple that the listening response is a key tool of good communication. Using this tool, the listener restates the message received from his or her partner ("What I heard you say was . . . ") and then asks if he or she heard correctly ("Did I get that right?"). When the speaker feels the message has been understood, then roles change and the listener gets to speak. Display the Listening and Understanding chart shown in Figure 6.6 (a copy of which is Poster B.17 in Appendix B) when you introduce and practice this communication skill. Use the top half of the chart on the basic listening response first, then expand to understanding later, as described below.

Explain the purpose behind listening skills to the couple before you model and have the couple practice these skills. You might say something like this:

Listening and Understanding

Listening
- Restate message received.
  "What I heard you say was. . . ."

- Ask if you heard correctly.
  "Did I get that right?"

- Get more information
  "Is there more?"

Understanding
- *"It makes sense that you feel the way you do."*

- *"That must make you feel. . . ."*

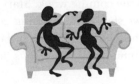

FIGURE 6.6. Listening and understanding skills.

"Listening may seem simple enough, but often it is not so easy, especially when you are discussing an important or sensitive topic from opposing viewpoints. When couples argue, the discussion often gets faster, louder, and more intense as emotions flare and both people try harder to make their points. Often people assume they know what message is being sent without really listening to what is being said. If you're thinking about what you want to say next, you are not listening to the speaker.

"To listen better we have to slow down the conversation. You don't have to agree with your partner to understand his or her point of view. I'm going to ask you to listen to your partner and say what you believe you heard him or her say. You may not get it right the first time. That's OK. Just try to really listen without judging or adding your own thoughts. You'll get a chance to talk, after you have understood what your partner had to say."

MODEL LISTENING FOR THE COUPLE

Next you model the use of listening skills, working with one of the partners. Discuss a positive or neutral topic, such as the weather or a local news event. First have the partner serve as speaker while you listen. Restate and check the accuracy of the message you received from the partner, using the formula from above (i.e., "What I heard you say was. . . . Did I get that right?"). When the partner affirms that you have heard the message correctly, you become the speaker and the partner tries to listen. Keep your statements brief and clear so that the partner does not become overwhelmed in the listener role. If the listener does not fully understand the major parts of your intended message, try again to send your message; repeat your attempts until the listener gets it right. Gently correct the listener, as needed, if they interject their own opinion before checking the accuracy of the speaker's message or if they fail to use the listening response formula.

HAVE THE COUPLE PRACTICE LISTENING IN SESSION AND AT HOME

Having the couple practice listening skills during the BCT session and at home is the next and most important part of teaching and learning this communication skill. Have partners take turns being the speaker and listener as they practice this skill together. The speaker should try to say something positive about the listener, such as an example from Catch and Tell, or something similar. The speaker should not talk about any issue that is "charged" or "heavy" at this time; there will be opportunities to do so later. The speaker should keep statements brief and stick with one topic to make the listener's job easier. Stress that the listener may need to clarify the speaker's message a few times before getting the message correct. The listener should not feel bad about doing this, and the speaker should try not to get frustrated when it occurs. Your job during this communication practice is to prompt each person to follow the guidelines on listening skills and to provide supportive and corrective feedback, when necessary.

When each person has practiced listening successfully in the session, then assign the same practice for completion at home in the coming week. Start them with positive or neutral topics that they discuss briefly. Usually we start by instructing couples to add the listening response formula when they do the Catch and Tell exercise each day. Over the course of BCT sessions, we gradually build up to longer communication sessions, in which they discuss more emotionally charged issues.

Two other components often are added to the basic listening response just described as BCT sessions progress. First, we try to move beyond very brief, often stilted exchanges to provide a more complete consideration of the speaker's topic. To do this we suggest that once the speaker has told the listener that he or she understood the message correctly, the listener should ask "Is there more?" The speaker may want to talk more about the topic, now that he or she feels heard by the listener. This process continues until the speaker feels like he or she has been heard fully by the listener; then the listener becomes the speaker. Second, we try to add deeper levels of listening and understanding to the couple's communication, as described next.

Listening and Understanding

Listening and understanding go beyond restating and checking the accuracy of the message to show that the listener understands the speaker at a deeper level and supports the speaker even when there is a disagreement. The listener shows understanding by communicating to the speaker that the speaker's thoughts and ideas make sense to the listener and that his or her feelings are valid. The listener also conveys understanding by showing that he or she understands the feelings behind what the speaker has said. Again, it is important to stress that understanding the speaker's opinions or feelings does not equal agreeing with the speaker.

You can help couples communicate understanding in the following way. Tell the couple that once the speaker states that the listener has gotten everything correct and there is no more he or she needs to say, the listener can show more understanding by making a statement, such as: "I can understand that" or "It makes sense that you feel _____ because?" Also, the listening partner can show more understanding by recognizing what the speaker is feeling and saying: "That must make you feel. . . ." When the speaker knows that the listener has not only heard the words he or she is saying but also recognizes that he or she feels a certain way, this experience can bring the couple closer and help create open, honest communication.

Once a couple has used the basic listening response successfully, you should move on to incorporate understanding. You may have to continue longer with basic listener skills for those with more strained relationships, until the couple becomes comfortable with practicing those new skills. If you don't feel the couple is ready to move on, then understanding skills can be left for later sessions. When you add understanding to listening skills, the process is the same as it was for the simpler skill. You model listening and understanding with one member of the couple, and then have the couple practice these skills under your guidance in the session, with further practice at home.

Next we turn to speaker skills, another key component of effective couple communication that we emphasize in BCT.

EFFECTIVE SPEAKING SKILLS: EXPRESSING FEELINGS DIRECTLY USING "I" MESSAGES

Table 6.6 provides the therapist checklist for introducing "I" messages to express feelings directly (from the checklist for session 5 of the 12-session BCT manual contained in Appendix A). Next we describe how the counselor completes each of these steps.

By expressing feelings directly, the speaker sends clear and direct messages that have a better chance of being received and understood by the listener. Expressing both positive and negative feelings directly is an alternative to the blaming, hostile, and indirect responsibility-avoiding communication seen in many substance abusers' relationships. Couples with sub-

TABLE 6.6. Therapist Checklist for Introducing "I" Messages

_____ Show "I" Messages Poster B.16 from Appendix B.
_____ Explain use of "I" messages to express feelings directly.
_____ Have partners take turns role playing expressing feelings directly.
_____ Assign home practice: Practice expressing feelings directly.

stance abuse problems often report a lack of effective communication. When communication patterns have deteriorated or broken down completely, conversations become loaded with negative expressions and exchanges that leave both partners feeling hurt and unheard. When partners become more aware of their feelings and learn how to express them effectively, healthier communication patterns emerge within the relationship.

Explain Expressing Feelings Directly Using "I" Messages

Introduce the skill of expressing feelings directly using "I" messages by restating that good communication happens when the speaker's intended message matches the message received by the listener (revisit Figure 6.1). Tell the couple that this skill will help them to get their point across more effectively when they are the speaker. Display the "I" messages chart shown in Figure 6.7 (a copy of which is Poster B.16 in Appendix B) when you introduce and practice this communication skill. Explain the purpose behind "I" messages before you have the couple practice these skills. You might start by saying something like the following:

"Becoming aware of feelings and learning how to express them are an important part of the recovery process. Although sometimes difficult at first, sharing feelings directly can bring you closer as a couple and rebuild trust in the relationship. When the speaker expresses feelings directly, there is a greater chance that he or she will be heard. The speaker says that these are his or her feelings, his or her point of view, not some fact about the other person. The speaker takes full responsibility for his or her own feelings and doesn't blame the other person for how he or she feels. This makes it easier for the listener to receive the

Expressing Feelings Directly Using "I" Messages

"I feel _____ [emotion]
when you _____ [behavior]."

- -

"I feel _____ [emotion]
when you _____ [behavior]
because _____ [specific reason]."

FIGURE 6.7. Expressing feelings directly.

intended message. The most important tool in expressing feelings directly is the use of 'I' messages. We will discuss and role-play the use of 'I' messages next."

Indicate that there are several advantages to using "I" messages: They ease tension, reduce defensiveness, encourage honest communication, and can help the speaker define a specific problem he or she is experiencing. Suggest that a person should consider using an "I" message particularly (1) when he or she wants to share feelings or thoughts without blaming, (2) any time there is a lot of stress in the relationship, and (3) when both partners are upset. Explain that partners can make "I" messages by using this simple formula: "I feel _____ [emotion] when you _____ [behavior]." Such statements encourage the speaker to slow down his or her speech and to choose his or her words carefully. "I" messages also help the person speak directly, using his or her own feelings, and encourage an open, honest discussion of feelings and behaviors. If an individual is able to express him- or herself directly, he or she is less likely to feel frustrated and misunderstood.

Couple Practices Expressing Feelings Directly Using "I" Messages

PRACTICE EXPRESSING *POSITIVE* FEELINGS DIRECTLY

After you explain the concept and answer any questions, it is time for the couple to practice using "I" messages. Partners should follow the simple formula displayed on the "I" messages chart (see Figure 6.7 above). Ask the partners to come up with at least two "I" messages each. These should be positive statements about something outside the relationship (e.g., "I feel happy when the sun is out") or something specific to the relationship (e.g., "I feel appreciated when you bring me flowers"). Allow partners an opportunity to share each of their "I" messages and provide corrective feedback, if necessary.

Once the partners become comfortable with this simple formula, you can add other components. By adding "because . . . " at the end, the speaker can tell the reason for feeling the way he or she did about the behavior in question. Such a statement follows this general format: "I feel _____ [emotion], when you _____ [behavior], because _____ [specific reason]." For additional practice using the expanded formula, ask the partners to build on their earlier statements or to create two more using the new formula. For example: "I feel excited when you plan a date for us because it shows me how much you care." Listen to the statements they make and provide corrective feedback, allowing each partner time to incorporate it and get the formula right.

After both members of the couple have demonstrated satisfactory use of "I" messages during the BCT session, assign home practice of this communication skill. Tell the couple that you would like them to have a communication session three times at home in the coming week to practice using the "I" message skill on a positive feeling. They should follow the guidelines outlined in the communication session chart (see Figure 6.5), which should be on display. You also may ask them to use other communication skills learned so far. For example, they might take turns being speaker and listener, with the speaker using "I" messages to express positive feelings directly and the listener using the listening response to restate and check the accuracy of the message received from the speaker. At the next BCT session, review their home practice (e.g., what worked, what seemed awkward) and have them practice the skill further to reinforce the learning. In other words, you follow the same steps in teaching the "I" messages skill that you use for all the communication skills in BCT.

PRACTICE EXPRESSING *NEGATIVE* FEELINGS DIRECTLY

We start work on effective speaking skills by focusing on expressing positive feelings directly. This follows the general BCT approach of starting with positives and later moving on to negative and charged issues. Teaching the couple how to express negative feelings directly follows the same format as just described for positive feelings. First, explain and give a few examples. Then ask the partners to practice making "I" statements about a negative feeling. This can be a negative feeling about something outside the relationship (e.g., "I feel irritable the next day when I don't get enough sleep the night before"), or it can be a negative feeling about something specific to the relationship (e.g., "I feel angry when you are late and don't call"). It can also involve explaining why the speaker is having a negative feeling (e.g., "I felt angry yesterday when you were talking with Jack because you used to do drugs with him, and I am afraid that contact with him could cause you to relapse"). After practicing under your guidance in session, couples practice at home, beginning with minor everyday problems that elicit low levels of negative feelings. Gradually couples progress over the weeks to discussing major "charged issues" about which one or both partners have strong negative feelings.

In helping couples learn to express negative feelings, you need to remember a number of additional points. First, you need to be considerably more active in your coaching of couples when significant negative feelings are involved. Observe partners closely as they take turns being speaker and listener. Interrupt if they go off topic or engage in unproductive negativity. If need be, facilitate the in-session practice by guiding each partner individually. Stand next to the person and quietly guide him or her with suggestions about how to convey feelings or respond as a listener. Also, you can take over for one of the partners and model the skill. You can defuse a speaker's negative feelings by using empathic listening to help the angry person feel understood. Once the partner feels heard, he or she generally becomes calmer, less upset, and more reasonable. Often it is better for you to use listening and understanding to convey empathy to an angry or hurt partner than to have the other partner try to do it when they are feeling attacked and defensive. Second, emphasize the "dos" and "don'ts" of communication chart (see Figure 6.4 above), particularly the "don'ts." Finally, try to prevent "negative carryover" from sessions in which one partner leaves the session still angry and continues to argue about the issue at home. Often there is a risk that negative feelings will escalate in such continued arguments. The next chapter describes methods for resolving conflicts and dealing with arguments to prevent escalation of negative feelings to dangerous levels.

CASE EXAMPLE

Bill and Marcy, a couple in their early 40s, started BCT after Bill had finished his fifth detox program for a chronic alcoholism problem. Although he had had a number of sober periods lasting 12–15 months each, he invariably followed a pattern of decline: He would start feeling confident that his sobriety was going well, slowly drift away from attending regular AA meetings, and then eventually relapse. At their fifth BCT session, they reported an argument from the prior week. Marcy had asked Bill if he was going to an AA meeting that night. Bill got angry because he felt she was checking up on him and monitoring whether he was doing his program. They didn't speak the rest of the evening.

When they discussed this argument in the BCT session, it became clear there had been a misunderstanding. Marcy had wanted to know so she could decide whether to visit her sister that evening, as she had planned. Marcy was uncertain because Bill had been feeling sick, so she thought he might not go to AA and instead might want her to stay around to make him some tea. After hearing this explanation, Bill apologized for getting angry. However, the therapist sensed that this argument reflected ongoing tension between them about Marcy's role in Bill's recovery. So the therapist suggested that they have a communication session to practice the listener and speaker skills they had learned to discuss this topic.

THERAPIST: I'd like the two of you to have a communication session to discuss your feelings about Marcy asking about AA meetings. Take turns being speaker and listener. Use the listener and speaker skills we've been working on. Let's start with you, Bill. *Could you first talk about any positive feeling you have on the topic. Then Marcy will tell you what she heard you say before responding to your feelings.*

BILL: Hmm. A lot of times I appreciate that little extra prodding about getting to a meeting and stuff, about doing this or doing that or something. Because I get lazy sometimes. But you've always been powerful in that respect with my sobriety. You make me want to do the right thing. You know what I'm saying?

MARCY: I hear you.

THERAPIST: Can you tell him what you heard him say and ask if you got it right. Let's see if you did hear him.

MARCY: What I heard you say was I help you by prodding you to go to meetings and wanting you to do the right thing.

THERAPIST: Ask if that's right.

MARCY: Is that right?

BILL: Yeah, just asking if I'm going to a meeting tonight, ya know?

MARCY: Because sometimes you can become lazy in that area and my question is supporting you?

BILL: Yeah, it helps me.

THERAPIST: Marcy, it's your turn.

MARCY: I didn't think you liked that. I didn't think you liked me opening my mouth about that kind of stuff.

BILL: Well . . . (*interrupted by therapist*)

THERAPIST: Bill, before you respond, tell Marcy what you heard her say and ask if you got her right.

BILL: OK. Marcy, I heard you say you didn't think I like it when you ask me about my meetings. Did I get you right?

MARCY: Yeah, that's right.

BILL: Well, I don't like you to beat it to death, but when you mention it, it's all right. A lot of times you get carried away. You make me feel like I'm not capable of doing something on my own sometimes. And then I get a little annoyed, and that's when I give you short answers. Do you know what I'm saying?

MARCY: Yes. That's why I go to Al-Anon. In order to take care of myself. I worry about you sometimes, and I put my two cents worth in. And sometimes you appreciate it—that's what I'm hearing you say—and sometimes you don't.

BILL: No, I always appreciate it. Just sometimes the way it happens, it loses its effectiveness when we get into an argument. All the good that came and then "poof," you know? You just get snappy. And then I snap back at you, and then we both get snappy. And then we go off and stop talking.

THERAPIST: It sounds like you're both learning something new right now about the interaction you have around meetings. It's supportive, up to a certain point. Maybe there's a simple request you could make of Marcy, telling her how you would like that support from her around meetings. And then we can see if it works for her. Because we don't want to lose the value of her support in that regard.

BILL: You mean, how I would want her to say something?

THERAPIST: Yeah. For example, "I would like you to support my going to meetings by asking me once if I'm going," or. . . .

BILL: Yeah. That would be it. Just, "Are you going to a meeting?" Or whatever, something like that and not, I don't know. You have a way about you that I don't know how to explain it. Just keep it short, you know what I'm saying?

MARCY: No, try to be a little clearer, honey.

BILL: Just casually mention it, jog my memory, like, if I'm thinking about doing this or that, just "don't forget about the meeting." And then let it go.

THERAPIST: OK. That's a good request. Let's see what Marcy heard you asking and then she can respond.

MARCY: In support of your AA attendance, you like when I casually ask "Are you going to a meeting tonight?" Is that what I heard you say?

BILL: (Nods.)

MARCY: And I always do that casually. That's what I say: "Are you going to a meeting tonight?"

BILL: Then it depends on what I say. If I say "I don't know," then it can get belabored.

MARCY: So you want me to ask you if you are going to a meeting and just leave it at that, is that right?

BILL: Yeah, and then just let me make up my mind. Chances of me going, I think, are greater if you just say something like that and then leave it alone.

MARCY: But are you going to answer me when I say that?

BILL: I might say "I don't know yet," or whatever. A lot of times when I say that, you say, "What do you mean, you don't know?" with that look on your face and my hair goes up. And then by the time we get through with this little dissertation, I say "Well, shit, I ain't going to the damn thing anyway now because I'm pissed."

THERAPIST: I'll show her.

BILL: Well, yeah, actually that's about what it gets to. The hell with it.

THERAPIST: So your request, Bill, might sound something like this: "I appreciate your asking me if I'm going, but no matter what my answer is, I'd appreciate if you'd leave it at that." Right?

BILL: Yeah.

MARCY: I need to hear you say that.

BILL: OK. You say something like, "Are you going to a meeting?" and I say whatever I say, and you just leave it there, even if it's just for a while, without getting into "Why aren't you going to a meeting?" or "Why don't you know if you're going to a meeting?" That type of thing—if we can avoid that part of it.

MARCY: So if you say "I don't know" after I ask you if you're going to a meeting tonight, you want me to say just "Oh, OK?"

BILL: Yeah. I'd probably give you something like "I don't know if I'm going to do this or do that."

MARCY: Yeah, we can try that.

FREQUENTLY ASKED QUESTIONS

- *Question 1*: Communication skills training starts with positive and neutral topics, then switches to real problems, first on less sensitive issues and finally working up to major charged issues. This does not seem realistic. People won't wait for such a logical approach. When they are upset about something, they want to talk about it then.

- *Answer*: In BCT we do not want to try teaching a communication skill using an emotion-laden topic because the emotion will interfere with the person's ability to learn the skill. Instead we have the couple learn and practice the skill on easier topics with less interfering emotion before trying the skill on more difficult topics. It's like learning to ski. You start on the beginner's slope. After you can ski and turn without problems on the beginner's slope, then you move to the intermediate slope. If you become skilled enough, you may progress to expert terrain.

However, this does not mean that you do not talk about emotionally charged topics until the middle or end of the course of BCT sessions. As indicated in the question, this would not be a realistic approach. When people are upset, they want, and may need, to deal with the issue then. This circumstance happens frequently in BCT sessions. The couple comes to the session upset over a conflict that occurred in the past week. Or there is an ongoing serious disagreement that cannot wait to be addressed until the couple becomes more proficient in communication. In such cases, the BCT therapist acts as a very active negotiator, problem solver, and guide to help the couple defuse the conflict or at least come to some temporary solution to the disagreement. The therapist does not coach partners to negotiate the solution "on their own" through back-and-forth communication using skills they have not yet fully learned.

To use the skiing analogy, consider the following situation. You get stuck at the top of the mountain in bad weather and the only way down is a steep expert slope, but you are an intermediate skier, at best. You don't want the ski patrol to coach you on how to improve your technique so you can ski down unaided. You want them to guide you down to safety.

- *Question 2*: You talked about filters, which are factors in each person that can block good communication because they distort how the listener interprets messages. One important filter was not addressed. This is the filter stemming from previous history with the partner and the thoughts and feelings that arise from that history. Could you discuss this type of filter more and how it is dealt with in BCT?

- *Answer*: Perhaps an example would help. Carl and Jenna were trying to repair their relationship in BCT after years of Carl's substance abuse, which had been particularly bad in the last 4–5 years. He had lost two jobs and had a DUI arrest. They had been separated twice. Just before they started BCT, Jenna had seen a lawyer about divorce. At their fifth BCT session, just a few days before a scheduled court hearing about the DUI charges, Jenna said she wanted to know the truth about the day Carl got the DUI. She said that he had given her two or three different versions of what had happened, and she wanted the truth. She said that when she had called off the divorce to try BCT after Carl's admission to detox, she had promised herself she was not going to put up with any more lying.

The counselor suggested they try to discuss this using their listening and speaking skills. With a lot of coaching from the counselor, they did surprisingly well, given the volatility of the topic. Carl told Jenna all that he could remember about events surrounding the DUI arrest. She was able to paraphrase what Carl had said but questioned whether he was covering up something by saying he couldn't remember a lot of what happened that night. Carl said he could understand why she might be skeptical. He admitted that he had lied to her on numerous occasions, trying to cover up his substance use and avoid arguments. He said he wanted to stay sober and be honest now. She wanted to believe him, but she wasn't completely sure she did.

Jenna's continuing skepticism and distrust were an example of a filter based on her experience with Carl. He had lied to her repeatedly, so now she was reluctant to believe what he told her, especially when they were arguing or in terms of events related to his substance use. The counselor pointed out that partial or total loss of memory was quite possible with a blood alcohol level (BAL) of .22, Carl's breathalyzer reading when he was arrested. The counselor also acknowledged that Jenna's skepticism and distrust were justified and understandable, given past events.

The counselor's initial response to Jenna's filter was to identify it and validate it: the typical BCT response the first time a filter is discussed. What else would the counselor do to deal with this filter? At later sessions, the counselor would ask her to be aware of this semiautomatic filter and try to question her negative interpretations of Carl's actions and communication now that he is pursuing recovery. The counselor probably would suggest that, if Carl's recovery continues, her distrust likely will lessen with time, though it may take many months. The counselor also might refer Jenna to Al-Anon for a fellowship of support from others struggling with similar issues. Finally, the counselor might have separate individual sessions with Jenna to let her tell the many details of their past history. Then she can pick those aspects she most wants to discuss with Carl during a couple session, with the counselor coaching them.

- *Question 3*: Some of the couples who are happy in their marriage often have a very hard time with communication skills training. They don't have issues or at least they don't admit to them. Many of these couples ask why they need to do these exercises. They don't find them valuable at all. Unhappy couples usually see the need for these sessions on communication. (This question comes from an experienced BCT counselor.)

• *Answer*: This is a great question that illustrates two points that may surprise those who are not familiar with BCT. First, why would happy couples with a substance problem take part in BCT? Can a couple really have a good relationship when one partner has sought help for a substance problem? Clearly, some couples with a substance abuse problem who say they get along fine have definite adjustment problems but do not want to admit them to each other or the counselor. However, many couples who say "we get along fine when he's not drinking or using" are giving an accurate picture. When we started doing BCT over 25 years ago, we assumed that all, or nearly all, alcoholism and drug abuse patients had serious relationship problems and could benefit from couples therapy to address these problems. Over the past two decades research on substance abusers' relationships has grown. Studies show that most substance abuse patients do have relationship problems, but the degree varies considerably: Some have very serious problems, and some score in the nonproblem range on relationship adjustment measures.[5] Also, we have changed our focus from couples therapy to alleviate relationship distress to BCT, which has dual goals of helping the patient stay abstinent and helping the couple get along better. Even patients without serious relationship problems can benefit from BCT's work to help them stay abstinent.

Second, BCT is a flexible approach. It can be tailored to the needs of the individual couple. Not all couples need all aspects of BCT to the same degree. In our outcome studies, we have delivered BCT in a standardized manner, with a similar sequence and content of BCT sessions, as specified by a session-by-session therapist manual, like the one shown in Appendix A. However, in clinical practice BCT can be applied flexibly. All couples generally get exposure to all BCT modules (i.e., recovery support, positive activities, communication skills, continuing recovery), but the relative emphasis placed on each module may vary. For happier couples, you might put less emphasis on positive activities and communication and more emphasis on the Recovery Contract and other supports for abstinence and on planning for continuing recovery. For unhappy couples with apparent conflicts, you might cover all modules of BCT fairly evenly because they need all parts of BCT.

SUMMARY

• Inadequate communication is a major problem for alcoholism and drug abuse patients and their spouses. BCT teaches the basic communication skills described in this chapter: effective listening and speaking, and use of planned communication sessions.

• Good communication exists when the intended message of the speaker matches the message received by the listener.

• Barriers to good communication include (1) filters that affect how the listener interprets the speaker's message; and (2) the "all-talk-and-no-listen" syndrome, in which both partners think they are right and are unwilling to listen to each other.

• A communication session is a planned, structured discussion used for in-session and at-home practice of communication skills. The couple talks privately, face-to-face, without distractions. Each spouse takes turns expressing his or her point of view, without interruptions.

• Effective listening includes both listening and understanding. The listener restates and checks the accuracy of the message received from the speaker ("What I heard you say was _____. Did I get that right?"). The listener shows understanding by saying that the speaker's ideas make sense and that his or her feelings are valid ("It makes sense that you feel _____ because . . . ").

- Effective speaking skills consist of expressing positive and negative feelings directly, using "I" messages: "I feel _____ [emotion] when you _____ [behavior] because _____ [specific reason]."

- Communication training in BCT starts with positive or neutral topics, then switches to real problems, first on less sensitive issues and finally working up to major charged issues. Before partners learn how to negotiate charged issues "on their own," the BCT therapist functions as a very active negotiator, problem solver, and guide to help the couple find at least temporary solutions to heated conflicts that arise.

- Spouse distrust based on the patient's past dishonesty is a common filter that makes the spouse reluctant to believe the patient now. Your first response is to identify and validate this filter. At later sessions, ask the spouse to be aware of this automatic filter and question the negative interpretations now that the patient is pursuing recovery. You also might refer the spouse to Al-Anon and have a few individual sessions in which the spouse reviews past history and picks those issues he or she most wants to discuss with the patient. Then the spouse brings the issues to a couple session, with you coaching the partners' interaction.

- BCT can be tailored to the couple's needs. For happier couples, you might emphasize communication less and the Recovery Contract, other supports for abstinence, and Continuing Recovery Plans more. For unhappy couples, you might cover all modules of BCT fairly evenly because they need all parts of BCT.

NOTES

1. Fals-Stewart and Birchler (1998); Fals-Stewart, Birchler, and O'Farrell (1999); O'Farrell and Birchler (1987).
2. Maisto, McKay, and O'Farrell (1995).
3. Many of the concepts and procedures to improve communication described in this chapter were based on John Gottman's couple's guide to communication (Gottman, Notarius, Gonso, & Markman, 1976) and Robert Liberman's book on BCT (Liberman, Wheeler, DeVisser, Keuhnel, & Keuhnel, 1980). Both of these books concerned couples without substance problems. We simplified and adapted these methods for couples with substance abuse problems.
4. These concepts on communication styles are based on the classic book on assertiveness by Alberti and Emmons (2001).
5. Fals-Stewart et al. (1999); O'Farrell and Birchler (1987).

7

Improving Communication, Part II
Resolving Changes, Conflicts, and Problems

The last chapter covered basic communication skills of effective listening and speaking and the use of planned communication sessions. This chapter presents more advanced communication skills of negotiating agreements for desired changes, conflict resolution, and problem solving. As described in Table 1.7 in Chapter 1, each of these more advanced skills is introduced for two sessions starting toward the end of the middle BCT sessions (i.e., session 7 of a 12-session format) and may be continued in later BCT sessions, depending on the particular needs of the couple.

NEGOTIATING RELATIONSHIP AGREEMENTS TO BRING ABOUT REQUESTED CHANGES

Many changes that partners want from each other may be achieved through the caring behaviors, rewarding activities, and communication skills taught in earlier BCT sessions. However, emotionally charged conflicts that may have caused considerable hostility between partners for years are harder to change. Relationships that have been damaged by substance abuse often lack partner willingness and ability to express needs or desires toward resolving such deeper issues.

The BCT module on relationship agreements instructs partners how to effectively express what they want from the relationship and successfully negotiate agreements that will initiate positive changes. When partners are specific and reasonable in their requests, and are able to compromise, they can successfully come to agreements to initiate changes that benefit both partners and the relationship. Helping couples negotiate relationship agreements to bring about requested changes involves three skills: (1) learning to make *positive specific requests*, (2) learning to *negotiate and compromise*, and (3) arriving at *agreements*.

In working to negotiate agreements, there are some general points that both counselors and couples should keep in mind. We encourage good-faith agreements in which each partner agrees to make his or her change independent of whether or not the spouse keeps their part of the agreement.[1] This agreement is not based on the promise "I'll do my part if you do yours" but instead reflects two people freely choosing to do something that helps the other. Each spouse volunteers to make changes needed to improve the relationship. It is key to remember that most requests can be fulfilled, at least in part, and that negotiation requires using all previously taught communication skills. Finally, negotiating—or meeting each other halfway—can have very positive benefits for the relationship.

Positive Specific Requests

The first step in helping a couple negotiate relationship agreements is to introduce the concept of positive specific requests. You might introduce the topic in this way:

> "To want change from your partner or change in your relationship is normal. However, asking for and negotiating for change is difficult in almost any relationship. When you are specific about, and reasonable in, the changes you want and are willing to compromise, usually you can agree on changes each of you will make to help you get along better. Let's start with learning how to make positive specific requests."

EXPLAIN POSITIVE SPECIFIC REQUEST CONCEPT

Display the Positive Specific Requests chart shown in Figure 7.1 (a copy of which is Poster B.18 in Appendix B) as you give this explanation. Reviewing this poster helps familiarize partners with the idea. Explain that all too often couples use a negative approach when they try to get the changes they want. Partners complain about what is wrong in their relationship and what they are not getting from it. Often they are vague and unclear about what they do want, and they may try to coerce, browbeat, or force the other person to change. Remind the couple that how they send a message is directly related to how it is received. BCT uses a positive

Positive Specific Requests

- <u>Positive</u>—what you want,
  not what you don't want.

- <u>Specific</u>—what, where,
  and when.

- <u>Requests</u>—not demands
  (which use force and threats),
  but rather requests, which have
  possibility for negotiation
  and compromise.

FIGURE 7.1. Positive Specific Requests chart.

approach to negotiate changes. In order to negotiate for desired changes, each partner must learn to state his or her desires in the form of positive specific requests. There are three parts to this skill: (1) *positive* refers to stating what the individual wants, not what he or she doesn't want; (2) *specific* refers to stating the when, where, and what of the desired change; and (3) *requests* leave an opening for compromise (i.e., they are not demands).

Next give examples of typical couple requests and have the couple practice identifying and writing their own positive specific requests. Figure 7.2 (a copy of which is Poster B.20 in Appendix B) contains a list of 10 sample requests that we display as a poster. Have the couple review this list and give their opinion about whether each item meets the positive specific request criteria. Of the 10 items listed, 1, 3, 5, 8, and 9 are positive specific requests. The other items do not meet criteria for a positive specific request. Items 4 and 7 are negative, meaning they say what the individual does not want rather than what they do want; they also convey a demanding tone. Having partners rewrite these negative requests so that they meet the desired criteria can help them understand this concept. The following are sample rewrites for items 4 and 7.

4. (Original) I would like my partner to stop bugging me so much.
4. *(Rewrite) I would like my partner, when she is angry, to ask me to sit down for a communication session no longer than 10 minutes to discuss her feelings.*
7. (Original) I would like my partner to stop spending all his time watching sports on TV.
7. *(Rewrite) I would like my partner to go for a walk with me after dinner each night.*

Items 2, 6, and 10 are not specific enough. However, note that most couple requests start at this level of vagueness. Your job is to help partners make their request more specific so that they can negotiate an agreement for change. The following are sample re-writes for items 2, 6, and 10.

Sample Couple Requests

I would like my partner to:

1. Kiss me when I come home from work.
2. Help out more around the house.
3. Tell me about his or her workday at dinnertime.
4. Stop bugging me so much.
5. Do the dishes on nights that I go to class.
6. Appreciate me more.
7. Stop watching sports on TV all the time.
8. Hold my hand while we watch TV.
9. Put his or her dirty clothes in the hamper.
10. Spend more time with our kids.

Items 1, 3, 5, 8, and 9 are positive specific requests.
Items 4 and 7 are negative.
Items 2, 6, and 10 are not specific.

FIGURE 7.2. Sample couple requests.

2. (Original) I would like my partner to help out more around the house.

2. *(Rewrite) I would like my partner to make dinner two nights a week and be responsible for keeping the bathroom clean.*

6. (Original) I would like my partner to appreciate me more.

6. *(Rewrite) I would like my partner to sit down with me for 15 minutes at bedtime and listen to me while I talk about things that are important to me.*

10. (Original) I would like my partner to spend more time with our kids.

10. *(Rewrite) I would like my partner to spend 20 minutes each night reading a story to the kids.*

A few common errors when dealing with couple requests are worth noting. Most couple requests start out like many of the original versions shown above: a request saying what the person wants but in rather general terms. Sometimes therapists push too quickly for partners to make the requests more specific, and sometimes they convey the notion that couples *should* be this specific or that there is something wrong when they are not so specific. This implied judgment can be a turn-off to the couple who may begin to view the therapist as a bit too pedantic and unrealistic. Another related problem is that the therapist or the couple may initially become hung up on the details rather than focusing on clarifying the underlying need or desire. Ideally, the specific request needs to satisfy the underlying need being expressed. Sometimes the therapist can tune into this subtler level. Other times the partners will discover this themselves when they find that completing an agreement did not produce the expected satisfaction.

HAVE EACH PARTNER MAKE HIS OR HER OWN LIST OF REQUESTS

After the couple understands the concept, ask each person to list five requests on the Positive Specific Request List you provide for this purpose. Figure 7.3 shows a sample list of requests (a blank version is Form C.14 in Appendix C). Suggest that their lists might include requests related to communication, money, children, household chores, leisure time and social activities, job, and so forth. They can complete their lists during a BCT session or for homework. Each should make his or her own list without consulting the other; they should not share their lists until they are in session with the therapist, who is available for coaching and conflict containment, if necessary. This process can be emotionally charged for many couples, especially those who have negative beliefs about changes in a relationship. Some individuals think that a request for change constitutes a criticism of the person, rather than being simply a request for a behavior change. Others believe that you cannot ask someone you love to change. BCT suggests that requests for change are a normal part of every relationship and are necessary to help two individuals meld their differences and build a stronger bond together.

Partners may add to their lists as time goes on. Those who fear conflict will list only minor change requests (e.g., "Squeeze the toothpaste from the end, not the middle, of the tube") at first. Later, as they gain confidence in their ability to negotiate changes, and as you encourage them to tackle more difficult issues, they may do so. The purpose of the list is to generate material that starts the process of negotiating specific changes each person agrees to make. Once each person has completed an initial list of five requests, the couple is ready to learn how to negotiate and compromise to reach an agreement that brings about desired changes.

POSITIVE SPECIFIC REQUEST LIST

It is not unusual for couples to talk about what is wrong and what they are **not** getting from a relationship. However, we are often vague and unclear when it comes to talking about what we **do** want. "Positive specific requests" is a technique that helps us effectively express our wants and desires to our partner.

Positive—say what you want, not what you don't want.
Specific—what, where, and when.
Requests—not demands, which use force or threats, but requests, which have the possibility for negotiation and compromise.

Make a list of positive specific requests. Requests might include things that would make you happier in your relationship and would make your life easier. Some areas to consider are communication, childrearing, money, leisure time and social activities, household responsibilities, sex, job, and independence.

Talk about plans for a family budget

Give some encouragement to our son to boost his self-esteem

Kiss me when I come home from work

Have dinner together as a family 3 nights a week

Do food shopping when I go to AA so we have more time to spend together

Take better care of himself (health and appearance)

Not swear at me when he gets angry

FIGURE 7.3. Sample list of positive specific requests.

Negotiation and Compromise

PARTNERS SHARE THEIR LISTS OF REQUESTS

Have each person share their list of requests, starting with what they feel are the most specific and positive items. Have them take turns reading one item at a time from their lists. Photocopy each person's list before the discussion starts. This way you will know what they are going to say and can judge whether either list contains major or sensitive issues that are likely to evoke a strong emotional response from the person's partner and be prepared to deal with such a response. As you review each request listed, give feedback on the degree to which the items meet the positive specific request criteria and help partners clarify and rewrite items as needed.

EXPLAIN THE NEGOTIATION PROCESS

Explain that negotiation and compromise can help couples reach an agreement in which each partner agrees to do things requested by the other. The idea behind negotiating and compromising is that most requests can be met, at least, in part. To help partners compromise on a stated request, instruct them to be flexible in terms of frequency, duration, intensity, or circumstance of what is being requested, rather than presenting the request in inflexible, all-or-none terms. For example, a husband might say he wanted "more time to work on my hobbies." This general, vague request should be translated into explicit dimensions of activity, such as when, how often, how long, and where. The husband might want to spend most evenings and Saturdays on his hobbies. The wife might feel this does not leave enough time for other important activities, including spending time with her. They might negotiate a compromise: He would spend an hour three times weekly after supper in the basement or garage working on his hobby of carpentry. The wife would agree not to complain about or interrupt the husband's free time on his hobbies. Thus, although the husband did not get as much time for his hobbies as initially requested, he did get much of what he wanted, including that his wife stopped complaining about his hobby time, and both were happier in the relationship.

COACH THE COUPLE TO NEGOTIATE AN AGREEMENT FOR REQUESTED CHANGES

Coach the couple as they have a communication session to negotiate one request that each person is willing to do for the other in the coming week. Start by asking each person to choose a request from the partner's list that he or she is willing to fulfill, at least in part, in the coming week. Having each person volunteer which of the partner's requests he or she is willing to address reduces the chance that the person will feel forced to do what the partner wants. Remind them to use the speaker and listener skills they have learned to make sure that they are stating their request clearly and that they are being heard correctly. Provide guidance as the partners work through a negotiation.

Work on getting an agreement for one person's request at a time. Consider a hypothetical couple. You decide to have the woman address one of her husband's requests first. She chooses a request from her husband's list to discuss. The husband states his request in a positive specific manner. When the wife has restated and checked the accuracy of her understanding of the husband's request, the negotiation process begins. The partners go back and forth, using their listening and speaking skills, until they reach a mutually satisfactory agreement about what the wife will do in the coming week to address the husband's request. Write what the wife agreed to do on the Negotiated Agreement sheet (Figure 7.4, which shows a sample negotiated agreement; a blank form is provided as Form C.15 in Appendix C). Next, repeat the process with the husband, who agrees to fulfill one of the wife's requests. Finally, carefully review the written agreement the couple has made for the coming week. Be sure that agreed-upon requests are specific enough (in terms of how often, how much, when, where, and with whom) so that each person fully understands what he or she is committing to in the exchange process. Agreed-to requests also should be realistic and reasonable. Overly optimistic promises make for a weak agreement with little chance of success.

The following dialogue from Liberman and colleagues[2] shows a therapist coaching Al and Mary when they try to negotiate an agreement for the first time.

> THERAPIST: Now that we've talked about and demonstrated how to use your communication sessions to make requests of each other, I'd like you to try it. You begin, Mary. Make a request. Then Al will tell you what he heard you say before responding to your request.
>
> MARY: It would make me feel good if you wouldn't turn away and read the paper or walk off when I try and tell you about my day at home with the kids.
>
> THERAPIST: Mary, you told him what you *didn't* want. What do you want him to do instead? Start again.
>
> MARY: It would make me feel important if you would listen to me once in a while when I try to tell you about my day.

NEGOTIATED AGREEMENT

During the session you negotiated one agreement to fulfill during the week. For your part of the agreement, you *volunteered* to fulfill one of your partner's requests, either in full or in part. Remember, this is voluntary on your part, out of the "goodness of your heart." Your partner also *volunteered* to fulfill one of your requests, either in full or in part. This agreement is not a matter of "I'll do mine only if you do your part" but instead reflects two people each doing something to help the other of their own free will.

I agreed to [be specific: what, when, how many times]: *Organize outstanding bills*
for rehab stay and figure out a plan to pay them

My partner agreed to: *Attend Al-Anon once a week*

Did I follow through with my agreement? [describe]: *Partly. I organized the bills,*
but I couldn't come up with a plan on my own. We need to discuss this.

Home Practice: During your communication session this week, negotiate another agreement at home. If possible, pick an item off your partner's list of requests that you would be willing to fulfill in full or part. Remember to use the Listening and Understanding techniques ("What I heard you say was. . . . Did I get that?")

I agreed to [be specific: what, when, how many times]: *Discuss plans for*
painting kitchen on Wednesday after supper

My partner agreed to: *Spend 1–2 hours Sunday straightening the basement*

Did I follow through with my agreement? [describe]: *Yes, I did.*

FIGURE 7.4. Sample negotiated agreement.

THERAPIST: Better.

AL: I hear you say that you would like me to listen to you when you want to tell me about your day.

THERAPIST: Is that what you said, Mary?

MARY: Yes.

THERAPIST: Now, it's your turn, Al. State how that makes you feel.

AL: I find it really upsetting to be greeted at the door with a long list of complaints about your day. I'm tired when I come home and need a few minutes to unwind.

MARY: Well, I'm tired, too, and . . . (*interrupted by therapist*)

THERAPIST: Mary, tell Al what you heard him say.

MARY: I heard you say that you don't like to listen to me complain when you first come home because you're tired and need some time to yourself.

THERAPIST: That's good, Mary. Now, state your request in more specific terms. How often, when, and for how long would you like Al to listen to you talk about your day?

MARY: I would like you to listen to me for about 10 minutes every day. I realize that you're tired when you come home, so maybe we could make it after dinner.

THERAPIST: Add how that would make you feel, why it's important.

MARY: It would make me feel as if I matter and as if what goes on at home is important to you.

THERAPIST: Good.

AL: I hear you say that you would like me to listen to you for 10 minutes every evening after dinner and that would make you feel as if you matter.

THERAPIST: Very good. Now, Al, you may respond to the request by agreeing or making a suggestion for more or less time or more or less often. You may also make a request for something in return. You mentioned something about time to unwind when you get home.

AL: I can understand how that would make you feel as if I'm not interested in you. I can try your plan to see how it works for a week. I come home from work very uptight, and I would like to have 15 minutes every day when I first come home to be left alone by the kids and everyone to unwind. I think that would put me in a better mood for the evening.

MARY: I hear you say that you would be willing to try this arrangement for a week and that you would like 15 minutes of uninterrupted time to unwind when you come home every day. I'll agree to that.

THERAPIST: It sounds like you have come to an agreement that you are both willing to try for 1 week. You will both be giving something and getting something. Report back next week on how it went.

Agreements

A number of BCT sessions can be devoted to negotiating written behavior-change agreements for the coming week, often with very good effects on the couple's relationship. During the sessions, progress on the prior week's agreements is reviewed briefly, including any suggested changes needed in the coming week. After completing agreements, with guidance from the counselor, the couple has a communication session at home to negotiate an agreement on their own and to bring it to the following session for review. A series of such assignments can provide a couple with the opportunity to develop skills in behavior change that they can use after the therapy ends.

Some agreements may be temporary and some may last longer. For example, many couples negotiate agreements about finances or children that allow the recovering substance abuser gradually to regain some part in decision making about these important family issues. A common agreement about finances is that one partner (usually the individual without substance abuse) will be the "family bookkeeper" who pays the bills and keeps the family accounts, but both partners will meet regularly to discuss the status of family finances and make joint decisions so that both are fully informed and involved. A common agreement for parents of preteen and teenage children is that they will maintain a "united front," meaning that neither will agree to a child's request about an important matter without consulting the other parent. Table 7.1 summarizes the steps in negotiating relationship agreements to bring about requested changes.

TABLE 7.1. Steps in Negotiating Relationship Agreements to Bring about Requested Changes

1. Explain positive specific request concept.
   - Wanting one's partner to change is normal, but negotiating it can be difficult
   - Give examples of typical couple requests.
   - Practice identifying and writing positive specific requests.
2. Have each person make their own list of requests.
   - Start with five requests, and add to lists later.
   - Partners complete lists in session or for homework.
3. Partners share their lists of requests.
   - Partners share their lists for the first time only with counselor present.
   - Can be emotionally charged if requests for change are viewed as criticism.
4. Explain the process of negotiation and compromise.
   - Most requests can be met at least partly.
   - Be flexible about how often, how long, and other details of an agreed-to request.
   - Meeting each other halfway can have major benefits for the relationship.
5. Coach the couple to negotiate an agreement for requested changes.
   - One person volunteers to fulfill (at least, in part) a request from partner's list.
   - Using listening and speaking skills, partners go back and forth.
   - Stop when both agree to a change the person will make in coming week.
   - Write down what the person agreed to do; be sure it is realistic.
   - Repeat the process with the other member of the couple.
6. Have couple carry out agreed-to actions in the coming week.
   - Each person agrees to carry out his or her change even if the other does not.

Case Example

Steve and Noreen were referred to the BCT program as part of Steve's aftercare plan following a residential alcoholism rehabilitation program. Steve and Noreen were in their early 40s, had been married 15 years, and had two teenage children. About 6 months earlier, the couple had separated, at Noreen's insistence, after Steve was fired from his job as a building supplies salesman for drinking and arrested for the second time for drunken driving. Steve refused to get treatment and continued to drink very heavily on a daily basis after the initial separation. Eventually Steve contacted Noreen, saying that he wanted to come home and to stop drinking for good. Noreen told Steve that she would consider giving their marriage "one last try" if he completed an intensive treatment program, established an aftercare plan that seemed reasonable, and remained abstinent. Initial sessions in the BCT program established a Recovery Contract with daily Antabuse use and regular AA attendance.

Once Steve had been sober for a while, the counselor started teaching negotiation skills to help them arrive at agreements for changes each wanted from the other. Steve and Noreen talked a lot in the BCT sessions about Noreen's unhappiness with Steve's not working and the consequent financial problems. Steve disliked Noreen's angry outbursts when she was feeling the financial pressures (e.g., when a creditor called). He also objected to her frequent questions about whether he had been looking for a job and what his prospects were of getting a job.

Steve and Noreen negotiated and successfully carried out a series of agreements about these issues. The first agreement was that they would have a weekly discussion in which Noreen would inform Steve about the current bills and Steve would review his job-hunting activities of the prior week and his plans for the coming week. Both agreed to use the communication skills they had been learning during this weekly discussion. Noreen further agreed to refrain from angry outbursts or other discussions about the money and unemployment problems; and Steve agreed to have a brief communication session about these issues during the week if Mary requested it. They made further progress in their weekly discussions at home and in their sessions with the BCT counselor. They wrote a joint letter to their creditors, explaining their situation, and arranged extended payment plans in most cases. After considerable discussion, Steve agreed to broaden his job search to include a much wider variety of positions. He also took a part-time job delivering pizza to provide some income while he continued his job search.

CONFLICT RESOLUTION

As partners work together in BCT toward relationship and lifestyle changes, old problems are bound to resurface and new ones are likely to evolve. As the couple begins to address emotionally charged issues and disagreements, conflict is inevitable. Conflict is a part of every close relationship. Conflict arises when two people have different thoughts or feelings about the same issue. A person can deal with conflict in one of three ways: using (1) an open and direct way, (2) avoidance and denial, or (3) verbal or physical aggression. Couples with a substance abuse problem often have very poor conflict resolution skills. The high levels of verbal and physical aggression not only hurt the adult members of these couples but also harm the children living in these homes. Children often witness their parents' arguments and violence. Helping couples as a part of recovery from substance abuse to address conflict effectively with respect, understanding, and fairness can improve life for the whole family.[3] Table 7.2 provides the therapist checklist for introducing conflict resolution (from the checklist for session 8 of the 12-session BCT manual contained in Appendix A). Next we describe how the counselor completes each of these steps.

An important goal of BCT is to help couples develop better skills for managing and resolving conflicts. Toward this end the BCT therapist educates partners on different methods for addressing conflict, explores how each partner currently copes with relationship conflict, and teaches the couple methods for successfully working through conflicts.

Educate the Couple about Types of Responses to Conflict

The first step in helping couples learn to manage and resolve conflicts is to educate them about responses couples commonly use to deal with conflict in their relationships. The goal is to help couples recognize negative, ineffective responses and encourage them to use positive, effective responses when addressing conflicts that arise in their relationship. You might introduce the topic in the following way:

TABLE 7.2. Therapist Checklist for Introducing Conflict Resolution

_____ Show *Responses to Conflict Poster B.21* from Appendix B.

_____ Explain that conflict is normal in every relationship. It's how we handle it that counts.

_____ Explain and discuss five types of responses to conflict: verbal aggression, physical aggression, flooding, avoidance and withdrawal, and verbal reasoning.

_____ Review couple's usual methods of addressing conflict in the relationship.

_____ Reassess risk of violence, if needed.

"At some point every couple experiences conflict. Conflict comes up when the two of you have different thoughts and beliefs about something that is important in your relationship. There are times when we don't agree with something someone is doing or saying because we look at the same situation in a completely different way. Such conflict may lead to an argument and increase tension in your relationship. Our goal is to learn how to manage and resolve conflicts successfully. Let's start by talking about the different ways people respond to a conflict situation."

Five common responses to conflict are verbal aggression, physical aggression, flooding, avoidance and withdrawal, and verbal reasoning. Only verbal reasoning is a form of conflict resolution—that is, a positive process in which two people work together to resolve problems or issues as they arise. The four other conflict responses generally are ineffective and not recommended. Display the Responses to Conflict chart shown in Figure 7.5 (a copy of which is Poster B.21 in Appendix B) as you describe and give examples of these five types of responses to conflict.

Responses to Conflict

Verbal Aggression: Commonly used when couple is frustrated and can't reach agreement; highly ineffective; causes more frustration and anger; doesn't lead to resolution.

Examples: blaming, name calling, swearing, yelling

Physical Aggression: Ineffective coping behaviors that hurt victim and relationship; common among couples with substance abuse.

Examples: slapping, hitting, biting, pushing, grabbing, shoving

Flooding: Person becomes overwhelmed with emotion and can't think clearly or speak effectively—like a car engine that won't start because it's been flooded with too much gas.

Avoidance and Withdrawal: Avoids discussing problems with his or her partner or withdraws from conflict by changing topic or leaving room; usually not effective if major relationship problems are not discussed.

Verbal Reasoning: Couple uses effective speaking and listening communication skills to resolve a conflict; both partners state their opinions; able to reach a compromise; typically leads to mutually agreed-upon solution.

FIGURE 7.5. Responses to conflict.

VERBAL AGGRESSION

Verbal aggression usually occurs when one or both partners become very frustrated and cannot reach an agreement about something that is causing them a problem. Acts of verbal aggression include yelling and swearing at the partner, calling the partner names, berating or putting down the partner's feelings, insulting the partner, and threatening physical harm to the partner. Verbal aggression is a common but a highly ineffective response to conflict. Someone who is using verbal aggression may think that this is the only solution to the problem. Typically, this conflict response style only causes more frustration and anger and does not lead to resolution of the conflict.

PHYSICAL AGGRESSION

Physical aggression includes throwing objects, pushing, grabbing, shoving, slapping, hitting, biting, choking, hitting with an object, threatening with a knife or gun, and using a knife or gun to hurt someone. Be sure to give some examples of less severe physical aggression, such as one partner shoving the other when they do not agree on an important issue, or one partner throwing a plate at the other when feeling frustrated. Although some forms of physical aggression are more severe than others, *all* forms are ineffective responses to conflict. All hurt the victim and damage the relationship. Also, children who witness such abuse and fighting may suffer emotional damage. Unfortunately, physical aggression in couples who report a substance abuse problem is common, with the majority of couples in treatment reporting at least one incident of physical aggression in the year prior to treatment.[4]

FLOODING

Flooding refers to a strong emotional response to a conflict situation in which an individual becomes emotionally overwhelmed and unable to process information or communicate effectively. The individual becomes "flooded" with emotions, like when a car engine is flooded with too much fuel and will not function properly. Overwhelmed with anxiety, fear, frustration, anger, or rage, the person can't think clearly or speak effectively. Taking a time-out, as described below, may help the emotionally or cognitively flooded person calm down and regain his or her ability to listen and speak effectively.

AVOIDANCE AND WITHDRAWAL

Avoidance and withdrawal occur when a person avoids discussing problems for fear that doing so might worsen the situation. Or a person withdraws from the conflict by changing the topic or leaving the room. Someone who responds to conflict this way may believe that problems are unpleasant and may clear up on their own, and that discussing them directly may make matters worse. Although this approach works sometimes, it usually is not effective in the long term if major problems in the relationship are not discussed.

VERBAL REASONING

Verbal reasoning is the one response to conflict that typically leads to conflict resolution. It involves using effective speaking and listening communication skills, such as those discussed in the previous chapter, in order to resolve a conflict. Both partners get a chance to state their opinions about the situation and are able to work toward a compromise. A couple applying verbal reasoning when facing a strong disagreement would not avoid the topic or heatedly argue about it. Instead, they would sit down and have a communication session about the problem, using the speaking and listening skills they learned in BCT.

REVIEW THE COUPLE'S USUAL METHODS OF ADDRESSING CONFLICT

After discussing different ways people respond to a conflict situation, take a few minutes to talk about what each person normally does when an argument or conflict occurs. It may be one of the five conflict responses just discussed or other behaviors. After both have identified one or more ways they deal with arguments or conflict, ask each to comment on which responses to conflict have been effective and which ones have been ineffective in the past. You can help them judge how effective a conflict response has been by asking a series of questions. Ask each to consider what effect this response usually has on the situation: Does it help the situation, seem to make the situation worse, have no effect, or cause problems in other areas? Also ask each person to consider how their partner typically reacts to this conflict response. Such questioning generally helps the person decide whether the behavior is an effective response to conflict in the relationship. This can be a sensitive topic, so you need to prevent each person from criticizing the other. Emphasize that this is time for each person to reflect on their own behavior, not a time to take each other's inventory.

REASSESS RISK OF VIOLENCE, IF NEEDED

This discussion may lead to some uncomfortable moments for the couple, especially if there have been high levels of ineffective responses to conflict in their relationship. Take a few minutes to assess how they are feeling. Ask if they have any concerns or comments about anything that was mentioned. Determine if they are ready to move forward to talking about coping skills for managing and resolving conflicts. In some cases, you will learn that verbal and physical aggression was more severe or more frequent in their relationship than they had reported during your initial assessment at the start of BCT. This discovery should prompt you to reassess the risk of partner violence and the suitability of the couple for BCT. Check that partners have not been hiding or minimizing verbal or physical aggression that has occurred since starting BCT. Remember that at each session, you review their BCT promises and inquire about arguments or problems they experienced in the past week. Most couples handle conflicts nonviolently while attending BCT, so it is rare to decide a couple is not appropriate for the therapy after attending for this many sessions. The typical response is to move forward to examine positive methods for managing and resolving conflicts.

Managing and Resolving Conflict

Although conflict happens in any relationship, many couples find that working toward solutions can be stressful, aggravating, and at times seem impossible. This is especially true for couples with a substance abuse problem. To help couples learn effective ways to resolve conflicts, BCT provides guidelines that can be followed and tools that can be used. Table 7.3 provides the therapist checklist for introducing managing and resolving conflict (from the checklist for session 8 of the 12-session BCT manual contained in Appendix A). Next we describe how the counselor completes each of these steps.

TABLE 7.3. Therapist Checklist for Introducing Managing and Resolving Conflict

_____ Hand out *Guidelines for Managing Conflict Form C.17* from Appendix C.

_____ Explain and discuss guidelines for managing conflict.

_____ Show *Time-Out Poster B.22* from Appendix B.

_____ Explain and discuss use of time-out to prevent conflict from escalating.

_____ Couple practices use of time-out in communication session on charged topic.

_____ Assign home practice: Use a time-out in coming week to reduce conflict.

GUIDELINES FOR MANAGING CONFLICT

Effective ways of dealing with conflict include all of the positive communication skills taught in BCT. So you will want to review key points briefly before looking at specific guidelines for dealing with conflicts. Remind the couple that if they start arguing, they should try to have a communication session in which they use the listener and speaker skills learned in earlier BCT sessions. The speaker uses "I" messages to state what he or she feels, thinks, or believes. The listener summarizes and checks the accuracy of what was heard and conveys understanding of the partner's feelings and beliefs. Implementing these communication skills help slow down the conversation so that partners can focus on each other's feelings and point of view. Because many conflicts center around changes one partner wants the other to make, remind partners of the following BCT suggestions for negotiating relationship changes:

- Use requests, not demands.
- Allow room for negotiation and compromise.
- Consider that even a partial change can have great benefits.

After this brief review of earlier communication skills, review the Guidelines for Managing Conflict shown in Table 7.4. (Form C.17 in Appendix C is a handout that elaborates on these guidelines.) Discuss each point on this handout with the couple and ask them which guideline would be most helpful to their relationship. These points are elaborated on the next page:

TABLE 7.4. Guidelines for Managing Conflict

- Be respectful.
- Use effective communication skills (especially on a "hot" topic).
- Maintain emotional control.
- Show willingness to understand.
- Communicate honestly and clearly.
- Be objective and avoid speculation.
- Request, don't demand.
- Focus on present and future, not the past.
- Look for balanced solutions that meet both partners' needs.
- Use active listening tools.

- Keep discussions respectful, even when feeling frustrated or hurt. Avoid using put-downs, name calling, or interrupting.
- Keep discussions on "hot topics" within a structured process. Make positive specific requests for such issues. Use a planned communication session or negotiation process.
- Maintain emotional control, even when feeling angry. Avoid yelling. Take a "time-out" (described below) if you cannot control your emotions.
- Show a willingness to understand. Use listening skills (e.g., "What I heard you saying . . . ") to help your partner feel understood and acknowledged.
- Communicate honestly and openly, using "I" messages. Holding back will only delay or complicate the resolution process.
- Be as objective as possible; avoid speculation, rumors, and assumptions.
- Express concerns in a constructive manner. Use positive specific requests, which typically are better received than a stance in which changes are demanded.
- Focus on future solutions rather than past blame. Keep in mind the promises made at the beginning of BCT.
- Look for solutions that meet both partners' needs.

These guidelines for managing conflict repeat many elements in the dos and don'ts of communication (see Figure 6.4, p. 120). Such repetition is an important part of BCT. It is needed to be sure that couples understand, and can actually apply, healthier, more positive ways of relating.

TIME-OUT: A TOOL FOR MANAGING CONFLICT

A time-out is a break requested by one or both partners to allow for calming down and clearing of thoughts and feelings so that the discussion does not escalate into an argument. A time-out is often used when the conversation is getting out of control or when emotions are running so high that flooding occurs, making it hard to continue. Often there is strong resistance to taking a time-out from the partner who is determined to discuss the issue immediately. He or she may believe that the partner taking the time-out is doing so just to avoid the issue, or worse, to shut him or her out. Therefore, we recommend that (1) when the time-out is requested, partners set a time to restart the discussion, and (2) the one who requests the time-out be the one who restarts the discussion when he or she is ready and able. These agreements help both partners get out of an ineffective discussion and restart one that is effective and includes a mutual goal of resolution.

When you explain time-out to the couple, display the Time-Out poster shown in Figure 7.6 (a copy of which is Poster B.22 in appendix B) for easy reference. Your explanation might go something like the following:

"When you are unable to slow down a conversation, you may need a break from trying to solve the problem or disagreement. This is when you use a time-out. A time-out allows you to take a break and step back so that you don't use verbal aggression or physical aggression to solve the problem. A time-out allows you to compose yourself, refocus, and restart the conversation when you are able to use the communication skills that will help you solve the problem. There are four parts to a time-out:

Time Out

Before: When discomfort or frustration in discussion first begins.

During: A "Time-Out" is requested. Couple separates to calm down and clear thoughts.

After: The "Time-Out" is over and discussion re-starts.

Resolution: A "Time-Out" increases chances of successful resolution.

FIGURE 7.6. Key points about "time-out."

"1. *Before*: If either of you gets uncomfortable or frustrated while discussing a problem and thinks it may lead to increased frustration, you should ask the other for a time-out. You might say, 'I'm getting uncomfortable. I want to take a 15-minute time-out. Once the 15 minutes is up, I would like to get back together and try to discuss this again.'

"2. *During:* Once you both agree to take a 15-minute time-out, go into separate rooms, relax, and try to get your mind off the argument by taking deep breaths, listening to soothing music, or whatever would help you to calm down.

"3. *After:* The person who requested the time-out should be the one who restarts the discussion. If things start to get tense again, ask for a second time-out. If things are still too tense, then postpone the discussion for an extended period of time. You might try talking again the next day or wait until your counseling session.

"4. *Resolution:* One or more restarts following a time-out usually result in a satisfactory resolution. However, because it is not possible for two people to agree about everything, when resolution by agreement and compromise is not possible, you should learn how to 'agree-to-disagree' as a way to resolve certain problems."

Next you can guide the couple in a communication session, putting to use all the skills learned to date, but with a specific focus on managing conflict and practicing the time-out skill. Ask the couple to choose a topic that involves a medium level of conflict, then observe the interaction carefully. Once the conversation comes to the point where you think a time-out would be helpful, intervene by saying, "I think a time-out would help the situation right now. Let's discuss how you would go about doing this." At this point, ask the partners what they would do to implement the time-out if they were at home. Having a plan for what to do during the time-out is important because a plan helps ensure that what each chooses to do is likely to reduce anger. Also a plan helps each person know what the other will do, so that he or she does not misinterpret the other's actions when upset. For example, partners might go to separate rooms, take a 5-minute walk, or practice deep breathing. After describing how they might do the time-out at home, ask the couple to use a time-out during the upcoming week, applying it to a real situation (perhaps an issue that arises during a communication session) or rehearsing in a practice situation. Their experience at home will be discussed during the next BCT session.

PROBLEM-SOLVING SKILLS

Often couples face problems that may not involve heated conflicts or desires for change but still cause a lot of stress when they remain unresolved. These problems range from family difficulties with children or extended family to external stressors that impact the relationship, such as financial or legal problems. Many times, the substance abuse itself has caused problems (e.g., unpaid bills, job losses). In addition, ordinary relationship problems may pile up and go unaddressed during periods of substance use. Even after abstinence is attained, problems are likely to continue. Unresolved problems caused by substance abuse can be overwhelming. Often partners disagree on solutions, or they don't know what to do, so they do nothing and try to avoid dealing with the problem. The problems remain unresolved and typically worsen.

Stressful unresolved problems create a risk for relapse. Problem solving requires the couple to be willing to recognize that a problem exists and to take steps to solve it. When people are under stress or abusing substances, they often focus on the "quick fix" and forget to look at all the options and long-term consequences of their choices. The S.O.L.V.E. problem-solving model helps the couple address a variety of problems, including relationship issues, finances, and childrearing. Use of the model will help the couple to develop or enhance the problem-solving skills needed to cope with stressors in their relationship.

Table 7.5 provides the therapist checklist for introducing the five-step model of problem solving (S.O.L.V.E.) (from the checklist for session 9 of the 12-session BCT manual contained in Appendix A). Next we describe how the counselor completes each of these steps.

TABLE 7.5. Therapist Checklist for Introducing the Five-Step Model of Problem Solving (S.O.L.V.E.)

_____ Show *S.O.L.V.E. Problem-Solving Model Poster B.23* from Appendix B.

_____ Introduce and discuss S.O.L.V.E. problem-solving formula.

_____ Therapist models using S.O.L.V.E. problem solving on an example problem.

_____ Hand out *Problem-Solving Example Form C.19* from Appendix C.

_____ Couple practices using S.O.L.V.E. on a problem of their own, with therapist coaching.

_____ Hand out *Problem-Solving Practice Form C.20* from Appendix C.

_____ Assign home practice: Couple has 30-minute communication session in which they use S.O.L.V.E. with a problem chosen in session.

Explain the S.O.L.V.E. Problem-Solving Method

Display the S.O.L.V.E. problem-solving model shown in Figure 7.7 (a copy of which is Poster B.23 in Appendix B) when you introduce and practice this communication skill. Explain the purpose behind problem solving before you have the couple practice these skills. You might start by saying something like the following:

> "Many couples find that problems developed or ignored during substance abuse often seem overwhelming in the early stages of recovery. Today we will introduce a new skill called S.O.L.V.E. This skill gives you a general problem-solving model that can help you work out a variety of problems, including finances and childrearing. You can use this skill for almost any personal or relationship problem you may face. In addition, S.O.L.V.E. is easy to learn and use in your daily life."

After this introduction, you should explain and discuss with the couple each of the following steps in the S.O.L.V.E. approach.

S—STOP, SLOW DOWN, AND SEE THE PROBLEM

The first step to effective problem solving is to stop, slow down, and identify the problem. It sounds like a simple thing, but in a situation that causes distress or when emotions are running high, reactions are not likely to be well thought out. Acting too soon can lead to further problems. Certain clues suggest a problem exists and that it is a good time to use this problem-

S O L V E

S   **STOP, SLOW DOWN, AND SEE THE PROBLEM**
  ✔ Is there a problem?
  ✔ What <u>exactly</u> is the problem?

O   **OUTLINE OPTIONS**
  ✔ Brainstorm: What can I do?
  ✔ What might work?

L   **LOOK AT CONSEQUENCES**
  ✔ Look at long- and short-term consequences.
  ✔ Look at positive and negative consequences.
  ✔ What will happen if I do this?

V   **VOTE**
  ✔ Evaluate consequences and eliminate bad choices.
  ✔ Which solutions have the most positive and least
    negative consequences?

E   **EVALUATE**
  ✔ How did it work?
  ✔ Did my choice solve the problem?

FIGURE 7.7. The S.O.L.V.E. problem-solving model.

solving approach. Such clues include bodily tension in the neck or other muscles, angry and agitated feelings and thoughts, or actions that show stress, such as slamming the door or avoiding a key person. Suggest to the couple that if they feel tense and overwhelmed or experience other distress signals indicating that there may be a problem, they should *stop* what they are doing, *slow down*, and take time to think about what the *problem* might be. A good way to slow down is to take a few deep breaths to help clear the mind so that it is easier to think. They can ask themselves: "Is there a problem?" and "What exactly is the problem?" Breaking the situation down this way and identifying one issue at a time often makes the problem seem more manageable.

O—OUTLINE OPTIONS

In this step, the partners brainstorm possible solutions for the problem. Try to get them to look at many different options, even if some may seem unlikely to succeed. At this stage, they should not criticize or evaluate the options. The point is to list as many possible solutions as they can think of, to look at the problem from different angles. What did they do about a similar problem in the past? What options have other people suggested? What other possibilities are there? Keep asking these questions until they run out of ideas. Suggest any ideas you might have. This exercise shows the partners that they have choices in how they decide to handle the situation and usually generates options they had not considered.

L—LOOK AT CONSEQUENCES

Next the couple reviews their list of options and considers the likely positive and negative consequences of each. Help them consider both the short- and long-term consequences for each option. Many people tend to focus only on what will happen in the short-term, because this is easier to see and quicker to figure out. Encourage the couple to slow down and look at the potential long-term consequences, because often the long-term consequences are most helpful in identifying the best course of action. Suggest that partners ask themselves "What might really work over the long term?"

V—VOTE

In this step, the partners evaluate the consequences of their choices, eliminate the less effective options, and identify a possible solution. As a couple, they rank the options and pick the one they think will be the most positive. Suggest that they ask themselves two questions: "Which choice has the most positive and the least negative consequences?" and "Which is better for us in the long term?"

E—EVALUATE

Finally, the couple takes action with the best option and then reviews the results. If the chosen solution does not appear to have worked after a reasonable period, partners should go back to their list and try another option. They may also choose to go through the process again, using what they learned on their first problem-solving attempt to guide them.

Have the Couple Practice Using the S.O.L.V.E. Problem-Solving Method

The goal of the S.O.L.V.E. problem-solving method is to give couples a basic tool they can use to work out a variety of problems. A couple needs to practice this skill to learn how to use it. First, present an example problem situation. You may want to use the example given on the Problem-Solving Practice sheet handout shown in Figure 7.8 to review the steps in the method. (See Form C.19 in Appendix C for this problem-solving example handout and Form C.20 in Appendix C for a blank version of the problem-solving form.) This example of a wife who is frustrated by warm orange juice may be described as follows:

PROBLEM-SOLVING EXAMPLE

S: Stop, Slow Down, and See the Problem
- Is there a problem?
- What exactly is the problem?

    Husband left OJ out 3 days in a row. Wife wanted some for breakfast, but

    she likes it cold, and now it is warm.

O: Outline Options
- Brainstorm: What can I do?
- What might work?

    1. Put ice in the glass and not tell husband that you were upset.

    2. Ask husband to put the OJ away from now on.

L: Look at Consequences
- What are the positive and negative consequences in the short run and long term?
- What will happen if I do each of the options?

    1. Husband will keep leaving OJ out. Wife may get too angry, end up yelling.

    2. Husband would know wife likes the OJ cold. He can change his behavior.

V: Vote
- Evaluate consequences and eliminate bad choices.
- Which solutions have the most positive and least negative consequences?

- *The second option seems better because it would bring positive results and*

    display effective communication.

E: Evaluate
- How did it work?
- Did my choice solve the problem?

    Husband now puts OJ away so wife feels satisfied. Also, wife is proud she

    used effective communication by letting husband know how she was feeling.

FIGURE 7.8. Sample problem-solving example.

"It's Saturday morning and you get up to find the OJ left out on the kitchen counter. This happens a lot. In fact, it's the third day in a row that your husband has left the OJ out. You wanted some for breakfast but like to drink it cold, and now it's warm."

Second, work with the couple on one of their own personal problem situations, allowing them to take more active roles in the exercise. Each partner may have a number of ideas to use for this task. Try to begin with a problem that is not too emotionally charged. This way, the partners can concentrate on how each step works rather than the emotional undercurrent. Work through the process one step at a time using the S.O.L.V.E. problem-solving model (see Figure 7.7 above), writing the process out on an easel board or sheet of paper. Your job is to keep the problem-solving process focused. Complete one step before moving on to the next. Give feedback and encourage the partners to use their communication skills as part of the problem-solving process.

Finally, partners should choose a problem to practice at home using S.O.L.V.E. In planning this home practice, it helps to choose a problem that is behavior-specific and not attributed to a personality factor. It is best to pick a recent stressor. Both partners should agree on the problem situation to be addressed. Avoid complex or emotionally charged topics when couples first practice problem solving at home on their own. Make sure the situation is not a combination of several problems. If it is, however, you can help the couple break it down and problem-solve one aspect at a time. They should set aside at least 30 minutes with no distractions to concentrate solely on this problem-solving task. Have the couples use a blank Problem-Solving Practice sheet (see Form C.20 in Appendix C) to make notes about the process. The couple should bring this worksheet to the next session for discussion. Once the couple understands the basic steps in problem solving, the therapist can spend many BCT sessions coaching the couple to use the S.O.L.V.E. process to find solutions to more difficult problems. The following case example illustrates this process.

Case Example

The case of Doug and Ginny illustrates a typical use of the problem-solving process to deal with a serious problem faced by a couple in BCT. Doug was a 38-year-old self-employed carpenter with a serious alcoholism and cocaine problem. He started BCT after undergoing his third detox program in 4 years when Ginny said that he could not return home unless he had a structured plan to help him stay abstinent after he left the detox program. After 7 weeks of BCT sessions, Doug was attending AA three times a week, had asked someone to be his sponsor, and was still abstinent. The BCT therapist had introduced the S.O.L.V.E. problem-solving method and the couple seemed to understand it.

At session 8, the couple reviewed with the therapist a list of problem areas in their relationship they had completed for homework. Both Doug and Ginny had listed financial problems as their most serious issue, and both said they wanted to work on these problems. Doug had worked less and earned less as his drinking and drug use progressed. Ginny had paid their daily living expenses from her job and by borrowing from her parents and from credit cards. They had not filed their income tax returns for the past 2 years, and they owed over $2,000 in back taxes from 3 years ago. As they discussed these problems, both became visibly tense and anxious. At one point Doug said he couldn't talk about the income tax problem any more; he knew people who had lost their home when the government forced the sale of their house to collect an unpaid tax debt. Talking about the taxes made him too nervous. He knew ignoring the problem would only make it worse, but he said he had no idea what to do about it. Just thinking about it left him feeling overwhelmed and guilty because his drinking had caused the financial problems. Ginny was more inclined to try to figure out a solution. The therapist suggested that they *not* discuss their financial problems in the coming week and that they plan to continue the discussion at their BCT session the following week.

At session 9, they reported not discussing their financial problems with each other, as agreed. Doug said he had thought about the tax problem during the week, nevertheless, and become upset. He was afraid he might drink over it, so he had talked about it with his sponsor. His sponsor reminded Doug that he had just celebrated 90 days of sobriety and overcome a number of problems in order to achieve this goal. The sponsor suggested that it might be better to try to deal with the problem. Doug said he was willing to start the problem-solving process, even though he was not sure he was ready to take any action steps. Ginny was fine with this approach, so the couple spent most of this session and part of the next outlining the following options, looking at the consequences of each, and ranking them in order of which option to try first.

1. Contact accountant who had done their taxes before they got behind and ask for advice.
2. Set up a payment plan with the government to pay the taxes they owed, like they had done once before.
3. Doug get a job on the weekend at a building supply store to earn money to pay taxes.
4. Ginny request overtime work on her job to earn money to pay taxes.
5. Ask Ginny's parents for a loan to pay their tax bill.
6. Wait until they caught up on their other bills and then tackle the tax problem.
7. Wait until the government contacted them about the unpaid taxes and unfiled returns.

Doug agreed to call the accountant but reported at the next session that he had forgotten to do so. The therapist coached Doug to call the accountant during the BCT session, and they set an appointment for the couple to meet with the accountant for advice.

With the accountant's help, and with continued coaching at BCT sessions, Doug and Ginny actually used the first four solutions to their problem. When Doug and Ginny met with the therapist for a follow-up appointment 2 years later, they reported that their payment plan for back taxes was almost finished. Doug also proudly reported that his continued sobriety had resulted in steady employment and that he was paying his taxes and filing his tax returns on time and no longer getting behind.

FREQUENTLY ASKED QUESTIONS

• *Question 1*: Each advanced communication skill described in this chapter—negotiating agreements for desired changes, conflict resolution, and problem solving—seems complex in its own right. Dealing with all these skills seems like it could be overwhelming for the couple and the counselor. Do you ever skip anything or not cover it in depth?

• *Answer*: Most couples benefit from all three advanced communication skill modules. However, depending on the couple's needs, you may wish to emphasize certain modules more than others. For example, moderate- and high-conflict couples may need more time spent on conflict resolution than would low-conflict couples. Couples struggling with many external problems may benefit from more time on the problem-solving module. Similarly, partners who have many desired changes to ask from each other may need more time spent on negotiating agreements for change.

- *Question 2*: In Chapter 4 you talked about the therapist helping the couple address stressful life problems in early BCT sessions to prevent early relapse. How is the later training in problem-solving skills in this chapter different from what you described earlier?
- *Answer*: Although early and later efforts both try to solve problems, they differ on the types of problems addressed and the methods used. Early BCT sessions deal with problems where some improvement can be made fairly quickly. Early on, the goal is just to resolve the problem, and the therapist often does much of the work coming up with possible solutions and intervening with people in the patient's environment. Later problem-solving efforts often address problems that are not amenable to quick action or solution. Such problems may be part of entrenched couple conflicts and disagreements, may have become chronic life patterns, or be complex in nature. In later problem-solving efforts, the therapist is active in suggesting and evaluating solutions but also tries to teach the couple a method they can use to solve their own problems.

- *Question 3*: Couples often ask why implementing these skills is such a slow and artificial process. They don't want to do the assignments because they find them boring and unnatural. A common couple question might be: "People really don't talk this way or argue this way. How can this way of talking really help me?"
- *Answer*: It is true that couples do not typically talk or argue this way. However, when a couple has struggled with problems in their relationship and has been unable to resolve them due to inadequate communication, then trying something new may help. Studies show that learning negotiating and problem-solving skills can help unhappy couples get along better and resolve many of their problems.[5] Also, studies show that couples who are taught these skills before they get married or in their early years together have happier relationships 5 years later and less chance of splitting up.[6] It also is true that, at first, using these skills seems unnatural and boring, slow and artificial. The bottom line is, partners have to put up with the drudgery to get the benefit of better communication and working out their problems. As they begin to apply the skills successfully to their relationship, they will be better able to judge whether the initial drudgery was worth the effort.

SUMMARY

- The last chapter covered basic communication skills of effective listening and speaking. This chapter presents more advanced communication skills of negotiating agreements for desired changes, conflict resolution, and problem solving.
- Most people have things they want their partner to change, but asking for and negotiating for change is difficult in almost any relationship. BCT teaches partners how to effectively express what they want from the relationship and successfully negotiate agreements that will bring positive changes. When partners are specific and reasonable in their requests and are

able to compromise, they can successfully come to agreements to initiate changes that benefit both of them.

- BCT helps couples develop better skills for managing and resolving conflicts. It explores how each partner currently copes with relationship conflict and educates partners on different responses to conflict, including verbal aggression, physical aggression, flooding, and verbal reasoning (the desired method). It teaches the couple methods for successfully working through conflicts, including use of a time-out to prevent anger from escalating.

- The S.O.L.V.E. problem-solving method gives couples a basic tool they can use to work out a variety of problems. It involves (1) seeing that a problem exists, (2) outlining options to solve the problem, (3) looking at the short- and long-term consequences of each option, (4) voting on the best option, and (5) evaluating the results of putting the best choice into action.

- Most couples benefit from all three advanced communication modules, but a couple's needs may suggest spending more time on one module than the others.

- At first couples find using these skills slow and artificial. However, studies show that learning these communication skills helps unhappy couples get along better and resolve problems. The bottom line: Couples have to put up with the drudgery to get the benefits.

NOTES

1. The concept of a "good-faith" couple agreement was taken from an article on this topic by Weiss, Birchler, and Vincent (1974) in the early days of using behavioral contracts as part of couples counseling. They encouraged each partner to make his or her change independent of whether or not the spouse keeps the agreement and without monetary or other rewards or punishments.

2. This dialogue of a therapist coaching a couple to make an agreement is taken almost verbatim from *Handbook of marital therapy: A positive approach to helping troubled relationships* (pp. 160–162), by R. P. Liberman, E. G. Wheeler, L. A. DeVisser, J. Keuhnel, and T. Keuhnel, 1980, New York: Plenum Press. Copyright 1980 by Plenum Press. Used with permission.

3. Material presented in this section on conflict was drawn from articles on (1) the Response to Conflict Scale (Birchler & Fals-Stewart, 1994), (2) the Conflict Tactics Scale (Straus, 1979, 1990; Straus, Hamby, Boney-McCoy, & Sugarman, 1996), and (3) partner violence in couple relationships of male and female substance-abusing patients (e.g., Chase, O'Farrell, Murphy, Fals-Stewart, & Murphy, 2003; O'Farrell & Murphy, 2002; O'Farrell, Murphy, Stephan, Fals-Stewart, & Murphy, 2004).

4. Chase et al. (2003); O'Farrell, Murphy, et al. (2004).

5. Shadish and Baldwin (2005).

6. Markman, Renick, Floyd, Stanley, and Clements (1993).

8

Continuing Recovery
Maintenance and Relapse Prevention

Most couples who attend BCT sessions faithfully experience a period of stable abstinence and get along better. BCT provides a supportive structure and encourages couples to engage in many actions that support recovery for the substance abuser and for the relationship. However, when the structure of the weekly BCT sessions ends, there is a natural tendency for backsliding. Many couples stop or decrease activities that supported recovery and find themselves vulnerable to relapse. It is critical to help couples maintain the gains they made in BCT and prevent or minimize relapse.

You need to plan for maintenance and relapse prevention before weekly BCT sessions end. As described in Table 1.7 in Chapter 1, planning for continuing recovery typically occurs in the last three weekly BCT sessions. This means you have to decide when a couple is ready to end weekly BCT sessions. Most couples are ready to stop weekly sessions after 3–6 months of consecutive abstinence and clear progress on their relationship problems have been achieved. Of course, this is an ideal that often is not attained. Many couples have to stop weekly BCT before reaching these clinically desirable milestones due to session limits dictated by health insurance or by a research study protocol. This need to stop weekly sessions prematurely in some cases is another reason to plan maintenance carefully and to reduce sessions gradually, rather than abruptly, as described in more detail below.

Once you have determined that weekly BCT sessions will be ending soon, start helping the couple prepare for this change. First, help the couple complete a Continuing Recovery Plan that specifies which aspects of BCT (e.g., trust discussion) they wish to continue. Second, anticipate high-risk situations for relapse and make an action plan to prevent or minimize relapse when faced with such situations. Third, continued contact for couple "checkup" visits every few months can encourage continued progress. Fourth, couples with more severe problems may benefit from attending 15 couple relapse prevention sessions in the year after weekly BCT ends. Finally, in the years after BCT, couples may need help with relationship issues in long-term recovery. Table 8.1 lists these BCT maintenance and relapse prevention interventions, which are described in this chapter.[1]

161

TABLE 8.1. Maintenance and Relapse Prevention

- Continuing Recovery Plan
- Action plan to prevent or minimize relapse
- Couple checkup visits for continuing contact
- Couple relapse prevention sessions
- Couple and family issues in long-term recovery

CONTINUING RECOVERY PLAN

Overview of Continuing Recovery Plan

It is important to plan for continuing recovery before weekly BCT sessions end. A good time to start is when there are two or three weekly BCT sessions remaining. The first step involves helping the couple complete a Continuing Recovery Plan. This plan specifies the activities partners agree to do to maintain abstinence and relationship recovery after the weekly couple sessions end. The couple chooses which behaviors from previous BCT sessions they wish to continue (e.g., daily trust discussion, communication sessions).

Table 8.2 provides the therapist checklist for introducing the Continuing Recovery Plan (from the checklist for session 10 of the 12-session BCT manual contained in Appendix A). Next we describe how the counselor completes each of these steps.

Ask the couple which interventions or behavior changes accomplished during BCT they found most helpful and might wish to continue. This is a good opportunity to focus on the many positive changes the couple has made and to compliment them on their hard work to make their lives together better. Figure 8.1 provides a Sample Continuing Recovery Plan (a copy of which is Poster B.24 in Appendix B). Review the sample plan displayed as a poster to familiarize them with the idea. Then consider each part of the BCT sessions they have completed and help them decide which they want to continue. Move slowly through each category of the plan and allow time for partners to record the items that are of particular importance to them on their own blank Continuing Recovery Plan (a copy of which is Form C.23 in Appendix C). Help the couple work together to make a plan that is specific, reasonable, and realistic. Remind the couple to be honest and realistic about how often (e.g., daily, weekly, monthly) they plan to do each activity. Begin discussing the Continuing Recovery Plan during a BCT session and have the couple discuss it further at home. Review and refine the plan at the next couple ses-

TABLE 8.2. Therapist Checklist for Introducing Continuing Recovery Plan

____ Show *Sample Continuing Recovery Plan Poster B.24* from Appendix B.

____ Review sample Continuing Recovery Plan to maintain abstinence and help relationship after weekly BCT ends.

____ Review non-substance-abusing partner's role in the continuing recovery plan.

____ Hand out *My Continuing Recovery Plan Form C.23* from Appendix C.

____ Conduct in-session practice in which couple completes a Continuing Recovery Plan.

____ Assign home practice: Discuss and refine Continuing Recovery Plan made in session.

SAMPLE CONTINUING RECOVERY PLAN

As part of my Continuing Recovery, I have checked the tools, activities, and skills I will practice and use to maintain sobriety and to continue to improve my relationship after weekly couples therapy ends.

1. Recovery Contract:

    _X_   Trust Discussion (daily)

    _X_   Take medication (_Antabuse_   ) during Trust Discussion

    _X_   Regular support meetings

        Tuesday 7 p.m. AA meeting—church

        Friday 8 p.m. AA meeting—church

        Saturday 9 a.m. NA meeting—treatment center

2. Positive Activities:

    ____   Catch and Tell

    _X_   Shared Rewarding Activities (_1_   ×/week)

    ____   Caring Day (____ ×/week)

3. Communication Skills:

    _X_   Communication Sessions (_1_   ×/week)

    ____   Listening and Understanding

    ____   "I" Messages

    _X_   Relationship Agreements (_review bills together weekly_   )

    ____   Problem Solving

    ____   Time-Out

4. Continuing Recovery Tools:

    _X_   Continuing Recovery Plan

    _X_   Action Plan to prevent or minimize relapse

    _X_   Couple checkup visits (every 2 months for 2 years)

    ____   Couple relapse prevention sessions (15 sessions in next year)

5. Other: _I will read from the Big Book before bed and go to gym 3x/wk._

We will focus on present and future and avoid arguments about past.

6. Partner's Role (completed by partner): _I will_

   a. Practice above skills with my partner to help our relationship.

   b. Take care of the kids on nights my partner goes to meetings.

   c. Go to Al-Anon 1x/wk on Monday 8 p.m. at church.

FIGURE 8.1. Sample continuing recovery plan.

sion, making any changes or additions needed. Finalize the plan no later than the last weekly BCT session.

Steps in Formulating Continuing Recovery Plan

First, discuss recovery tools directly related to maintaining abstinence. Generally, we encourage couples to continue the Recovery Contract that has been working for them for at least another 6 months and often longer. So if they have been doing a daily trust discussion with Antabuse taking during BCT, we generally suggest they continue this routine. Similarly, if AA or Al-Anon has been part of their recovery plan during BCT, we encourage them to continue these activities on a regular basis.

Second, discuss which aspects of positive couple activities and communication skills they would like to continue. Couples often choose to continue shared rewarding activities and communication sessions. Some couples also choose to continue specific relationship agreements that they made in BCT. For example, partners may decide to continue agreements about how to deal with their finances or their children.

Third, discuss the continuing recovery tools they plan to use. These tools include this Continuing Recovery Plan and an action plan to prevent or minimize relapse, as described below. It also may include periodic contacts for regular checkups or for systematic couples relapse prevention sessions, both described below.

Fourth, ask if there are any other rituals or routines they have found to be helpful and might want to continue. These could be related to substance abuse recovery or self-care. Examples include reading the Big Book or other 12-step or related inspirational literature, listening to relaxation tapes, practicing meditation, participating in regular exercise, and talking with one's sponsor in depth at least weekly. Examples of specific relationship recovery rituals or activities include going to church together, going out to breakfast on Saturdays, a sit-down family dinner with no TV or other distractions at least twice weekly, and saying "I love you" when leaving in the morning. Some couples may choose to continue one or more of the promises for relationship recovery (i.e., focus on present and future, don't argue about the past; don't threaten breaking up impulsively in anger; no violence or threats of violence).

Finally, ask what role the non-substance-abusing partner will take in the Continuing Recovery Plan. Discuss how this partner plans to support the substance abuser in his or her recovery. Much of the partner's support will come from taking part in the recovery and relationship tools already chosen for the Continuing Recovery Plan. Some partners will choose additional supportive activities, such as caring for the kids when the substance abuser goes to a 12-step meeting. Also consider what the non-substance-abusing partner will do for self-care: for example, attending Al-Anon meetings, engaging in regular exercise, planning time just for oneself, and so forth.

Case Example

The case of Gerard and Cathy illustrates the process of creating a Continuing Recovery Plan. In their early 40s, they had been together for 12 years. Gerard's severe alcoholism and cocaine problem had led to two arrests, a job loss, and a 9-month separation in the year before they started BCT to give their relationship one last try. They faithfully came to BCT sessions and did most of the recommended activities in BCT, despite many struggles and difficulties. A few weeks before weekly sessions were scheduled to end, they reviewed their experience in BCT. After careful discussion of each element on the Continuing Recovery Plan sheet, Gerard and Cathy said they wanted to continue four activities that had been particularly helpful.

The first was the Recovery Contract that had helped Gerard to stay sober and Cathy to reinvest in the relationship. Continuing the daily trust discussion and daily Antabuse taking for another 6 months was something both of them decided to do to prevent relapse. Gerard also decided to continue attending AA meetings at least three times a week for the next 6 months. The second was planning weekly enjoyable activities together, including going to the movies, watching television or a video together at home, going for walks, and eating out. The third was to hold communication sessions at least weekly because during BCT they had started talking more and they wanted to continue this practice. They also wanted to continue their weekly discussions about finances, an agreement they had negotiated during BCT. Finally, they wished to maintain a focus on the present and future. Both agreed that after many years together, it was all too easy to destroy their hopes for happiness now by dwelling on the hurts and disappointments of the past.

Cathy planned to take care of the kids when Gerard went to his AA meetings. She also resolved to continue her own weekly Al-Anon meeting and to take a lunchtime walk at work to reduce stress. They also decided to schedule checkup visits with the BCT counselor every 2 months for the next 2 years. A major goal of the checkup visits (see below) was to help them stick with their Continuing Recovery Plan. Figure 8.1 displays the Continuing Recovery Plan formulated by Gerard and Cathy. (See Poster B.24 in Appendix B for this sample plan and Form C.23 in Appendix C for a blank version of the plan form.)

ACTION PLAN TO PREVENT OR MINIMIZE RELAPSE

Next help the couple anticipate high-risk situations for relapse and make an action plan to prevent or minimize relapse when faced with such situations. The action plan has three parts, as described in Table 8.3. The first is to provide a framework for talking about relapse. The second is to identify high-risk situations and early warning signs for relapse. The third is the action plan itself for how to prevent drinking and drug use and how to minimize the length and negative effects of any substance use that occurs.

Table 8.4 provides the therapist checklist for introducing the action plan (from the checklist for session 11 of the 12-session BCT manual contained in Appendix A). Next we describe how the counselor completes each of these steps.

TABLE 8.3. Action Plan to Prevent or Minimize Relapse

- Give framework for discussing relapse.
  - Fire drill analogy.
  - Continuing recovery process.
- Identify high-risk situations and early warning signs.
- Formulate and rehearse plan to
  - Prevent relapse.
  - Minimize length and negative effects of substance use, if it occurs.

TABLE 8.4. Therapist Checklist for Introducing the Action Plan

____ Use fire drill analogy to introduce action plan to prevent or minimize relapse.

____ Help couple identify high-risk situations and warning signs likely in next few months and decide plan of action to deal with them.

____ Show *Sample Action Plan Poster B.25* from Appendix B.

____ Hand out *My Action Plan Form C.25* from Appendix C.

____ Help couple decide plan of action if substance use occurs.

____ Show *Sample Partner's Action Plan Poster B.26* from Appendix B.

____ Hand out *Partner's Action Plan Form C.26* from Appendix C.

____ Review partner's role in action plan (includes safety plan to avoid violence).

____ Assign home practice: Discuss and refine action plan made in session.

Provide a Framework for Talking about Relapse

FIRE DRILL ANALOGY

Providing a framework for talking about relapse is very important because many couples find such discussions upsetting. Often, couples worry that talking about relapse means that relapse is inevitable. Others may think that such talk subtly gives permission for drinking or drug use. This is particularly the case when discussion turns to what to do to minimize drinking after the first drink has been taken. Marlatt and Gordon's[2] fire drill analogy can provide a reassuring framework for discussing relapse. Taking steps to prevent a fire (e.g., removing oily rags or old paint cans stored near the furnace) does not mean that a fire is inevitable. Having a fire drill to practice what to do in case of fire is designed to save lives by being prepared for quick action. Once a fire has started, the goal is to put out the fire as quickly as possible to minimize damage. None of these aspects of fire prevention and fire safety implies that fires are inevitable or in any way desirable. In fact, just the opposite is the case. The fire drill analogy makes sense to most couples and helps them start discussing what to do to prevent or minimize lapses and relapses.

CONTINUING RECOVERY PROCESS

Discuss the process of continuing recovery with a focus on the couple's strengths and what has been learned in BCT. We assume that everyone has strengths, stressors, and problems in their lives that will most likely continue well into the process of recovery. This focus helps couples recognize that they have skills and strengths to draw upon when facing the inevitable challenges of substance abuse and relationship recovery. Explain the process of continuing recovery. Let the couple give their input and ask questions. You might begin like this:

"Nobody plans to relapse, but we know it does happen. It helps to look at relapse as a process. It is something that occurs over time, not as an isolated event. Relapse is possible no matter how long you have been in recovery.

"You are in a different place now than when you were actively using or just starting counseling. We are confident that the skills you have learned will better equip you to handle the stress that comes with everyday living. You made a Continuing Recovery Plan of skills, tools, and strengths you intend to use in your process of recovery.

"High-risk situations do not have to lead to relapse. At any point in the process, you can use your strengths and skills to maintain a drug- and alcohol-free lifestyle. Next we will make an action plan that will help you anticipate things that may put you at risk for relapse and devise a plan to help prepare you."

As you describe the continuing recovery process, stress each of the following points:

1. *The partners are in a different place now than before their recovery process began.* Help each member of the couple recognize gains and improvements he or she has made during BCT. The goal is to enhance their confidence and help them feel more empowered as they face the challenges of continuing recovery.

2. *There are differences between a lapse and a relapse.* Marlatt and Gordon[2] introduced the distinction between a lapse and a relapse. A "lapse" refers to the singular occurrence or act of substance use following a period of abstinence; a "slip" is another word for a lapse. The concept of a lapse or a slip is meant to help those in recovery realize that if they have one drink or one substance-using episode, it does not mean that they "blew it." They do not have to return to heavy, regular substance use. Rather, they can view the lapse as a mistake or an ineffective coping response, get back on track, and return to abstinence immediately.

A relapse is the "full return to the former behavior"[3] after a period of improvement. For many substance abusers, the term "relapse" indicates that the person has returned to substance abuse, has "blown it," and is doomed to continue substance abuse. With this thinking, the substance abuser often decides that because he or she have already "blown it," they might as well keep using, thus reverting back to the former state of substance abuse.

3. *The relapse process can be interrupted at any point and coping strategies implemented to get back on track.* Most substance abusers and their partners initially interpret a lapse as permission to use substances every so often. As long as things are not too bad, no one wants to make waves. On the other hand, to many a relapse means that all is lost and there is no hope for complete abstinence. Couples need to understand that recovery can resume at any point—and the sooner the better, before too much damage has been done.

4. *Steps can be taken to increase the chance of resisting relapse.* A person's thoughts and feelings play a big part in his or her ability to avoid or cope with high-risk situations. An individual needs to recognize warning signs such as feeling angry or thinking that one drink won't hurt anything. Then he or she can use coping skills to avoid entering into a high-risk situation and thereby avoid using substances.

5. *It is important to develop a plan ahead of time.* If a person can identify high-risk situations and plan how to avoid them, chances of staying substance free are greater. If a person has a plan for what to do if he or she uses, there is less risk that a lapse will turn into a relapse. It is better to have a plan and not have to use it, than not to have a plan and need it.

Anticipate High-Risk Situations and Warning Signs of Relapse

After establishing a framework for discussing relapse, the next step is to help the couple identify high-risk situations and warning signs of relapse. To begin this process, explain the concepts of *high-risk situations* and *early warning signs* to the couple.

HIGH-RISK SITUATIONS

Explain that high-risk situations can include any people, places, moods, and physical or psychological signs that are possible triggers to a lapse or relapse. A high-risk situation influences a person's thoughts and feelings to make it more likely that he or she will drink or use drugs. A high-risk situation might involve driving by an old neighborhood where the person formerly used drugs. Another example would be stopping by the bar in which the person used to "hang out" to "just get a soda." Other examples include having an argument with the partner or attending a friend's wedding. These situations are high risk because alcohol or drugs are easily available or may be an escape from the pain and frustration of an argument.

WARNING SIGNS FOR RELAPSE

Explain that warning signs can be related to a change in a person's behavior, attitudes, feelings, thoughts, or any combination. These warning signs do not necessarily mean that the person is going to use. However, they can alert a person to changes he or she is experiencing that may eventually lead to use. The following examples of each type of warning sign help couples think of things that apply to their own situation:

1. *Behavior changes*—include behaviors such as skipping self-help meetings, smoking or eating more in response to feeling stressed, or stopping in a bar to have a soda.
2. *Attitude changes*—include slipping into a negative attitude or not caring about recovery any more.
3. *Changes in feelings or moods*—include strong feelings such as anger, depression, frustration, or sudden feelings of euphoria.
4. *Changes in thoughts*—include thinking about using alcohol or drugs, thinking that one drink won't hurt, or remembering only the fun times connected with using.

Formulate the Action Plan

Finally, help the couple formulate their action plan. This plan has two parts. The first part involves planned actions in response to risky situations and warning signs to prevent substance use. The second part involves planned actions to minimize negative effects if use occurs. There are separate action plans for the substance abuser and for the partner. However, both members of the couple take part in making each plan, and both agree to the final plans made. Figure 8.2 presents a sample action plan for the substance abuser (a copy of which is Poster B.25 in Appendix B). Figure 8.3 presents a sample action plan for the partner (a copy of which is Poster B.26 in Appendix B). Review the sample plans displayed as posters to familiarize partners with the idea. Then move slowly through each category of each plan and have each person complete their own blank action plan forms (copies of which are in Appendix C; see Form C.25 for the substance abuser and Form C.26 for the partner).

ACTION PLAN FOR HIGH-RISK SITUATIONS AND WARNING SIGNS

Have the couple list high-risk situations (triggers) they anticipate facing in the next 6 months. Reviewing events that led to relapse in the past and incidents linked to strong urges during

SAMPLE ACTION PLAN

1. High-Risk Situations and My Plan of Action:

High-Risk Situation	Action
Court date	Attend a meeting before and after court.
Pay day	Arrange for direct deposit or have my partner deposit my check.
Family wedding	Remind friends and family I can't drink or use drugs (even "just this once").

2. Warning Signs and My Plan of Action:

Warning Signs	Action
Sleeping too much	Get back on regular schedule by attending morning meetings.
Thinking one drink won't hurt	Remember that my last relapse started this way. Call my sponsor.

3. Action Plan If Use Occurs:

Goal	Action
Stay Safe →	I will try not to argue with Nancy if I am under the influence.
Act Quickly →	I will call someone within 48 hours if I drink or use.
Get Help →	I will call my AA sponsor or Sally, my BCT counselor.

4. Support Network—If I Feel an Urge or Have a Lapse, I Will Call:

Name	Phone #	Other Phone #
My sponsor	555-1234	555-2468 (cell)
Sally (my BCT counselor	555-4321	
AA local central office	853-0388	

5. Other Helpful Activities: _Go for a ride in the country._
Ride my bike or take a walk when I feel stressed out.

FIGURE 8.2. Sample action plan.

SAMPLE PARTNER'S ACTION PLAN

1. Warning Signs:

Partner isolates.
Partner starts losing his temper a lot.

2. Action I Will Take If I Notice Warning Signs:

Ask to go to a meeting with my partner.
Ask for a Communication Session with my partner to tell him my concerns.
Plan a Shared Rewarding Activity to reduce stress.

3. Action Plan If Use Occurs:

Goal	Action
Stay Safe →	*I will avoid getting into an argument if my partner comes home drunk. If an argument starts, I will leave the house. I can go to my sister's house until it is safe to return home. I will not confront my partner about his use while he is drunk or high.*
Act Quickly →	*I will wait no more than 48 hours to call someone if he drinks.*
Get Help →	*I will call Sally, my BCT counselor, or my Al-Anon sponsor.*

4. Support Network:

Name	Phone #	Other Phone #
My sponsor	*555-1234*	*555-2468 (cell)*
Sally (my BCT counselor)	*555-4321*	
Al-Anon	*567-8342*	

FIGURE 8.3. Sample partner action plan.

BCT may help partners generate a useful list. Work with the couple to come up with a reasonable and realistic plan to cope with these situations. It can help to give an example such as the following:

> *High-risk situation*: Court date to determine if I will go to jail for barroom assault charge.
> *Plan of action*: Attend a self-help meeting before and after court; ask my sister to come with me to court.

Next, have partners write down the plan of action for each situation. When possible, the safest plan is to avoid the situation (e.g., stay away from people and places where substance abuser used to buy drugs). When the person cannot avoid the situation, then a planned coping response may be needed (e.g., drink club soda and stay with partner at a job-required social function).

Consider warning signs of relapse and repeat this process with the couple. Ask them to write down warning signs that led to use in the past and ones they think may lead to use in the future. Suggest that they think in terms of changes in behavior, attitude, moods, and thoughts. Typical examples include angry outbursts, spending more time alone, and thinking that one drink won't hurt. Next, have them write down specific ways each of them can try to prevent relapse if they notice the warning signs. For the substance abuser, prevention actions might include calling his or her sponsor, recalling problems caused by prior relapses, going to a meeting, or having a communication session with the partner. There is a separate action plan for the non-substance-abusing partner for a number of reasons. The partner often notices changes in the substance abuser's behavior before the substance abuser does, leading to quicker action to prevent relapse. The partner, having noticed a warning sign, might call the substance abuser's sponsor, talk with the partner about the changes noticed, ask if the partner would like to go to a meeting, or attend his or her own support meeting. Be careful that planned actions by the spouse to deal with perceived danger signs and fears do not produce couple interactions (e.g., nagging, accusing) that can unwittingly lead to relapse.

ACTION PLAN IF USE OCCURS

In the second part of the action plan, the partners decide what each of them will do to deal with any drinking or drug use that might occur. The goal is to minimize the length and negative consequences of the use episode. We give couples three guidelines for their plan: (1) stay safe, (2) act quickly, and (3) get help.

The suggestion to *stay safe* refers to the risk of conflict and violence in couples when the substance abuser drinks or uses drugs. It is only natural that the partner becomes angry if the substance abuser drinks or uses drugs. However, arguing with an intoxicated person can lead to conflict and, possibly, violence. Therefore, we encourage all couples to plan to avoid arguing when the substance abuser is under the influence of alcohol or drugs. The spouse specifically agrees not to confront the substance abuser when the substance abuser is intoxicated or hungover. If an argument does erupt or if the spouse becomes afraid of what might happen, usually the plan is for the spouse to leave and stay with a friend or relative until the situation improves. This discussion needs to be treated delicately. Pose these suggestions as a way to keep both members of the couple safe and free from unwanted conflict that they could regret later.

The suggestion to *act quickly* refers to the need to intervene early, at the beginning of a relapse episode. Often substance abusers and their partners wait until the drinking or drug use has reached dangerous levels again before acting. By then, additional damage may have been done. A typical scenario is that the substance abuser drinks or uses drugs on one occasion and then not again for a few days or a few weeks. The spouse may feel that "it isn't too bad yet" or think "I'm waiting to see what happens. He knows I don't want him to drink." Meanwhile the substance abuser is feeling that he or she can handle drinking or using drugs because it has not gotten out of hand so far, and the spouse doesn't seem too upset. Before long, the substance use has grown more frequent and more intense, with imminent or actual problems. The fire analogy may make this point more vivid to couples. You might say something like the following:

> "We've been talking about how you need to act quickly if use occurs. Consider again how a relapse is like a fire. A small fire gets bigger if it is not put out. Counting on a fire to burn itself out is risky. The fire may just keep on raging, gaining strength as it goes along. Or it may burn itself out but only after destroying what was in its path. So unless you want to wind up back where you started, it is better to nip a relapse in the bud. Getting substance use stopped quickly should be a top priority."

The suggestion to *get help* refers to how difficult it can be for a person to think clearly and act sensibly when faced with substance use, especially after he or she has worked hard to stay abstinent. Talking to someone else who is more objective and not immediately affected can help. Calling a sponsor or the BCT counselor is the most common action plan that couples choose for getting help. It is very important that both members agree on this plan in advance so that the spouse feels that he or she has the substance abuser's permission to call someone for help. It can reduce the feeling that such a call is an act of disloyalty, a betrayal of sharing their problems with an outsider.

SUPPORT NETWORK AND OTHER ACTIVITIES

For the last parts of the action plan, ask each partner to make a list of persons whom he or she could call to support the decision to be drug and alcohol free. This list could include sponsors, group members, the BCT counselor, or supportive friends or family. When faced with a high-risk situation or urges to use, a good coping method is to call someone for support. This person should be someone who can be called in an emergency and who can listen well and steadfastly encourage abstinence. Finally, ask partners to make a list of other activities that have helped in the past to deal with urges and cravings or with relationship stress or other problems. Examples might include listening to relaxing music, taking a hot bath, going for a walk, going to the gym, or jogging. A handout on helpful hints for continuing recovery is given out and reviewed at this time. Figure 8.4 presents this handout (a copy of which is Form C.22 in Appendix C).

A COUPLE'S PERSPECTIVE ON THE ABSTINENCE VIOLATION EFFECT

You also need to prepare the couple for how to deal with possible negative emotional reactions if the patient uses. Marlatt described the *abstinence violation effect* (AVE) in which any substance use is viewed by the substance abuser as complete failure, paving the way for a full

CONTINUING RECOVERY HELPFUL HINTS

☞ Continuing recovery is a process. It can change. You can change. You can add ideas as you learn and grow.

☞ You are in a different place now. You bring with you new skills and experiences to deal with high-risk situations.

☞ Reach out and call someone from your support network. Plan to deal with any effects of the lapse.

☞ Remember to do your regular daily inventory to check for high-risk factors.

☞ Be alert for high-risk factors and plan to take action to reverse the effects.

☞ Make a commitment to be active in your recovery.

☞ A lapse or relapse tells you that there is a hole in your Continuing Recovery Plan. Go back and check it out. Add to it. Make it more specific.

☞ A lapse can be part of the learning process. Learn more about your high-risk factors. Decide what coping skills you will use next time to cope without using.

☞ When you can, avoid a particular high-risk factor, and if not, use one of your coping strategies.

☞ Don't just plan—act. Do it. Try it.

☞ Your confidence will increase when you successfully cope with high-risk situations.

FIGURE 8.4. Handout on Continuing Recovery Helpful Hints.

relapse.[2] Spouses often experience their own version of an AVE. Many couples view taking part in BCT as their last hope. They feel that if they can get the drinking or drug use behind them, than their relationship and their lives, in general, would be far better. When the patient drinks or uses drugs during or after BCT, the spouse is extremely disappointed. Although such emotions are understandable, they can easily turn into a couple-based AVE. More specifically, without proper preparation or planning, spouses may view the lapse as a signal that the relationship is doomed and/or that their time and effort in BCT were wasted. Spouses often think that substance use means that the patient is not committed to the relationship and does not care about the spouse or family. This highly stressful couple dynamic around substance use creates further tension in the home, setting the stage for a progression to full relapse.

We also have observed a couple-based AVE of sorts when a couple experiences a major conflict without the patient using. Couples who take part in BCT often have the unrealistic expectation that once the patient achieves abstinence, the problems in the relationship will be largely or fully resolved. Often couples find out that some problems in their relationship are independent of the substance use. They may have ignored these problem while they were coping with the drinking or drug use. They also may find that problems caused by substance abuse (e.g., distrust, resentment, anger) have a life of their own even after the substance use has stopped. Major arguments can bring these issues to light and lead to significant disappointment. Conflicts can lead many couples to conclude that BCT failed and that the BCT activities designed to improve the relationship really didn't work. Again, without proper planning or preparation, couples can very quickly resort to negative relationship behaviors (e.g., poor communication, distancing) after a conflict.

So, how can AVEs be minimized? In BCT we tell couples that an AVE is a fairly common reaction to the patient's substance use or an intense argument by the couple. More importantly, as described above, we ask partners to make specific plans for what they will do if substance use or major arguments occur, including how to minimize and manage the negative thoughts and emotions of an AVE.

COUPLE CHECKUP VISITS FOR CONTINUING CONTACT

The partners have chosen a plan for continuing activities to promote recovery, and they have made an action plan of what they will do to prevent or minimize relapse. What can you do to help the couple stick with these plans when weekly BCT ends? Couple checkup visits for continued contact with you every few months can encourage continued progress.

Content, Reasons, and Schedule for Checkup Visits

We suggest continued contact with the couple for checkup visits at regular, and then gradually increasing, intervals. We recommend that you continue these contacts for 5 years after a stable pattern of recovery (i.e., 3–6 months abstinence) has been achieved. Use this ongoing contact to monitor progress and assess follow-through on the plans they made for continuing recovery. At each checkup visit, specifically review the Continuing Recovery Plan and the action plan they made at the end of weekly BCT sessions to see if they are using these plans and whether any changes need to be made. Provide ongoing support and problem solving for concerns that develop over time. Also evaluate if there is a need for additional therapy sessions to deal with new or unresolved problems. Staying in regular contact means that they are more likely to call you between planned checkups if they have a problem. However, you must take responsibility for scheduling and reminding the couple of follow-up sessions so that continued contact can be maintained successfully.

Explain the reason for continued contact over a long period. Substance abuse is a chronic health problem with a high rate of recurrence. It requires active, aggressive, ongoing monitoring to prevent or quickly treat relapses for 5 years or more after an initial stable pattern of recovery has been established. The follow-up contact also provides the opportunity to deal with couple and family issues that appear after a period of recovery (see below).

How often should checkup visits be scheduled? A typical schedule of checkup visits would be every 2–3 months for the first 2 years, then every 6 months for the next year, and yearly thereafter. Some couples initially need more frequent contacts after weekly BCT ends. Then gradually increase the time between contacts as you and the couple feel increasingly confident in their coping abilities. Such couples generally are those who have more severe problems or who have had trouble during the weekly BCT sessions. These couples may benefit from a planned, systematic schedule of 15 couple relapse prevention sessions in the year after weekly BCT, as described below. Table 8.5 summarizes the key points of couple checkup visits for continuing contact.

TABLE 8.5. Couple Check-up Visits

- Every 2–3 months for 2 years, then every 6 months, then yearly to 5-year follow-up.
- Start after 3–6 months abstinence.
- Counselor schedules and reminds couple.
- Couple can call for unscheduled meetings.
- Checkup visits help the counselor to:
  - Assess use of Continuing Recovery Plan.
  - Monitor couple's progress.
  - Provide ongoing support and problem solving.
  - Evaluate need for additional treatment.

Deciding How Much Help a Couple Needs

DIFFICULTY DECIDING IF A COUPLE IS "DOING ENOUGH"

Helping a substance-abusing individual and his or her partner decide how much help they need to sustain their recovery after weekly BCT ends can be difficult. In our experience, very often people could benefit from more tools and supports than they think they need. Logically, it might make sense to continue everything the couple has been doing during BCT because it has been working, and they will be stopping the weekly BCT that presumably is an important support. One could even argue that activities should be *added* to replace the support received from BCT, which is being withdrawn. However, frequently couples want to reduce, not increase, efforts to promote recovery. Couples frequently start BCT after a crisis, and their motivation to do whatever it takes is high. By the end of BCT, things usually have been going well for a while and the crisis has receded into the background, leading to reduced motivation to pursue multiple activities for recovery. Parenthetically, this tendency underscores the need to make a solid Recovery Contract with as many tools as possible in the early weeks of BCT because couples are very unlikely to add things later.

BASIS FOR RECOMMENDATIONS

When faced with these concerns, we generally recommend any additions to a couple's recovery plan that we think would be useful. This step involves a process of negotiation and education with the couple. We consider the balance between risk factors and coping factors in deciding what, if any, additional recovery tools to recommend.

Risk factors present challenges that must be addressed to maintain abstinence. Those who have more severe and more chronic substance abuse and relationship problems and more problems of other sorts (e.g., medical, psychiatric, job, financial, social) face higher risk factors. Similarly, those whose environments contain higher levels of ongoing stress and more frequent exposure to high-risk situations face higher risk factors. Coping factors constitute resources that can be used to deal with risk factors without relapsing. Those who have coped successfully with recent problems and plan to use more recovery tools after BCT have higher coping factors.

Couples facing more risk factors need more coping factors. For such couples, we are likely to recommend, as the end of weekly BCT draws near, that they reconsider tools they had rejected for their Continuing Recovery Plan. The following brief case examples show how this process works.

CASE EXAMPLES

First, consider *the case of John and Martha*. John was 45 years old with a very serious, long-term alcohol problem that had caused serious marital, job, and health problems. He was a physically dependent drinker who drank throughout the day, every day, in large quantities—between 1.5 to 2 pints of liquor daily. He sought help after his wife left him, he was fired from his job, and he had a withdrawal seizure. Once John sought help, his wife and his boss both agreed to give him "one last chance" to get sober. During BCT, their Recovery Contract included a daily trust discussion with Antabuse taking, which the couple implemented faithfully. John refused to go to AA, saying that he was "turned off" by its spiritual aspects. They took part in the positive, relationship-focused parts of BCT, but to a lesser degree. They were rather estranged due to many years of John's drinking and their 3-month separation before BCT. Also Martha held back from reconnecting with John because she feared he would go back to drinking after a few months, as he had done in the past. For their Continuing Recovery Plan after BCT, they agreed to continue the daily trust discussion and quarterly checkup visits. John wanted to stop the Antabuse; he did not think he needed it any more and said he would consider going back on it if he had a serious relapse. Martha was upset that John wanted to stop the Antabuse. Given their disagreement, they asked the counselor what she recommended.

In evaluating the proposed recovery plan, the counselor concluded that they had many risk factors, not the least of which was John's style of drinking. Once he began to drink, he drank heavily and within a few days was back to drinking to ward off withdrawal symptoms. He had never stopped drinking soon after restarting, while still at a low level. If he went back to daily heavy drinking, both his marriage and job were in serious jeopardy. In terms of coping factors, his coping level during BCT had been good; he had resisted urges to drink on a number of occasions. However, he usually had attributed his success to knowing he was on Antabuse and would get sick if he drank. In terms of planned recovery tools, John was stopping both BCT and Antabuse at the same time, with little to replace them. Coping factors did not seem strong enough, given the many risk factors. The counselor explained this perspective to John and Martha and recommended that John stay on Antabuse for 6 more months. The counselor also suggested they attend 15 relapse prevention sessions (see below) in the next year to deal with their continuing relationship issues. After lengthy discussion and "thinking it over" at home in the week before the last BCT session, John agreed to the recommended plan.

Second, consider *the case of Duane and Aretha*. It is interesting to note how the recovery plan recommended by the counselor for Duane and Aretha differed from the prior case, even though many aspects of the two cases were very similar. Duane was 39 years old with a long-term, serious problem with alcohol and crack cocaine. He drank most days but had not become physically addicted to alcohol. His heaviest drinking occurred in binges when he took time off from work to "party." These binges almost always led to his using crack cocaine and often to staying away from home. He had very similar marital and job problems as did John, in the prior case. He also had legal problems; he was on probation for a year due to a drug-related arrest that had occurred the week before he sought help. Duane's Recovery Contract during BCT was the same as John's, above, except that Duane also went to AA. For their recovery plan after BCT, Duane and Aretha agreed on the daily trust discussions; three AA meetings a week, with regular contact with his sponsor; and quarterly checkup visits. Duane wanted to stop the Antabuse, as had John. He, like John, did not think he needed it any more. Aretha wanted Duane to stay on the Antabuse. She was confident that he would not drink on the Antabuse, and if he was sober, she did not worry about cocaine.[4] Given their disagreement, they asked the counselor what she recommended.

In evaluating the proposed recovery plan, two important differences from the prior case led the counselor to make somewhat different recommendations. The first difference was on the risk side. Although both cases had high risk factors, Duane's drinking pattern suggested that if he started drinking, there might be more time to intervene before it got too bad. His past relapses had occurred when he started drinking just a little to test if he could handle it, and gradually built up over a few weeks to a month before drinking very heavily again and turning to crack. The second big difference was on the coping side. He had a strong connection with AA and planned to continue it. When he had coped with strong urges to drink during BCT, he had attributed his success to "thinking the drink through" and considering the bad things that would happen if he drank. On some occasions he called his sponsor to ask for help. These were active coping efforts, rather than just relying on the Antabuse. The counselor explained these points to Duane and Aretha and recommended letting Duane try to stay clean and sober without the Antabuse. The counselor also suggested that the couple agree to two other points: first, that Aretha would call the counselor immediately if she suspected drinking and second, that Duane would seriously consider going back on Antabuse if he drank.

COUPLES RELAPSE PREVENTION SESSIONS

Some couples need more frequent contacts initially after weekly BCT has ended. Such couples generally are those who have more severe problems or who have had trouble during the weekly BCT sessions. These couples may benefit from a planned, systematic schedule of 15 couples relapse prevention (RP) sessions in the year following weekly BCT.

A recent study tested couples RP sessions for maintaining change after BCT. The study compared patients with alcoholism who participated in 15 additional couples RP sessions in the year after weekly BCT, with those who did not. In the 3 years after starting BCT, male alcoholics who got RP after BCT had more days abstinent, used the trust discussion with Antabuse more, and maintained improved marriages longer than those who got BCT alone. The benefit of getting the added RP was most apparent among patients with more severe drinking and relationship problems.[5] The RP sessions described here are based directly on this recent study.

As described earlier, BCT typically consists of weekly couple sessions over a 3- to 6-month period. Couples RP sessions consist of 15 couple sessions scheduled at gradually increasing intervals in the year following weekly BCT. Couples RP sessions aim to (1) maintain gains achieved during weekly BCT, (2) deal with problems that are still unresolved or that emerge later, and (3) prevent or minimize relapse. Table 8.6 provides an outline of the content and schedule of RP sessions. Finally, we suggest that couples have regular checkup contacts for the next 4 years after the RP sessions have ended.

**TABLE 8.6. Key Points about Couples Relapse
Prevention Sessions**

- Help couple maintain gains achieved in BCT.
  - Refine plan of BCT behaviors to continue.
  - Monitor use of Continuing Recovery Plan.
- Use skills learned in BCT to deal with:
  - Relationship and other issues still unresolved.
  - New problems that emerge later in recovery.
- Create action plan to prevent or minimize relapse.
  - Review relapse risk situations and warning signs.
  - Refine action plan, as needed.
  - Minimize time and effects of any substance use.
  - Use relapse as a learning experience.
- Recommended frequency and scheduling of RP sessions:
  - 15 sessions in year after weekly BCT ends
  - 6 sessions every 2 weeks for first 3 months
  - 4 sessions every 3 weeks for next 3 months
  - 3 sessions every 4 weeks for next 3 months
  - 2 sessions every 6 weeks for last 3 months
  - Maintain regular checkup contacts for next 4 years.

Maintaining Gains Achieved in BCT

The first goal of the RP sessions is to help the couple maintain the relationship and recovery improvements they made in the weekly BCT sessions. Reviewing and refining the couple's Continuing Recovery Plan is the main method used to achieve this goal. This process begins at the initial RP sessions.

INITIAL COUPLES RP SESSIONS

Hold the first RP session with the couple 2 to 3 weeks after the last weekly BCT session. Begin this session with a brief review of events since the last BCT meeting. Find out if there have been any substance use episodes or serious conflicts or problems. Serious problems, although rare at this point, must be given priority when they do occur. In most cases, the session quickly turns to orienting the couple to the RP sessions, reviewing their Continuing Recovery Plan, and considering issues to address in upcoming RP sessions.

Orient the couple to the RP sessions by explaining their purpose and schedule. Providing a handout with the information in Table 8.6 helps. Explain how they can reach you for phone or in-person crisis contacts between regularly scheduled sessions. Emphasize that the goal is to prevent or minimize substance abuse relapse and serious relationship problems. Urge the couple to make the crisis contact as early as possible in the development of a substance use episode or relationship crisis so that they can avoid further deterioration.

Reviewing and refining the couple's Continuing Recovery Plan, formulated toward the end of BCT, occupy most of the initial RP session. Go over successes and problems in sticking to the plan so far. Discuss any changes that either partner wants to make in the plan. Be sure that the couple is still committed to the plan. Explain that you will review how well they kept to the plan at the start of each RP session, right after you review any substance use or strong urges to drink or use drugs that occurred. Continue refining the couple's plan during later RP sessions, as needed.

Issues to address in upcoming RP sessions are the final focus of the first RP session. Often this topic is deferred, or at least not completed, until the second RP session. Dealing with such issues and problems are considered in more detail next.

Dealing with Unresolved and Emergent Problems

The second goal of the RP sessions is to help the couple deal with unresolved problems or those that emerge in the year after BCT. During the initial RP sessions, help the couple identify unresolved problems either in the relationship or related to maintaining sobriety that they wish to discuss. Explain that many couples use the RP sessions to discuss sensitive or longstanding problems that they felt uncomfortable raising earlier. You can suggest topics based on your knowledge of the couple's concerns during BCT. Couples often discuss the substance abuser's efforts to regain important roles in the family that were lost through substance abuse. Other typical concerns include adolescent or young adult children, intimacy, and responses to various stressful events. The section below on long-term recovery ("Couple and Family Issues in Long-Term Recovery") gives more details on the types of relationship concerns typically raised by couples during RP sessions.

A number of methods can help the couple deal with unresolved problems or those that emerge during the RP sessions. Have the couple apply the skills they were taught during BCT. Try communication, negotiation, and problem-solving skills from BCT. Ask the couple to have a communication session about the problem under consideration during your meeting with them and to continue talking about it at home. During this discussion, partners speak one at a time, without interruptions, using the listening and speaking skills learned in BCT to discuss possible ways to deal with the problem. Negotiation and compromise to reach agreements about continuing conflicts also are used frequently in RP.

Preventing or Minimizing Relapse

The third goal of the RP sessions is to prevent or minimize relapse. Achieving this goal consists mainly of going over and upgrading the couple's action plan. It also involves dealing with any drinking or drug use that occurs in the year after BCT.

REVIEWING AND UPGRADING THE COUPLE'S ACTION PLAN

Typically the action plan the couple developed during BCT needs to be expanded and upgraded. BCT devotes only a limited amount of time to this plan. RP sessions allot more time to cover the plan in depth and to use the plan on an ongoing basis. Review the high-risk situations and warning signs for relapse that the couple identified in BCT. Add new items, as needed. At each RP session, go over risk situations and danger signs faced by the patient since the last session and coping methods used to deal with them. Also examine their planned course of action for dealing with future risk situations. Give particular attention to their plan for dealing with a lapse or relapse to be sure it is sound. Help the couple rework these plans, as needed. However, all of this is still *planning*. The strength of the RP sessions is that they go beyond relapse planning. In RP couples actually put their plans into practice when they are faced with real high-risk situations or warning signs for relapse and with actual, not just possible, relapses.

DEALING WITH DRINKING OR DRUG USE WHEN IT OCCURS

In the year spanning RP sessions, many couples experience an episode of drinking or drug use by the substance abuser. Again, this is one of the advantages of the extended RP sessions. When couples go through a relapse during RP, it tests their action plan while they still have a counselor who can help them cope with a relapse.

Your first aim is to minimize the length and negative effects of the relapse. If one of the partners calls you soon after substance use starts, as specified in most action plans, it is easier to nip the problem in the bud. Of course, couples often wait until drinking or drug use has reached dangerous levels again before they contact you. Once you find out that substance use has occurred, try to get it stopped. Help the couple decide what to do to stop the substance use and keep it stopped (e.g., meet with you right away, restart recovery medication, go to more 12-step meetings, enter a detoxification unit).

Your second aim is to help the couple use the relapse as a learning experience by engaging in an in-depth investigation of the triggers that led up to the relapse. Ask partners to come up with solutions (other than substance use) for similar future situations. Also, ask them to weigh the impact of the relapse:

- How long did the relapse last?
- What negative effects did it have?
- How did it compare with prior relapses?
- What would they do differently in the future to prevent or minimize a relapse?

For these couple discussions about relapse to be successful, you must be extremely active in defusing hostile or depressive reactions to the substance use. Stress that relapse does not mean total failure and that uneven progress is the rule rather than the exception.

Typical Format of RP Sessions

Certain aspects are part of all RP sessions, whereas others change over the 12 months of RP. Begin nearly all sessions by reviewing any substance use or strong urges to drink or use drugs that have occurred since the last session. Also at each session go over the couple's Continuing Recovery Plan, with an emphasis on activities to prevent drinking and drug use and promote abstinence. Other parts of each session depend on the specific areas that are the focus of that phase of the RP sessions (e.g., problem solving, action plan) and on significant events in the couple's life at the time. The RP sessions are less structured than the earlier BCT sessions. Much of BCT focused on teaching the couple skills to deal with their problems. RP sessions stress applying these skills to deal, in depth, with ongoing couple problems. RP sessions do not have a rigid session-by-session format, but rather a set of goals and procedures that are flexibly applied. In later RP sessions gradually reduce the control and structure you provide to the sessions. As the time between sessions increases, try to decrease partners' dependence on you and increase the responsibility they assume for their own progress, with less input from you. Spend the final few sessions reviewing the lessons that have been learned and considering what they plan to do to maintain their progress.

Regular Checkup Visits for 4 Years after RP Sessions End

As noted, we recommend that couples have checkup visits for 4 years after the RP sessions end. This ongoing contact with the couple through a 5-year follow-up is a very useful method to monitor progress, assess compliance with planned maintenance procedures, and evaluate the need for additional RP sessions. We discussed these planned checkup visits earlier in this chapter.

COUPLE AND FAMILY ISSUES IN LONG-TERM RECOVERY

Many substance abusers continue to have relationship problems even after a period of stable abstinence has been established. Couples receiving maintenance contacts in the months and years after the end of regular BCT sessions often present such problems. Other couples who achieved abstinence without couples therapy may seek help for relationship problems at a later date. Either way, it is useful to consider types of problems typically seen in long-term recovery and guidelines for dealing with such situations.

Types of Relationship Issues Commonly Seen in Long-Term Recovery

Although a wide variety of issues can present difficulties to couples during long-term recovery, a number of concerns and life patterns predominate. First, difficulties in role readjustment occur when the spouse resists the substance abuser's efforts to regain important roles in the relationship (e.g., disciplinarian to children, equal partner in money decisions) that were lost through substance abuse. Nearly all couples with a serious substance abuse problem face this problem early in the recovery process. BCT helps many couples resolve these problems. However, some couples, especially those who do not participate in couples therapy in early recovery, may get stuck on the role readjustment issues and seek couples therapy later for this problem. Second, problems with children—especially communication and behavior management with adolescents, or the substance abuse problems of adolescent and young adult children—frequently become a focus during long-term recovery. Third, couples often present problems with sex and intimacy[6] somewhat later in recovery, after many of the most severe hardships due to substance abuse have been repaired and roles have started to restabilize. Finally, couples during the recovery process seem particularly vulnerable to stresses created by critical transitions in the family life cycle (e.g., children leaving home), external life change events (e.g., job loss), or developmental changes in any of the family members (e.g., midlife crisis).

Guidelines for Dealing with Relationship Issues in Long-Term Recovery

The relationship issues just described are by no means unique to couples with a substance abuse problem. Concerns about roles and control, adolescent children, intimacy, and responses to stressful events are common complaints of couples for whom alcohol and drugs are not part of the problem. However, when couples with a substance abuse history request help for such issues during long-term recovery, you must consider two factors not evaluated with other couples.

First, determine if a relapse is imminent so that necessary preventive interventions can be instituted immediately. Even if there is no imminent threat of relapse, be sure that the substance-abusing individual is getting the help he or she needs to stay abstinent, especially during the stress of relationship problems. Do not assume because the person has been abstinent for an extended period that his or her current sobriety supports are sufficient or that relapse is an unlikely event. For BCT, abstinence from alcohol and drugs remains the first priority, in both early and later recovery, before attempting to help the couple with other problems.

Second, determine each person's view of the connection between the earlier substance abuse problem and the current relationship difficulties. Partners may think that the substance abuse problem caused the current problems or that there is little or no connection. Each person's opinion is important because it will determine what he or she thinks needs to be done to solve the relationship problems. You also need to carefully assess whether or not you share the couple's view. Couples often continue to attribute difficulties in their relationship to the previous substance abuse problem, rather than to their current life situation. A few case examples illustrate these points.

Case Examples

THE CASE OF JEFF AND BERNICE

Jeff had achieved 12 years of sobriety after a serious alcohol problem, through AA for himself and Al-Anon for his wife Bernice. Jeff had stopped regular AA meetings a few years earlier, but Bernice remained a regular Al-Anon participant. They sought couples counseling after Jeff became involved in a romantic relationship with a coworker. Bernice attributed her husband's relationship to his "alcoholic personality." By this she meant that although he was not drinking, Jeff was still lying and sneaking around, like he had done to conceal his drinking years earlier, and that the relationship was a substitute for the drinking. She insisted that he return to regular AA attendance, a demand that Jeff opposed.

In a separate interview, Jeff said that he had no desire to drink. He remembered vividly the job, health, and relationship problems caused by his drinking and had no intention of going back to that. Although he no longer went to AA, he still talked with his old sponsor periodically and would contact him if he felt tempted to drink. His sponsor had suggested that he seek couples counseling. He said he still loved Bernice and did not love his coworker, with whom he had been infatuated but not sexually involved.

Further assessment provided other important information. In the past year Bernice had started to work outside the home, leaving less time for special meals and other attention that Jeff liked. In addition, Jeff's job had become much more stressful, requiring him to work evenings and Saturdays, and the long hours made him quite irritable. These changes disrupted evening and weekend activities previously enjoyed by the couple. In response to Jeff's irritability, Bernice withdrew affection and communication, choosing to use her Al-Anon friends for support instead. When Jeff turned to the woman at work, the couple's problems got much worse. Note that the counselor did not accept Bernice's blaming Jeff's affair on his alcoholic personality (after 12 years of sobriety) or her insistence that he return to regular AA attendance. The counselor explained his view of their problems to the couple this way:

> "A lot of changes, mainly from job pressures, took you away from each other in the past year. You both felt rejected and pushed each other away. Jeff gave in to the attentions of the woman at work who was having problems at home. This hurt you a great deal, Bernice, but Jeff still loves you. He wants to make your marriage work again. I don't know if returning to AA is the solution. I suggest you consider some counseling together as a couple to see if you can work out your problems."

Bernice reluctantly agreed to try counseling. During a few months of couples counseling, Jeff and Bernice gradually rebuilt their relationship. Jeff convincingly ended the relationship by asking for a job transfer to another location. He told Bernice how sorry he was. They started making time for each other and reconnecting through some of the BCT exercises (e.g., Catch Your Partner, shared rewarding activities). Both felt their relationship was back on solid ground.

THE CASE OF BOB AND ALICE

Bob had 5 years of sobriety following a rehab program and 6 months of BCT sessions with his wife Alice for his serious alcohol dependence problem. They now had yearly couple sessions to review current status and renegotiate an Antabuse contract. Alice called for help when Bob refused to participate in the Antabuse observation, despite their agreement, and threatened to drink and to end the marriage. Contact with Bob revealed that he was still taking Antabuse, although he would not give Alice the satisfaction of knowing this. A few crisis intervention sessions revealed the factors that had precipitated the marital crisis. Serious sexual problems had concerned the couple for some time. Bob's 50th birthday was approaching, and he wanted to have more sexual fulfillment and closeness in the marriage or the freedom to seek it in a new relationship "before it's too late." In addition, the couple had a mentally ill son in his early 20s who, in the previous year, had shown that he was not going to be able to support himself or to live outside a sheltered setting.

Bob was not in danger of relapsing and intended to stay on Antabuse. Interestingly, both Bob and Alice blamed their sexual problems and their son's emotional problems on Bob's alcoholism. They had become very estranged during Bob's many years of alcoholic drinking and had separated for a year before he went to rehab. Although they had reconnected in many ways during the earlier BCT sessions, sex had remained infrequent, with little affection, and Bob had started to have difficulty maintaining an erection when they did try to have sex. Their son's disability, according to Alice, was the result of Bob's lack of time with his son when he was a child and the family turmoil from Bob's alcoholism. Bob defended himself, saying that it wasn't all his fault, but he also blamed himself for his son's problems. Both had been emotionally devastated as they began to realize in the past year that their son was severely impaired and probably would never be "normal."

They agreed to 6 weeks of couples counseling to address the crisis and then reevaluate whether additional counseling was needed. Most of the time was spent discussing their son, because he was their most distressing concern. Early in high school he had started smoking marijuana, drinking, doing poorly in school, withdrawing into himself, and getting arrested for minor offenses. More recently he had developed psychotic symptoms and was hearing voices; he had been admitted to a psychiatric hospital, then discharged to a partial hospital program for psychiatric patients. The couples counselor questioned whether their son's upbringing was the main cause of the son's problems. The counselor indicated that mental health experts no longer blamed parents' inadequacies for the development of such serious mental illness problems, thinking instead that internal chemical imbalances may be more responsible. The counselor encouraged them to talk with the social worker at their son's treatment program. Bob and Alice joined a family psychoeducation group at the treatment center, where they learned more about mental illness and decreased their self-blame further. After 6 weeks they declined the offer of more couples counseling to work on improving their sexual satisfaction. There was no longer any talk of drinking or marital breakup. They were working together to try to help their son and to accept the reality of his limitations.

FREQUENTLY ASKED QUESTIONS

• *Question 1*: The extended relapse prevention (RP) sessions seem so useful that it raises the question of why you wouldn't want to offer them to all patients after they complete BCT. You suggest using RP sessions for patients with more severe problems. Why not have this be part of regular treatment?

• *Answer*: Based on the outcome research data,[6] your suggestion would make sense. In our study of RP sessions, we found that the patients who received RP after BCT had more abstinence and happier relationships than patients who only got BCT. However, the subgroup of patients with more severe drinking problems got the most added benefit from the additional RP. So the study findings support both giving RP to all patients and only to those with more severe problems.

Also, the therapists in the outcome study really liked doing the RP sessions. They saw the patients and their spouses for 20–24 weekly BCT sessions and then 15 RP sessions over the next year, for a total of 18 months. The additional RP allowed therapists to work with couples on problems that surfaced later or that had not yet been addressed due to time constraints or couple reluctance. Most important, therapists were able to help many patients deal with one or more relapses and get back on track during the extended treatment.

The two main reasons for not making RP sessions a part of regular treatment for all patients are cost and acceptability to patients. Many health insurance plans will not cover such extended treatment, and without at least partial insurance payments, many patients cannot afford to pay for the extended RP sessions out of pocket. Even when cost is not a barrier, some patients do not want to continue couple sessions for a variety of reasons. They may think they do not need the extra sessions, or it may be a matter of the inconvenience of getting to the sessions. They were both willing to put up with the inconvenience and the stress of attending BCT sessions in the beginning when their problems were intense, but they may no longer be willing to do so now that their problems have lessened. Some patients may have a covert plan of trying a return to a lower level of substance use—something they know the counselor will not endorse. Given these problems with cost and acceptability of extended RP sessions, less intensive maintenance interventions are needed. In this chapter we suggested periodic checkup sessions on a less frequent schedule than the RP sessions. Prearranged periodic phone calls initiated by the therapist also can help.

- *Question 2*: What do you do if the substance abuser does not follow through with what he or she agreed to do on the action plan? What if the substance abuser relapses but refuses to call his or her sponsor or the BCT counselor, as he or she agreed to do? What are the options when a couple is no longer seeing a BCT counselor?
- *Answer*: This is a really good question that reflects a very common clinical dilemma. The answer is that the spouse should do what he or she agreed to do in the action plan if the patient used. This might include not arguing when the patient is under the influence, calling the BCT counselor, and talking with an Al-Anon sponsor. The spouse should act quickly and let the patient know that the spouse has followed through on his or her part of the action plan (except for cases in which doing so could create risk of violence). In other words, the spouse should keep the commitments he or she made, regardless of what the patient does or does not do. The answer is based on BCT's good-faith–individual-responsibility approach. As described in Chapter 1, each member of the couple freely chooses to make needed changes in their own behavior, independent of whether or not the partner makes corresponding changes in behavior.

The question also may reflect circumstances in which the spouse feels helpless when faced with a mate who is continuing to drink or use drugs and making no effort to seek help, as agreed in the action plan. The spouse may think that what behaviors agreed to in the action plan will be of little help and therefore initially decides not to follow through. Often the spouse tends to think in all-or-none terms when considering options for reacting to a using partner. Either the spouse puts up with the patient's continued using or makes the patient leave and they get a separation. The spouse may not be ready to kick out the substance-abusing partner and may have learned not to make idle threats of separation. So the spouse does little or nothing, which the patient may interpret as passive acceptance of substance use. The spouse waits and watches, hoping that the patient will decide to stop on his or her own. The patient continues drinking or drugging and the relapse gets worse, finally leading to some behavior the spouse finds quite unacceptable. *Then* the spouse acts, but at that point a damaging relapse has occurred. Again, the spouse is not to blame for the relapse or for its continuing unabated; the patient is. However, if the spouse does not keep the commitment made in the action plan, then he or she has not done his or her part to deal with the substance abuse problem of the patient.

- *Question 3*: You recommend continuing checkup visits for 5 years after the end of weekly BCT sessions. This seems unrealistic. Other treatment programs for substance abuse usually do not have such extended follow-up contacts. Is this a necessary part of BCT?
- *Answer*: We consider continuing checkup visits for 5 years after the end of weekly BCT sessions to be a recommended, not a required, part of BCT. How realistic such long-term contacts are depends, in part, on cost and on patient acceptance, as already discussed in the first question about RP sessions. Like other chronic conditions (e.g., hypertension, high cholesterol), serious substance abuse problems benefit from long-term, if not lifelong, monitoring and attention. Most substance abuse treatment providers would agree with the preceding statement. Most providers believe that substance abuse is a chronic, relapsing disorder, but the

treatment system does not reflect this belief. Currently the U.S. treatment system is organized to provide acute episodes of care over fairly short time frames. Hopefully, this less-than-ideal situation will change.

SUMMARY

- Most couples who attend BCT sessions faithfully show substantial improvement. However, when the structure of the weekly BCT sessions ends, there is a natural tendency for backsliding. Therefore, it is critical to help couples maintain the gains they made in BCT and prevent or minimize relapse.

- The Continuing Recovery Plan specifies activities to do to maintain abstinence and relationship recovery after weekly couple sessions end. In this plan the couple chooses the behaviors learned in previous BCT sessions they wish to continue (e.g., daily trust discussion, communication sessions).

- Next the couple anticipates the high-risk situations and warning signs for relapse they may encounter and makes an action plan for how they will prevent or minimize relapse when faced with such situations. If the patient relapses but does not follow through with the agreed-to action plan, the spouse should still follow through with his or her part of the plan.

- After weekly BCT ends, couple checkup visits with the counselor for an extended period can encourage continued progress. These ongoing contacts provide a structured setting in which partners can review their success with continuing activities to promote recovery and with their action plan to prevent or minimize relapse.

- Couples who have more severe problems or who had trouble during BCT may need more frequent contacts initially after weekly BCT ends. These couples may benefit from 15 RP sessions in the year after weekly BCT to (1) maintain gains achieved during weekly BCT, (2) deal with problems that are still unresolved or that emerge later, and (3) prevent or minimize relapse.

- When problems with cost and/or patient acceptance limit use of extended RP sessions after BCT, less intensive maintenance interventions are still needed. Checkup sessions on a less frequent schedule than the RP sessions and prearranged phone calls initiated by the therapist also can help.

- Many substance abusers continue to have relationship problems even after a period of stable abstinence has been established. We considered types of problems typically seen in long-term recovery and provided guidelines for dealing with such situations.

NOTES

1. We adapted work on maintenance and relapse prevention in behavior therapy and addictions for use with couples. Much of this chapter is based on the concepts presented in Marlatt and Gordon's (1985) classic work on relapse prevention, Whisman's (1990) work on maintaining treatment gains, and O'Farrell's (1993b) chapter on a couples approach to relapse prevention.
2. Marlatt and Gordon (1985).

3. Quote is from page 32 of Marlatt and Gordon (1985).

4. Kathleen Carroll and colleagues have shown that Antabuse increases both alcohol and cocaine abstinence among patients who frequently combine alcohol use with cocaine use (Carroll et al., 2000, 2004).

5. For details on these research findings, see O'Farrell, Choquette, and Cutter (1998), and O'Farrell, Choquette, Cutter, Brown, and McCourt (1993).

6. For some research on sexual adjustment problems, see O'Farrell, Choquette, Cutter, and Birchler (1997). For clinical guidance on dealing with common sexual problems seen in couples therapy, see McCarthy and McCarthy (2002, 2003).

9

Challenges in BCT, Part I
Separated and Dual-Problem Couples

The preceding chapters described how to use BCT with the majority of couples you will see. Now we want to focus on challenges in BCT. This chapter shows how to use BCT with potentially suitable couples who are separated or in which both members have a current substance abuse problem. The next chapter examines couples with partner violence, providing an in-depth rationale for using BCT with these couples and extended case examples; it also covers other common clinical problems encountered in the course of BCT. Table 9.1 lists the challenges in BCT covered in these two chapters.

TABLE 9.1. Challenges in BCT

- Separated couples
  - Couples living apart when you first see them
  - Couples who separate after starting BCT
- Dual-problem couples
  - Both partners have a current substance problem
  - Treatment when *both partners* want to change
  - Treatment when *only one partner* wants to change
- Intimate partner violence
  - Rationale for using BCT with violent couples
  - Excluding couples with very severe violence
  - How BCT prevents violence
- Other challenges
  - Resistance to home practice, behavioral rehearsal, and other aspects of BCT
  - Couples who come to session angry
  - Psychiatric comorbidity
  - Clinical impasse
  - Reading level
  - Sexual issues and affairs

188

COUPLES WHO ARE SEPARATED WHEN YOU FIRST SEE THEM

Couples who are separated present a challenge to BCT. Generally BCT requires the couple to live together and to work daily to see if substance abuse and relationship problems can be improved. Separated couples generally cannot provide the daily support and commitment so critical to BCT's success. The following guidelines and case examples should help you, as a BCT counselor, deal with couples who are separated when you first see them. A later section addresses couples who separate after starting BCT.

Guidelines for Couples Living Apart Initially

The initial session for a couple who is separated follows the same guidelines used with all couples inquiring about BCT, as described in Chapter 2. You also must get more in-depth information about the separation. For example, you will need to know if there is a restraining order that prohibits contact, because it will have to be removed or modified before further couple sessions can occur. Most important, you should try to clarify what, if anything, could lead to a reconciliation and a mutual willingness to work on the relationship. Both are needed before you can proceed with the standard BCT program.

Separations initiated by the spouse to provide a "trial period" for the substance abuser to demonstrate that he or she wants, and can maintain, sobriety are relatively common. You need to find out what specific changes are desired to make the relationship viable. Spouses frequently state that the patient stopping substance use is necessary for the relationship to improve. Also, you should clarify what signs, in addition to sobriety, the spouse will use to determine if it is safe to attempt a reconciliation. Many couples enter BCT as a "last chance" to save their relationship. However, for some separated couples, one partner may be uncertain about whether sobriety or other changes will make a difference. For these couples too much damage may have been done to the relationship for it to continue, and they would not benefit from BCT. However, most separated couples you will see are ambivalent about the relationship but not ready to end it. Often you can see such couples for initial couple sessions while they remain living apart to develop a plan for them to resume living together. Once the couple has reunited, BCT proceeds as with other couples.

Your meetings with the couple while they are separated should seek to develop a realistic basis for reconciliation. Before reconciling, the couple need a plan to address the problems that led to the separation. Partners need to have clear and realistic expectations about what will be different when they reconcile that will prevent their relationship from breaking down again. They also need to have begun the process of putting planned changes into practice. Some couples may want to reconcile too soon, before the patient has a plan to support abstinence and before the couples understand the changes needed to promote relationship happiness. This is particularly true for younger relationships in which positive feelings can be rekindled more easily. However, rekindled feelings and promises for change may not be sufficient for a successful reconciliation. Sometimes you may ask partners to stay apart a little longer so that they can have a better chance of long-term success. Don't forget that leverage for change is highest when the couple is still separated. The patient may be more willing to start recovery activities (e.g., Antabuse, AA) suggested by the spouse or therapist while they are still separated than after they reconcile. Importantly, patients often continue these sobriety supports once they start them. Whereas some separated couples develop a realistic basis for reconciling after a few couple sessions, other couples take longer to reach this goal.

Many couples (especially those who have been separated more than a few weeks) will need more extensive counseling while they remain separated. If the partners are willing, a *structured separation therapy*[1] may help them decide if they wish to reconcile or stay separated. This approach involves a time period during which they definitely do not reconcile but spend preplanned time together ("dates") at least twice weekly. We usually suggest that partners stay apart *at least* 6 weeks while having weekly couple sessions. They agree not to discuss if or when they will reconcile during their planned times together. This agreement avoids the undesirable situation in which one person badgers and pleads with the other to reconcile each time they are together. Often you can use some of the BCT methods during this structured separation counseling. The partners' preplanned dates follow the guidelines for shared rewarding activities; that is, they try to have fun together, and they keep discussion of relationship problems to a minimum. Catch Your Partner and caring days also can be part of the couple's dates. Some couples do the trust discussion, not necessarily on a daily basis, but when they see each other and in between by phone. You need to help the patient develop a strong individual program (e.g., attending 12-step meetings and individual counseling, developing new sober friends) to strengthen his or her commitment to abstinence. Be sure that the spouse knows about the steps the patient is taking to deal with the substance abuse problem. Seeing the patient taking action to stay abstinent may build confidence in the spouse that recovery is possible. Finally, a major focus of the couple sessions is to define and begin to implement a realistic plan for changes needed before reconciliation. When the planned time apart is nearly elapsed, help the partners decide whether they are ready to reconcile or whether they need to negotiate another period of continued separation. Table 9.2 summarizes key points about dealing with couples who are living separately when you first see them.

Case Examples of Couples Living Apart Initially

BOB AND LISA: BRIEF COUPLES SESSIONS LEAD TO RECONCILIATION AND BCT

Bob and Lisa were in their early 30s with a 2-year-old daughter and had been separated 10 days when they first saw the BCT counselor. When Bob was arrested for DUI on his way home from work, Lisa told him not to come home until he got help for his drinking problem. Bob had been staying at his mother's house, calling Lisa daily and pleading to be allowed back home.

TABLE 9.2. Couples Who Are Separated When You First See Them

- Separations to change substance abuser are common.
- *Structured separation therapy* may help some couples.
  - Couples stay apart for a designated time period.
  - Couples go on two "dates" per week to reconnect, but do not discuss reconciling (takes pressure off reluctant partner).
  - Therapist finds out what changes are desired before reconciliation.
  - Therapist helps partners develop realistic plan for reconciling.
  - Therapist starts some BCT methods with them while they are separated.
  - Therapist does standard BCT once they are back together.

He had not had a drink since being arrested, and he made an appointment to go with her to the BCT program. Lisa insisted they go to the first BCT session before she would let him return home. Bob had not kept his promise to get help earlier when they were apart a few days over another alcohol-related incident.

Bob's pattern had been to drink daily, starting on his afternoon work break, on the way home in his truck, and at home until he went to bed. On the weekends he drank most of the time. His father was active in AA and had been sober for many years, whereas his alcoholic brother was still drinking and in the middle of a bitter divorce. Both Lisa and Bob's father had been urging him to stop drinking and get help for some time.

In the first session, when the counselor asked their requirements for reconciliation, Lisa said she wanted Bob to stop drinking and get help to stay sober. When he didn't drink, they got along fine. Bob just wanted to come home. He missed his wife and little girl and hated sleeping on his mother's couch. He acknowledged his drinking problem and that he wanted help to stay sober. The counselor suggested that Bob attend two AA meetings in the coming week, at least one with his father, and that he see the clinic physician to be evaluated for Antabuse. After Bob agreed to these suggestions, the counselor suggested that the couple not reconcile until the following week, after Bob had had a chance to follow through on these steps of getting help for his drinking. Bob was upset at this suggestion. He had come to the appointment tonight, as Lisa had asked, and now he wanted to go home. The counselor explained how easy it is to for people to put off getting the help they need. She stressed that another week away from home, although inconvenient and disappointing, was a small price to pay to give them and their daughter the best chance of a positive future together. The counselor stressed that this was her suggestion but that, of course, they would have to decide what to do. Lisa said that she would like it better if Bob waited to come home. Bob reluctantly agreed to stay apart until their next week's BCT session, but he insisted that he would not continue BCT if he did what was asked of him and the counselor again suggested postponing their reconciliation.

At the next session, Lisa announced that Bob had been back home for 2 days, after he had kept his AA and Antabuse commitments. They had a long talk in which they recommitted to their relationship and to using BCT to make things better. So the counselor began standard BCT sessions now that Bob and Lisa had reconciled.

LOU AND LESLIE: BRIEF COUPLES SESSIONS WITHOUT RECONCILIATION

Lou and Leslie were in their early 40s, married 4 years (second marriage for both), and separated 3 weeks when they first saw the BCT counselor. Lou was staying with his brother, and Leslie was at home with her three teenage children. Leslie insisted on the separation when Lou violated a "house rule" by having alcohol and cocaine in their home. Despite Lou's pleading and objections, Leslie had no intention of reconciling quickly. The BCT counselor suggested a four-session evaluation to learn more about them, their prospects for reconciliation, and their suitability for BCT.

When the couple had first met, Lou was not drinking or using cocaine, but he started up after a few months of marriage. He also overused prescribed medications, including opiates, barbiturates, and tranquilizers, for a series of painful medical problems. He had undergone three detoxes during their marriage. Lou was vague about his substance use before he met Leslie, saying that his first marriage had broken up because of incompatibility, not from his addiction problems.

When asked about requirements for reconciliation, Leslie said she wanted Lou to get long-term residential treatment and stay clean and sober for at least a year before returning home. She felt that their relationship problems were due almost entirely to his substance abuse. Lou angrily refused to consider her requests, stating that her uncaring attitude and unrealistic demands for "perfection" were the reasons the marriage would not work. The couple sessions were quite volatile, with a great deal of anger on both sides. Their limited contacts between sessions also were very strained.

Session 3 was particularly intense. Leslie said that she had new evidence of Lou's unwillingness to change and be honest. His sister had called to say that she "should know the truth" about Lou. The sister recounted Lou's history of alcohol and drug problems, starting at age 17, that included many lost jobs, a failed marriage, and a year in jail on drug charges. He had been mainly abstinent when the couple met because he had just gotten out of jail 6 months earlier. Lou responded defensively, saying that he had been dishonest because he didn't think Leslie would have married him if she knew the truth. Leslie's attitude now showed he had been right. Now he was convinced their marriage was "over." The counselor tried unsuccessfully to reign in the angry escalations, so she met with each person individually for 15 minutes. She reminded them that at the next session she would sum up the results of their meetings.

Session 4 was structured to review the past three sessions and their current situation, give feedback and recommendations, and discuss options. First, the counselor met with each person separately for 15 minutes, during which she shared the following impressions. They did not agree on what was needed for reconciliation. They seemed very angry and unable to talk constructively, even with the counselor present to intervene. They did not appear to have a mutual desire to improve their relationship. Lou and Leslie each agreed that these observations were basically correct. Then the counselor met with them as a couple and reviewed the same information she had discussed with them individually. This couple session did not escalate into arguments or blaming, as in previous sessions. They remained calm, with an air of seriousness and quiet resignation. They agreed with the counselor's observations, as they had when alone.

Both were strongly urged to seek counseling, Leslie to address the stress of the separation, and Lou for ongoing substance abuse treatment—preferably more intensive and long-term care, including a sober residence. They were encouraged to continue a trial period of separation before considering reconciliation, given their intense conflict when together recently. Finally, the counselor invited them to return for couples counseling in the future if, after a period of addressing their individual issues, they felt they could work together productively.

Phone check-ins a week later revealed that both were coping adequately. Each expressed relief that they were no longer trying to reconcile. At her in-person follow-up interview 2 weeks later, Leslie said that she and her kids were doing fine, and she did not want additional counseling. At his follow-up, Lou declined more intensive substance abuse treatment, opting to continue his weekly outpatient counseling. At this time the couple's case was closed because they remained separated and each person was getting the help they wanted.

LARRY AND BARBARA: EXTENDED SEPARATION THERAPY WITH RECONCILIATION AND BCT

Larry and Barbara were in their late 40s, married for 16 years, and had been separated a year, with little contact, when they first saw the BCT counselor. For the past 2 months Larry had been living in a halfway house, going to AA five times a week, going to substance abuse counseling, and staying abstinent. He hated the halfway house and wanted to return to living with his wife. After twice weekly Al-Anon for 2 years, Barbara was skeptical about reuniting.

The clinical history showed that Larry's drinking had caused marital and job problems for many years, but 5 years ago the situation got much worse. After his mother died and he retired on disability (for back problems) from his job as a firefighter, he started drinking all day every day. He drank, watched TV sports, and slept. Barbara had him committed to treatment. In the next 3 years he was in four more treatment centers, always going back to drinking within a month of leaving the center. Finally, about a year before their first couple session, when Larry was kicked out of a treatment program for drinking, Barbara had said she wanted a separation.

At their first session, Larry wanted to go home right away, pointing to his regular AA attendance, individual counseling, 2 months of sobriety, and his dislike for living conditions at the halfway house. To consider reconciliation, Barbara wanted Larry to (1) have achieved 6 months of sobriety with a convincing plan for staying sober, (2) get a job or some regular structured activity to occupy his time, and (3) do things together and communicate as a couple. They agreed to a compromise suggested by the counselor: They would stay apart at least another 2 months while they participated in couple sessions to see if they could rebuild their relationship. After this time period, they would revisit the issue of reconciling.

The couple sessions included twice weekly dates on which to reconnect as a couple. At first Larry used their dates to argue for coming home right away, complaining about his living conditions and stressing his commitment to recovery. Barbara responded by recounting the many problems he had caused and lies he had told when he was actively drinking. Their dates became less tense when they followed the counselor's suggestion not to bring up negatives from the past or decisions about the future. In couple sessions, the counselor coached them to communicate about the damage alcoholism had done to them and their family and their concerns about problems that might happen if they reconciled. Catch Your Partner also was made part of their dates. During their dates, they did the trust discussion and he told her what AA meetings and counseling sessions he had attended. Eventually they did the trust discussion daily by phone.

After 2 months they reevaluated their situation, as planned. Larry had been sober for 4 months, very active in AA and counseling, and they were more comfortable spending time together after their extended separation. Barbara still wanted to make their reconciliation contingent on 6 months of abstinence and a job or other activity. The counselor suggested that they might start spending weekends together because they were progressing well and Larry had been trying to find work. A few weeks later, Larry got a part-time job at a supermarket, and they reconciled. They continued BCT sessions for 6 more months, with periodic follow-ups for 2 years and continued to do well.

COUPLES WHO SEPARATE AFTER STARTING BCT

Guidelines for Couples Who Separate after Starting BCT

Although separations after starting substance abuse counseling are much less common among patients who participate in BCT than those who receive only individual counseling, some couples do separate during and after BCT. A separation often occurs after some progress has been made. In some cases a relapse may lead to separation. For other couples, progress on relationship and recovery goals may fall below expectations. As a BCT counselor, you can help such couples deal with separation in a way that is least hurtful to all involved.

When a couple separates, try to avoid a number of common counselor mistakes. First, do not assume that the separation will be permanent. Even when one or both partners are very angry and it seems as if their relationship is over, they may change their minds in a few days or a few weeks. Take a wait-and-see approach to most separations. Being separated may have different meanings for different couples and different meanings for the same couple at different times. Temporary separations in substance abusers' relationships to motivate change or to reevaluate commitment may be more common than in the general population, where most separations end in divorce.[2] Second, try not to side with one person over the other, even though one member of the couple may want you to validate his or her decision to separate. Doing so would limit your ability to resume your role as their couples counselor if the couple reconciles or asks for help again. Third, do not stop counseling sessions when the couple separates. Just because the couple is separated does not mean that counseling is over. Rather, the nature and focus of counseling changes.

Generally when a couple separates, you should continue separate individual contacts by phone and in person with each member of the couple. Once the separation has lasted more than a week, your role and goals change. You should explain these changes to each partner. Before the separation, you tried to help both members of the couple improve their relationship. After the separation, your goal is to promote the individual well-being of each member of the couple and minimize the negative impact of the separation, while they decide what they want to do about the future of their relationship. Support the patient's sobriety. Reach out to a patient who has relapsed and arrange needed help (e.g., detox) or just stay in contact to let the person know that help is available when he or she wants it. Help patients who have not relapsed identify actions (e.g., attending more meetings, returning to individual counseling) to prevent relapse during this very stressful period. Also be sure that the spouse has the emotional support he or she needs. This support may involve periodic sessions with you, referral to a mental health counselor, or support from friends, family, and Al-Anon. Continue regular contacts until the situation has stabilized and both partners seem to be getting the help they need to cope with being separated, or until they no longer want you to be in touch with them. Leave the door open to return to see you if they want help in the future. Table 9.3 summarizes key points about dealing with couples who separate after they start BCT.

TABLE 9.3. Couples Who Separate after Starting BCT

- Do not assume that the separation will be permanent.
- Try not to side with one person over the other.
- Continue counseling, with changed focus.
  - Individual well-being of each partner is primary, not helping them to improve relationship as a couple.
  - Use individual sessions and contacts to help each person and refer for other help, as needed.
  - Try to minimize negative impact of separation.
- Be available if they want more couples counseling.

Case Examples of Couples Who Separate after Starting BCT

BEN AND KATE: THEY SEPARATED BUT EVENTUALLY RECONCILED

Ben and Kate were in their late 30s, married 8 years, with two young children. They started BCT after Ben's third detoxification from alcohol. The first 6 weeks of BCT sessions seemed to go well. Ben took Antabuse daily during their trust discussion and went to two AA meetings each week. Kate was relieved to see Ben pursuing sobriety and was starting to believe that things might be different this time. One unresolved problem area was Kate's belief that Ben gambled too much. Ben denied gambling, telling Kate that he had stopped buying lottery tickets and stopped betting on sports. Then Ben, who worked as a computer salesman, had to attend a convention in Reno, Nevada. The plan for the trip was that Ben would call nightly to do the trust discussion, go to an AA meeting if he felt he needed it, and not gamble.

They missed the next BCT session, after Ben's return from his business trip. When the BCT counselor called to inquire about the missed session, Kate said that they were not coming to couple sessions any more. They were separated. She had thrown Ben out when she discovered that he had drunk and gambled heavily on his trip. He did not make the first planned daily call, and his speech was slurred when he did call. She looked at bills in his desk and found material showing other recent gaming activity. So he had lied to her about not gambling any more. She also found out that in the week before he left for the trip, he had faked taking the Antabuse. Ben had planned to drink and gamble on the trip. She felt betrayed and very angry.

The BCT counselor invited Kate to a session by herself to review what had happened. At first Kate refused. She had made up her mind that the marriage was over and did not want the counselor to try to talk her out of this decision. She reluctantly agreed to the session when the counselor explained that she would not try to convince her to stay in the relationship. Now that they were separated and Kate thought it probably would be permanent, the counselor's role was to help her and Ben, as individuals, cope with the separation as best they could, not to try to push them to stay together. At the individual session, the counselor asked how Kate was coping. Kate felt she was doing OK. She had support from her immediate family and from two close friends, including her sponsor from Al-Anon. She declined the counselor's offer to provide or refer her for individual counseling to help sort through the difficult decision to end her marriage. She did agree that the counselor could call her periodically to see how she was doing.

Ben called the counselor to say he was sleeping on the couch at his brother's house. He confirmed what Kate had said about his drinking, lying, and gambling. He readily accepted the counselor's invitation for an individual session, at which he asked the counselor to intervene with Kate to take him back. The counselor refused, explaining that her role, now that they were separated, was to help each of them as individuals, not to try to help them reconcile unless that was what they both wanted. The counselor suggested that Ben should focus on himself and deal with his serious alcohol and gambling problems. Recovery from these problems would help him deal with his own life and be a better divorced father to his kids. The counselor saw Ben for an individual session every few weeks. Ben was deeply troubled that his lying and problems were causing his family to break up. He admitted that he had a gambling problem and went to his first Gamblers Anonymous (GA) meeting. He also increased attendance to four AA meetings a week, joined a group, and got a sponsor—all of which he had been unwilling to do earlier. In retrospect, he confided that earlier he had been focused more on placating Kate than on his own recovery.

Periodically the counselor placed separate calls to Ben and Kate to see how they were doing. After about 3 months Kate called the counselor to say that she and Ben had decided to reconcile. They wanted to restart BCT sessions. For the next 18 months, they faithfully attended BCT sessions, at first weekly and then less often. During this time, Ben stayed sober and did not gamble, with regular help from AA and GA, and they successfully rebuilt their relationship.

JOSÉ AND MARIA: PERMANENT SEPARATION AS A GOOD OUTCOME

José, age 43 and divorced for 6 years after an 18-year marriage, had two teenage sons who lived with his ex-wife. Maria, age 26, had been divorced for 3 years after a 4-year marriage without children. She worked in an insurance office. He had managed a building supply store during his early 30s, when abstinent for 5 years, but had worked at various construction jobs since then. José saw a poster about the BCT program during an inpatient stay for detoxification from heroin and cocaine. His recent pattern was to stay clean for 10–12 months. Then, after conflicts with people in his life or other types of stress, he would start using cocaine, followed by heroin to come down from the cocaine. Daily drug use would continue for a few weeks to a few months, ending when he sought detox because he was physically sick and emotionally exhausted.

José and Maria had met 18 months earlier at a church group for divorced individuals. They had moved in together and talked about getting married. Then they separated for 2 months during José's drug binge, when he lied repeatedly, stole money from Maria to buy drugs, and stayed away from home for weeks. When starting BCT, José had just moved back with Maria. They were still planning to marry but had not set a date.

As part of the BCT assessment, the counselor weighed violence risk carefully in both joint and separate sessions. Both reported that, even when not using drugs, José became loud and intimidating when angry and on one occasion had broken an object. However, Maria denied being afraid that he would hit her or that he had ever hit or threatened to hit her. She also said, in a private session, that she would call the police if she felt threatened. She had called the police when he was high on drugs during his earlier binge, and they had escorted him from the house. Both promised nonviolence, and the counselor reviewed this promise at each couple session.

José's Recovery Contract included the daily trust discussion with Maria and weekly urine screens, but he refused to attend 12-step meetings or to take recovery-related medication. The first four couple sessions went as planned. With help from the counselor, they did the Recovery Contract and kept the promises faithfully. José reported no major urges to use, had all clean urines, and now had over 2 months of abstinence. He got a job on a construction crew. The couple also was starting to communicate better, have fewer arguments, and were discussing their plans for marriage.

Then things began to deteriorate over the next few weeks. José stayed clean from drugs but he lost his job. His foreman felt José was bossing other men on the crew and causing tension on the job site. Financial stress and Maria's uncertainty about his reliability led to increased arguments at home and in the couple sessions. Session 7 was the worst. José was very angry that Maria was unwilling to set a wedding date. He was counting on them getting married and his two teenage sons coming to live with them. He felt betrayed, saying that she had led him on. He stormed out of the session after about 20 minutes, refusing to return. The rest of the session was spent with Maria alone, planning for her safety. She continued to contend that she did not fear he would hurt her, and that she would call the police, if necessary. Over the next few days the counselor tried to reach them by phone to see how they were doing after the tumultuous session. Finally, Maria called to say that they had separated and she had gotten a temporary restraining order. José had continued to argue the day after their session. When he broke a picture of the two of them and started threatening her, she went to a neighbor and called the police. She did not think that José had used drugs when she last saw him, but she was not sure where he was currently.

Maria accepted the offer of individual sessions and met with the counselor for five weekly sessions. The counselor explained that her role, now that they were separated, was to help each of them as individuals, not to try to help them reconcile unless that was what they both wanted. The sessions focused on what Maria could do to keep herself safe from possible harm from José. The counselor supported her decision to extend the restraining order for a year and suggested that Maria ask a friend to accompany her to court. The counselor also suggested that police should escort José when he retrieved his belongings. In addition, they discussed Maria's options for seeking support from church members and friends and for getting a roommate. Maria tried Al-Anon but was uncertain whether she would continue, preferring the support of friends from church. The counselor gave her names of two therapists in the community in case she wanted to consider longer-term issues related to the men she picks in her life. After the five sessions, Maria reported that she was relieved she had ended the relationship and felt happier than she had in many months, so the counseling ended.

The counselor also tried repeatedly to reach José. A week and a half after the last couple session, José called back. He confirmed Maria's account of their breakup and said how shocked and bitter he was because he had thought they were going to get married. He denied drug use and any intent to contact or harm Maria. He wanted to see the counselor for individual sessions but had no transportation to get to the appointment. They agreed to regular phone contact until José could get to the clinic in person, but he never returned the counselor's calls. About 3 weeks later, José was admitted to the detox unit, reporting a 2-week binge on cocaine and heroin. The BCT counselor visited José in the detox to see how he was doing. Although still bitter over the breakup, José understood that the relationship was over. His drug use and the restraining order had violated his probation, so he was court-mandated to a 90-day residential treatment program after detox. At this time the couple's case was closed because they were permanently separated, and each person had received the help they needed.

Successful Sobriety and the Bankrupt Relationship

In some cases, even though the substance abuse patient remains abstinent, the relationship is no longer viable. We call this "successful sobriety and the bankrupt relationship" and consider "breaking up without breaking out" a major accomplishment. The couple may have grown apart or one partner may be unwilling to set aside the past hurts. Whatever the reason, facing the emptiness and inevitable dissolution of the relationship often precipitates a dangerous crisis. Often there has been a strong tendency to blame the substance abuser for relationship problems. At this time there may be a strong push for the substance abuser to relapse to provide a convenient reason for the relationship breakup. As a counselor, you can try to help the couple confront separation and divorce without the substance abuser failing again and becoming the convenient scapegoat for the breakup. If the couple can separate without the substance abuser relapsing, the substance abuser's future relationship with his or her children may be preserved. It also may help both members of the couple gain a more realistic assessment of the basis for their divorce, thus reducing the intense and lengthy bitterness that accompanies many relationship breakups. To achieve this goal, you will need to follow the suggestions given above for helping couples who separate after BCT (e.g., seeing each partner separately, strengthening the patient's sobriety supports, promoting arrangements that are least destructive for all involved).

DUAL-PROBLEM COUPLES:
UNDERSTANDING THEIR TREATMENT NEEDS

Dual-problem couples are those in which both members have a current substance abuse problem. These couples present a special challenge to BCT, which relies heavily on support for abstinence from a non-substance-abusing partner. When both members want to stop drinking and drugging, the use of standard BCT, with some modifications, generally is workable. However, when one or both members of the couple lack motivation to change, special methods to increase motivation may be needed to prepare couples for BCT. The following guidelines and case examples describe how to adapt BCT for use with dual-problem couples.

Role Conflict, Role Modification, and Dual-Problem Couples

BCT builds and uses the strength of the relationship as a curative mechanism in the reduction or elimination of drinking or drug use. Thus, BCT assumes that there is sufficient support within the relationship for abstinence, particularly from the non-substance-abusing partner. The foundation of this support for change is conflict. More specifically, chronic and excessive drinking or drug use by a spouse is not compatible with fulfilling the role of being a good relationship partner. Efforts to meet the demands of both roles creates "role conflict," in which the role of being an alcoholic or drug abuser is inconsistent with the role of being a good spouse or partner.[3] In turn, partners seek change to resolve this conflict in one of three ways.

First, the partners may dissolve their relationship; in our experience, many substance-abusing patients entering treatment who are not married or cohabiting were in such a relationship at one time. Second, the substance-using partner may quit drinking or using drugs; BCT helps the partners meet this goal. Third, when both partners drink or use drugs, we often see another option of resolving role conflict: what we call "role modification." More specifically, partners in these couples resolve or otherwise avoid potential conflict by changing the very nature of their relationships to accommodate their drinking and drug use. When taking a clinical history, we often find that, at some point in the couple's relationships, only one partner abused drugs or alcohol, and the role conflict was resolved by the other partner initiating or increasing his or her use. Indeed, it is very common for drug-abusing men to introduce illicit substance use to their female partners. In turn, these couples often form drinking or drug use partnerships in which substance use becomes an important shared recreational activity. Thus, among couples in which both partners drink or use drugs, there is often implicit or explicit support for substance abuse. Conflict can arise when one partner seeks substance abuse treatment, often as a result of an external mandate.

Options for Treating Patients Who Are Part of a Dual-Problem Couple

Many married or cohabiting patients who seek substance abuse treatment are involved in intimate relationships with individuals who also have current problems with drugs or alcohol. This is particularly true of women who seek substance abuse treatment, the majority of whom have male partners with alcohol or drug problems.[4] Such patients are part of what we call a dual-problem couple. Given the scope of the problem, counselors need treatment options for these patients.

There are three approaches for treating patients who are part of a dual-problem couple. The first approach is to provide individual treatment to the patient who has sought help. Such treatment tries to strengthen the patient's motivation and supports for recovery and to teach the patient how to deal with pressures from the partner to drink and drug. Unfortunately, patients in these couples usually have fairly poor outcomes with individual treatment. If the patient successfully reduces or eliminates his or her substance use, the relationship often dissolves. In most cases, however, the treatment-seeking partner fails to stop drinking or using drugs, and the relationship survives. Treatment focused on one partner, particularly in an outpatient setting, usually will not have sufficient impact to overcome the influence of living with a husband or wife who encourages the patient to use. Residential treatment that is followed by a period of living in a substance-free setting may have a better chance of helping the patient achieve abstinence, but if the patient returns to an unchanged home environment, the risk of relapse is very high.

The other two treatment methods involve a couples-based approach. The second approach can be used when both members of the couple are motivated to change. It involves standard BCT with some minor modifications, as described in the next section. The third option, for use when only one partner is motivated to change, involves trying to increase motivation for change as preparation for BCT. This final approach is described later in this chapter.

DUAL-PROBLEM COUPLES: WHEN BOTH PARTNERS WANT TO CHANGE

Guidelines for BCT When Both Want to Change

Standard BCT, as described in this book, can be effective with dual-problem couples when both members are motivated to change.[5] If both members want to stop drinking and drugging when they first see the counselor, or if this mutual decision to seek abstinence can be attained during the first few couple sessions, then BCT generally is workable. Substance-focused BCT methods require some minor adjustments, however. You negotiate a Dual Recovery Contract with a joint trust discussion daily, along with other recovery activities for each person (partners do not have to do exactly the same recovery activities). Relationship-focused activities to increase positive activities and improve communication proceed according to standard BCT. Maintenance activities also proceed accordingly. However, some themes and issues are more frequent and more intense in these dual couples. Blame is a big issue—blame for who has the worst problem or blame for using (e.g., "I only used because you did"). Competition and criticism are also major issues that often focus on arguments about who is doing recovery the right way. Partners criticize each other because they each may be pursuing recovery in slightly different ways. For example, the person who calls his or her sponsor daily criticizes the partner who does not contact his or her sponsor so often. These couples benefit from BCT's emphasis on individual responsibility and constructive communication.

Sue and Gene: BCT with a Dual-Problem Couple When Both Want to Change

Sue and Gene were in their mid-30s, married 16 years, with three children ages 5–11. Sue was referred to the BCT counselor after a hospital detox for very heavy daily drinking, plus cocaine use three or four times per week and regular marijuana use. She also used and overused prescribed tranquilizers (benzodiazepines) prescribed by her family doctor for stress. At the first couple session, the counselor learned that Gene had similar substance problems, except that his alcohol use was not quite as heavy, so he had not gone through detox. Both had decided to "quit for good" to try to get their kids back.

They had lost custody of their three children a month earlier, when Gene was arrested for drunk driving. Sue and the three kids were in the car, and Sue also was obviously intoxicated. They had been out partying at their local bar on Friday night, had picked up the kids from a friend's house, and were driving home. The police made a complaint of suspected child neglect and endangerment to social services. Investigation and interviews of neighbors and family revealed that both Sue and Gene frequently drank and used cocaine or marijuana when caring for their kids. Social services placed the children with Sue's parents for 6–12 months, with the possibility of regaining custody if Sue and Gene got treatment and stayed abstinent.

Sue and Gene came to BCT sessions weekly for 6 months. With the counselor's help, they set up the Dual Recovery Contract shown in Figure 9.1. (Forms for the Dual Recovery Contract and calendar are in Appendix C; see Form C.28 for contract and Form C.29 for calendar.) In this contract they agreed to (1) do the daily trust discussion, in which each promised the other to stay abstinent that day, (2) take Antabuse daily together, (3) attend 12-step meetings three times weekly, and (4) undergo weekly urine screens. As shown on the Recovery Contract calendars in Figure 9.1, they were pretty faithful to the contract, once they got accustomed to it after the first few weeks. Neither of them drank while in weekly BCT.

About 5 weeks after starting BCT, Sue used cocaine on Friday night when she went to the local bar with a girlfriend. She reported this usage at the next BCT session, and her urine taken that session was positive for cocaine. They agreed in session that both the bar and the girlfriend were high-risk triggers for using that they should both avoid. However, the following Friday found them both in the bar. They had decided to go together and had pledged to each other not to drink or use cocaine but just to socialize, watch TV sports, and play pool. They planned to help each other if either was tempted. Once at the bar, they ran into the girlfriend who had given Sue cocaine the previous week. When it was offered to them, they didn't refuse but told each other "we'll just do a line each." They stuck to this limit. However, the next night they went to the bar again, and this time they each used multiple lines of cocaine.

At the following BCT session they discussed this relapse. At first they each blamed the other. Gene blamed Sue for going back to the bar and for giving in to her girlfriend's influence. Sue blamed him for not stopping her from using cocaine, for not being stronger himself. Then the counselor suggested that they analyze their mutual relapse: the triggers that had led to it, damage impact, and things learned for the future. They reflected that this level of use was not nearly as much as they had used before starting BCT. However, they were heading back to

DUAL RECOVERY CONTRACT

In order to help with their recoveries _Sue_ and _Gene_ _____ agree to the following.

Sue 's Responsibilities	_Gene_ 's Responsibilities
☒ DAILY TRUST DISCUSSION	
• States intention to stay substance free that day (and takes medication _Antabuse_ if applicable).	• States intention to stay substance free that day (and takes medication _Antabuse_ if applicable).
• Thanks partner for recovery efforts and support.	• Thanks patient for supporting his or her recovery.
• Records these actions on calendar.	• Records these actions on calendar.
☒ FOCUS ON PRESENT AND FUTURE, NOT PAST	
• Agrees not to mention partner's past substance abuse or fear about future use outside of counseling sessions.	• Agrees not to mention partner's past substance abuse or fear about future use outside of counseling sessions.
☒ WEEKLY SELF-HELP MEETINGS	
• Commitment to 12-step meetings: _AA mtgs_ 3x/wk	• Commitment to 12-step meetings: _AA mtgs_ 3x/wk
☒ URINE DRUG SCREENS	
• Urine drug screens: _Weekly at_ couple sessions	• Urine drug screens: _Weekly at_ couple sessions
☐ OTHER RECOVERY SUPPORT	
•	•

EARLY WARNING SYSTEM
If, at any time, the trust discussion (with medication, if taking it) does not take place for 2 days in a row, we will contact (therapist/phone #: _Dr. Tim O'Farrell 123-456-7899_) immediately.

LENGTH OF CONTRACT
This agreement covers the time from today until the end of weekly therapy sessions, when it can be renewed. It cannot be changed unless all of those signing below discuss the changes together.

Sue Jackson

Gene Jackson

Timothy O'Farrell Ph.D.
Therapist

_9 / 3 / xx_
Date

DUAL RECOVERY CONTRACT CALENDAR

☐ ✓ = Trust Discussion Done
☒ ⊘ = Trust Discussion with Medication (_Antabuse_)
☒ A = AA or NA Meeting
☐ N = Al-Anon or Nar-Anon
☒ D = Drug Urine + or –
☐ O = Other

FIGURE 9.1. Contract and calendar for a dual-problem couple, Sue and Gene.

201

their old pattern, with use on weekends escalating into use during the week. They realized that they would not get their children back if they continued in this pattern. Someone might see them in the bar and report them to social services—which would be quite damaging.

This relapse was a turning point for Sue and Gene. Realizing how close they had come to "starting the madness again," as Gene put it, they became more committed to their recovery. They planned specific activities for Friday and Saturday evenings, starting with an AA meeting together on Friday evening. Sue called the girlfriend to say that she wouldn't be going to the bar or using drugs, that she wanted to get her children back. Gene called the woman's boyfriend and delivered the same message. They each decided to get a sponsor and to socialize more with sober friends. They also benefited from relationship-focused parts of BCT, especially work on communication. Now that they were both abstinent, conflict between them was pretty low. They had not realized how much alcohol and drug use had caused problems between them. Their bitterest arguments and a few occasions of minor violence had always occurred when both were under the influence of alcohol and cocaine.

After 6 months of weekly BCT, Sue and Gene returned to see the counselor for quarterly checkups for 2 more years. Both stopped Antabuse soon after weekly BCT sessions ended, but both continued AA, gradually decreasing to one meeting a week. They also continued the trust discussion daily for over a year. A few months after BCT, they regained custody of their children, for which they were extremely grateful. Gene stayed abstinent, except for a few isolated days of cocaine and marijuana use in the first year after BCT. Sue also stayed abstinent until midway in the second year after BCT. An occasional glass of wine with her old girlfriend progressed quickly to a 5-day relapse of heavy drinking and daily cocaine use. Gene convinced her to enter a 3-day detox, after which they saw the BCT counselor for two crisis sessions. Sue reinstated three-times-per-week attendance at AA meetings and the daily trust discussion and went back on Antabuse for 2 months. After this relapse, she stayed abstinent.

At their final checkup visit 2½ years after starting BCT, they reflected on their lives together. They had met in high school when both were part of a group of teens into binge drinking and experimenting with drugs. Looking back, what had started as teenage fun-seeking had developed into an adult lifestyle of abusive drinking and drug use that led them to act irresponsibly in many ways. They had not thought too much about their behavior before the DUI arrest, because their friends also were into heavy drinking and drug use. They were still embarrassed and ashamed that they had lost their kids temporarily. However, they were grateful they had changed to a sober lifestyle—a change they might not have made without losing the kids. Now ages 8–14, their children were heading into the teenage years—something that scared the parents a little, given their own teenage history. The counselor recommended a class for parents of teenagers at a local church and invited Sue and Gene to return for future couple sessions, as needed.

DUAL-PROBLEM COUPLES:
WHEN ONLY ONE PARTNER WANTS TO CHANGE

The patient who enters treatment and is living with a partner who is not motivated to stop using presents a real challenge for BCT. If we assume that a major barrier to conducting BCT with such couples is an absence of motivation to change in one or both partners, then an intervention designed specifically to address lack of motivation to change should be a particularly appropriate prelude to BCT with these couples. Two substance abuse treatment approaches explicitly target motivation enhancement: motivational interviewing and contingency management. In preliminary work, we have combined each of these with BCT when working with dual-problem couples, with some positive effects.

Motivational Interviewing

Motivational interviewing (MI), developed by Miller and Rollnick and modified for use with at-risk couples by Cordova and colleagues,[6] is an empirically validated clinical approach designed to actively facilitate people's intrinsic motivation to change. Miller and Rollnick[7] define MI as "a client-centered, directive method for enhancing intrinsic motivation to change by exploring and resolving ambivalence." Ambivalence about both substance use and the relationship is likely in dual-problem couples because such couples are particularly likely to experience both the benefits and costs associated with continued usage and with contemplating change. For example, one benefit of continued substance use is often the role it plays as a central part of intimate relating. The potential loss of that source of connection between partners may diminish both partners' motivation to change, despite a variety of substance-abuse-related problems they may be experiencing.

MI can be used to actively facilitate partners' willingness to change by working with partners to perceive the discrepancies between what they are doing now (e.g., substance abuse) and what each partner cares most deeply about when contemplating his or her future (e.g., their own, their partner's, and their children's health). Rather than confronting the partners' ambivalence to change, MI can be used to help partners discover that their most cherished values are incompatible with the choices they are currently making. Further, MI can be used to help partners discover their own ability as individuals and as a partnership to pursue change successfully, particularly in the context of a proven treatment such as BCT, which can help them come together as effective teammates on the path to shared recovery. A number of well-controlled studies have demonstrated the efficacy of MI interventions with alcohol-abusing individuals.[8] What makes MI particularly compelling as a possible adaptation for using BCT with dual-problem couples is the substantial evidence that MI works well as a prelude to other treatments—even treatments with very different theories of change. In addition, Cordova and colleagues have demonstrated that MI can be easily adapted to couples work and facilitate measurable and sustained improvements in relationship functioning.

In sum, a couples-based MI approach can be added as a prelude to BCT for dual-problem couples to prepare them to work together during subsequent BCT. Once both partners are committed to change, then you can use BCT for the dual-problem couple, as described above. In our preliminary work, the combination of MI and BCT has shown some positive effects, particularly with couples in which both partners drink. To date, we have had less success with MI plus BCT with couples in which both partners use illicit drugs, whom we have found to be very difficult to engage in treatment and to establish any substantive period of abstinence.

Case Example of Motivational Interviewing with BCT

Kathy was a 33-year-old married white female referred to outpatient alcoholism treatment by her family physician. During her intake interview, Kathy reported that she began drinking regularly in her early 20s but did not view her alcohol consumption at that time as problematic.

She had met her husband, Don, at a local bar, when she was 25 years old and married him 2 years later. She reported that Don had always been a "heavy drinker," noting that he went out drinking with coworkers 3–4 nights per week and had been doing so since the beginning of their relationship. In an effort to stay close to him, Kathy reported that she would go out with her husband and his friends to bars 2–3 nights per week, but after a while felt that she was "in the way." During the last 2 years, she began drinking by herself, in the home, on an almost daily basis, consuming four to six drinks per occasion.

Kathy expressed significant concerns about escalating conflict with her husband during the last year, who often referred to her as a "drunk" and a "fat slob." Kathy sought a treatment referral from her physician because she and Don were considering having a child. She felt she was "unfit" to be a mother because of her excessive drinking. She had made several attempts to stop on her own, but with little success. Because her husband was also a regular drinker, alcohol was stored in the house and the refrigerator. She also drank in response to feeling lonely and when she had conflicts with Don.

Don was asked to come to a family assessment session as part of Kathy's intake evaluation. Kathy's description of Don's drinking behavior was fairly accurate. Although he did not view his drinking (or Kathy's) as a problem, he did express concerns about his deteriorating relationship with Kathy and whether they would make "good parents" if they were to have a child, which he also wanted. He described his own childhood as "miserable—my parents were drunks and fought like cats and dogs." He eventually agreed that Kathy should, in fact, stop drinking in the short term and generally improve her health if she was going to get pregnant.

We provided Kathy and Don with feedback on what the assessment had revealed about their drinking behavior and their relationship. Both partners were diagnosed as being dependent on alcohol and as having substantial relationship problems. Although Don did not view his drinking as problematic, both partners agreed that their relationship was an unhappy one and was something they both were motivated to address before having a baby. We also told Kathy and Don that they had significant problems with conflict resolution, deficits in communication skills, and a lack of mutual caring behaviors. They were given information about the typical relationships of couples with alcohol problems and the difficulties faced in addressing relationship problems when one or both partners have an active drinking problem. Lastly, we emphasized options available to them to address the issues identified, including couples therapy.

Kathy and Don agreed to participate in couples therapy to address their problems. Kathy also received individual alcoholism treatment to address her drinking. Don agreed not to drink during their participation in couples therapy because of concerns that to do so might interfere with success of the intervention, but he did not commit to abstinence after couples therapy was completed. He also was unwilling to engage in individual treatment to address his alcohol dependence, and this was not a requirement for his participation in couples therapy. Don did agree to remove alcohol from the house to support Kathy's effort to remain sober.

As Kathy and Don spent more quality time together, partly due to completing assignments given to them during couples therapy, both reported decreased desire to drink. Their relationship gradually improved over time. Both partners remained consistently abstinent during and after completion of couples therapy. Kathy got pregnant several months after completion of couples therapy. Long-term follow-up interviews revealed that both partners were happy with their new family, and both partners remained sober.

Contingency Management

We have seen greater success with contingency management (CM) approaches when both partners use illicit drugs. In general, the central tenets of CM treatment are to provide tangible reinforcement when a specified target behavior occurs and to withhold reinforcement when the behavior does not occur. In substance abuse treatment, these reinforcers often take the form of vouchers, which can be exchanged for retail goods. Target behaviors are often the submission of drug-free urine samples, session attendance, homework completion, and so forth. A series of studies has demonstrated that CM procedures, as an add-on to other types of counseling, are more effective than standard treatment, disease-model therapy, or behavioral counseling without CM, in terms of session attendance, number of drug-free urine samples provided during treatment, and retention in treatment. CM techniques have been shown to be effective in enhancing treatment and reducing drug use of every population tested thus far, including opioid-dependent patients in methadone maintenance programs and outpatient detoxification, patients entering drug-free treatment programs following detoxification, and patients who abuse marijuana, benzodiazepines, and alcohol. Although greatly underutilized in community-based settings, CM techniques are very powerful and effective interventions for substance abuse.[9]

We have been using CM with dual-drug-abusing couples as a method of external motivation to engage both partners in BCT. Partners receive vouchers for attending sessions and providing drug-free urine samples and breath tests that do not reveal recent alcohol use. This approach has been particularly effective with couples in which only one partner is entering treatment and is living with a partner who is not motivated to stop using. Typically, we ask the partner who was not initially entering treatment to participate in an assessment session. During this assessment session, we emphasize that it is very difficult for anyone to maintain stable abstinence if he or she is living with a partner who is actively using. Thus, we propose to both partners that they attend sessions and provide breath and urine samples three times per week. We also tell them that they need not be motivated to cease their drug use to participate, but they will only obtain vouchers for attending and for providing breath and urine samples that indicate no use. During the couple sessions, we use elements of MI, combined with standard elements of BCT, to motivate partners to work collaboratively on being drug and alcohol free.

Results for CM as a prelude to BCT, although preliminary at this time, have been very promising and are the best outcomes we have observed for dual-substance-abusing couples.[10] Although the mechanism of action by which CM helps couples change their behavior has not been studied formally, it has been our experience that the external motivation (i.e., the vouchers) for these partners to cease using drugs and alcohol allows them to make decisions about their relationship and other aspects of their lives while being abstinent at the same time. These couples report that they rarely have had this opportunity because they have not both stayed abstinent for any length of time in the past. These couples come to realize that they can, in fact, remain abstinent and gain confidence that this may be possible for the long term, even in the absence of reinforcers.

Case Example of Contingency Management with BCT

Janice was a 28-year-old African American women who was referred to outpatient treatment for cocaine dependence as part of the conditions of her court-ordered probation. According to her probation officer, Janice had been arrested for shoplifting. She later admitted to her probation officer that she regularly used crack cocaine. She also said that she wanted to have children but needed to stop using drugs before becoming pregnant. The probation officer noted that Janice was living with (but not married to) a long-time significant other, Ron, a 29-year-old African American man, but the probation officer knew very little about him.

During her intake interview at treatment entry, Janice described a 5-year history of problematic cocaine and alcohol use. She reported that Ron had introduced her to crack, and she soon developed a drug-using partnership with him in which regular cocaine use became the couple's primary recreational activity. Janice reported that she had tried to stop using crack on several occasions, but Ron continued to use in the home, dooming her efforts on each occasion. Now Janice was very motivated to stop using because continued use of cocaine (and evidence based on urine screening results) would result in a probation violation and incarceration. However, she believed strongly that her efforts would fail again if Ron continued to use. She emphasized that she loved Ron, had nowhere else to go, and was not ready to consider moving out of the home.

Janice's counselor contacted Ron and invited him to come in with Janice for what was referred to as a "relationship checkup." The counselor emphasized that Ron was not entering treatment, but that the treatment team wanted to get his views on his relationship with Janice. During the assessment, Ron admitted to smoking crack regularly. He said he planned to quit eventually, but he was not motivated to stop using now. Ron recognized the problems this created for Janice and the consequences she faced if she continued to use. He expressed some remorse but was not willing to move out of the home or commit to stop using crack.

Janice's primary counselor described the CM couples treatment to the couple. It was emphasized to Ron that he did not have to be motivated to stop using, but that he would receive vouchers that could be exchanged for goods and services with local merchants only if he provided clean urine samples for cocaine three times per week and attended couples sessions with Janice. The vouchers would increase in value as they attended consecutively scheduled sessions and provided consecutively clean urine samples. Vouchers would go back to their initial values if the person did not provide a sample at a scheduled point, missed a scheduled couples therapy session, or if the urine sample revealed cocaine use. Janice took part in the voucher program under the same conditions. She also received individual counseling as well as couples therapy. Ron was only asked to take part in the couples program, with the notion being that he was supporting Janice's treatment effort. Both agreed to participate.

The partners initially attended scheduled sessions for couples therapy and urine collection. Ron expressed surprise on several occasions that staff did not "browbeat" him to enter treatment or to go to support groups. After 4 weeks, the couple missed a conjoint therapy session and both missed a scheduled urine collection; the value of the vouchers was reduced, as agreed. The couple continued to attend conjoint sessions and provide clean urine samples for 8 more weeks. After completing the couples CM sessions, Ron entered individual-based treatment for himself. As part of their respective individual-based treatments, the voucher program was continued with Ron and Janice for an additional 8 weeks. Ron reported that he was now motivated to quit. He and Janice started attending local Cocaine Anonymous meetings. After completing outpatient treatment, the partners did not, of course, receive any more vouchers. Yet both Ron and Janice reported that they were clean and sober during the follow-up interviews conducted periodically in the year after leaving treatment.

Table 9.4 summarizes key points about treatment options for dual-problem couples.

TABLE 9.4. Dual-Problem Couples

- These are couples in which both members have a current substance abuse problem.
- They are a challenge to BCT, which relies on support for abstinence from a non-substance-abusing partner.
- They often encourage each other to use, and one may resist the other's efforts at recovery.
- Treatment options when both partners are motivated to change:
  - Use standard BCT with minor modifications.
  - Negotiate a Dual Recovery Contract.
  - Increase positive activities and teach communication.
  - Deal with competition, criticism, and blame.
- Treatment options when only one partner is motivated to change:
  - Individual treatment for willing partner—possibly residential treatment followed by substance-free housing.
  - Increase motivation as a prelude to BCT by using motivational interviewing or contingency management.

FREQUENTLY ASKED QUESTIONS

- *Question 1*: With couples who are separated when they first see you, it seems like you advocate a reconciliation so that the couple can do BCT. Many separated couples would be better off to stay apart. It seems like you try to get them to reunite, even when they shouldn't.
- *Answer*: We did not intend to convey the impression that we necessarily advocate reconciliation when a couple is separated. In our view, it is not our role to advocate or advise on whether or not partners should reconcile. Our goal is to help each person be clear about what he or she needs to see happen in order to consider reconciling. We also try to help the couple make a sound agreement and a solid plan that gives an attempt at reconciliation the best chance of being successful. Then the couple can decide whether to try a reconciliation. Although much of our work is focused on helping couples improve their relationships, we try not to impose our beliefs about staying together or splitting up on couples.

- *Question 2*: All the case examples you gave of dual-problem couples involved women who had sought help at a substance abuse treatment program. These women had male partners at home who had substance abuse problems. What about the other way around—men who seek treatment and have female partners at home with substance abuse problems?
- *Answer*: In our experience, the clinical guidelines and treatment procedures we described for these dual-problem couples apply similarly when it is the man who has sought help. However, many more of the dual-problem couples we have seen have been those in which the woman sought help. This is not surprising. The literature[11] shows that female substance abuse patients are considerably more likely to have heavy drinking or drug-abusing male partners than male substance abuse patients are to have heavy drinking or drug-abusing female partners. In our own studies,[12] nearly 70% of married or cohabiting substance-abusing women entering treatment had male partners with alcohol or drug problems, in contrast to only 20% of women partners of male alcoholics seeking treatment.

SUMMARY

- Couples who are separated when you first see them may benefit from a few exploratory sessions or more extended structured separation therapy to find out if they are committed enough to the relationship to use BCT.

- When couples separate after starting BCT, you should maintain contact with each person to promote individual well-being, minimize negative impact of the separation, and be available if they want more couples counseling.

- Dual-problem couples are couples in which both members have a current substance abuse problem. Research on treating such couples is still in the early stages, but we offer some tentative suggestions.

- When both partners are motivated to change, you can use standard BCT with minor modifications. Negotiate a Dual Recovery Contract and proceed with BCT as usual.

- When only one partner is motivated to change, try to increase motivation of the reluctant partner by using motivational interviewing or contingency management as a prelude to BCT. If this does not work or is not practical, provide individual treatment for the willing partner.

NOTES

1. Stuart (1980) suggested this type of structured separation therapy.
2. McCrady (1983); O'Farrell, Harrison, Schulmeister, and Cutter (1981).
3. For more details on role incompatibility theory as applied to couples with a substance abuse problem, see Fals-Stewart, Birchler, and O'Farrell (1999).
4. For instance, in the Winters, Fals-Stewart, O'Farrell, Birchler, and Kelley (2002) study examining the effects of BCT on drug-abusing women and their non-substance-abusing male partners, nearly 70% of married or cohabiting substance-abusing women entering treatment at the recruitment site had male partners who had alcohol or drug problems.
5. A recent study found that outcomes (after BCT) for couples in which both partners had a current alcoholism problem and both wanted to change were similar to outcomes obtained for couples in which only one member had a current alcoholism problem (O'Farrell, Fals-Stewart, & Murphy, 2003; Schumm, O'Farrell, Murphy, and Fals-Stewart, 2006).
6. Cordova, Warren, and Gee (2001); Gee, Scott, Castellani, and Cordova (2002).
7. Miller and Rollnick (2002), p. 25.
8. For a review of literature on the effectiveness of motivational interviewing, see Burke, Arkowitz, and Dunn (2002).
9. For reviews of literature on the effectiveness of contingency management in substance abuse treatment, see Higgins, Heil, and Lussier (2004) and Petry and Simcic (2002).
10. Gorman, Klostermann, Fals-Stewart, Birchler, and O'Farrell (2004).
11. Jacob and Bremer (1986); Wilsnack and Beckman (1984).
12. O'Farrell, Fals-Stewart, Murphy, and Murphy (2003); Winters, Fals-Stewart, O'Farrell, Birchler, and Kelley (2002).

10

Challenges in BCT, Part II
Violence and Other Issues

This chapter examines the use of BCT for couples with a history of partner violence. It provides an in-depth justification and an extended consideration of clinical methods for using BCT with these couples.[1] It also covers other common clinical problems encountered in the course of BCT, such as resistance and psychiatric comorbidity.

JUSTIFICATION FOR USING BCT WITH VIOLENT COUPLES

Throughout this book we have described using BCT with substance-abusing couples who have a history of intimate partner violence (IPV), unless the violence was very severe. At first glance, using BCT with couples with a history of IPV seems controversial. Many say you should not use couples therapy when there is partner violence. IPV is one of the most emotionally charged public health issues of our times, so we want to make our position clear. This section justifies using BCT with violent couples. Later sections clarify the BCT exclusion criteria based on very severe violence and summarize the aspects of BCT that aim to prevent violence.

Types of IPV

Before exploring IPV among couples seeking BCT, it is important to describe the different forms partner violence can take. IPV often is treated and discussed as if all cases of it were the same or very similar. However, physical aggression between intimate partners varies greatly along such dimensions as (1) the type and severity of aggression (e.g., a push vs. an injury-inducing beating); (2) frequency (a single push vs. repeated episodes of pushing and grabbing over an extended time frame); (3) emotional and physical impact (i.e., aggression that induces

209

fear and/or causes injury); and (4) intent of the perpetrator (planned threat or use of force to intimidate and control the partner vs. an impulsive act arising from frustration in an argument).

Johnson (1995)[2] put forth a helpful model of IPV that captures these distinctions. He described two types of IPV that appear to be conceptually and etiologically different. One type, "patriarchal terrorism," is what comes to mind when we think about men entering domestic violence treatment programs or women seeking help and refuge at shelters. Patriarchal terrorism consists of severe male-to-female physical aggression (e.g., punching, beating, threatening with weapons), with less severe female-to-male violence occurring in these episodes primarily as self-defense. For the female partner, patriarchal terrorism is marked by a high likelihood of physical injury and increased fear of the male partner. The distinctive feature of this severe type of IPV is that the man's aggression serves the purpose of dominating and controlling the female partner.

The second type of IPV, referred to as "common couple violence" or "situational violence," consists of partner aggression that is mild to moderate in severity and often engaged in by both the male and the female partner. It is less likely to cause fear in, or endanger, the female partner. It also is less likely to be used as a form of control. Common couple violence, as the name implies, is far more typical than patriarchal terrorism. As we will see, this less severe form of violence characterizes couples starting BCT.

Unfortunately, the dialogue and debate about treatment for IPV implicitly or explicitly center almost exclusively on patriarchal terrorism. Standard domestic violence interventions for court-mandated male batterers evolved as an effort to treat this form of IPV. This stance makes sense: The intervention model fits batterers' severe violence problems. The problem with assuming that all IPV is similar and requires an intervention based on the patriarchal terrorism model is that less severe forms of violence may be helped by other methods. For example, couples therapy, which is contraindicated for very severe violence arising out of patriarchal terrorism, may be effective with less severe violence.

Table 10.1 summarizes key points about the differences between patriarchal terrorism and common couple violence.

TABLE 10.1. Two Types of IPV

Patriarchal terrorism

- Involves very severe male-to-female violence (e.g., punching, beating).
- If woman is violent, it is usually in self-defense.
- Woman likely to be injured and to fear the man.
- The man uses violence to dominate and control the woman.
- This severe form of violence typifies men entering court-mandated batterer intervention programs and women seeking help at shelters.

Common couple violence

- Violence is mild to moderate severity (e.g., pushing, grabbing).
- Often both the man and woman engage in violent acts.
- Less likely to injure or scare the woman.
- Less likely to be used as a form of male control; more often arises from frustration in an argument.
- This less severe form of violence characterizes couples starting BCT.

IPV among Substance-Abusing Couples Starting BCT

Next we examine research about BCT and IPV. Some of this work was mentioned very briefly in Chapter 1, but a detailed examination is needed to show the strong evidence supporting the use of BCT with couples who have a history of IPV. The following statistics come from two recent studies of male and female alcoholic patients starting BCT. In the first study[3] of 303 male alcoholic patients and their nonalcoholic female partners, 60% of the men had been violent toward their female partner in the year before BCT; conversely, 64% of the women had been violent toward their male partner. These rates were over 5 times the comparison sample rate of 12%. In the second study[4] of 103 female alcoholic patients and their nonalcoholic male partners, 64% of the men had been violent toward their female partner in the past year, and 68% of the women had been violent toward their male partner.

What do these data on IPV among couples seeking BCT mean? In interpreting the data, we draw on our experience with over 2,500 alcohol- and drug-abusing couples in our research projects and clinical programs. First, and most striking, the prevalence of violence among these couples is very high. If we eliminated couples who had recent IPV from BCT, most patients would not qualify for the therapy. This would be a most unfortunate circumstance because BCT has proven more effective than standard individual substance abuse counseling. Excluded patients would not receive the (documented) greater benefits of BCT, including better abstinence, happier and more stable couple relationships, better child functioning, and, as we shall see below, *greater reductions in IPV*.

Second, the type of partner aggression reported by couples starting BCT was more akin to the less severe common couple violence than to patriarchal terrorism. Most of the violence reported was of mild to moderate severity, with the most frequent violent acts being pushing, grabbing, or shoving while arguing. In most of these couples both the male and female partner engaged in violence. Less than 2% of couples were excluded from these studies of BCT because (1) the woman was afraid of the man or (2) the violence was so severe as to constitute a high risk of physical injury to the woman (two markers for patriarchal terrorism).

Third, our records across multiple substance abuse treatment programs show that very few patients who seek BCT have been mandated by the courts to complete a domestic violence intervention program. Moreover, although most domestic violence programs will admit nonmandated patients, we have found that very few substance-abusing patients will accept a referral to these programs. In addition, patients who do accept the referral and attend the violence program without a court mandate typically drop out.[5] As mentioned earlier, domestic violence programs are designed for the patriarchal terrorism form of IPV and for participants mandated by the criminal justice system. In contrast, substance abuse patients starting BCT engage in less severe violence and are very rarely mandated to a domestic violence intervention program.

Finally, female-to-male IPV is very common in couples starting BCT. Among couples in which only the male partner abuses alcohol or drugs, the woman may push, grab, or slap the man out of frustration at the man's continued substance use or relapse. Among couples in which the female partner abuses alcohol or drugs, women often report that when they are intoxicated, they argue and initiate physical aggression with their male partners. Both of these situations can set the stage for reprisals by the man (either immediately or at a later time).

We are not saying that female-to-male aggression is equivalent to male perpetration of aggression. The consensus in the domestic violence literature is that male-to-female, as compared to female-to-male, violence is more damaging and disruptive. Men's greater physical size and strength make the risk of injury and potential for continued intimidation much greater for male-perpetrated domestic violence. Negative health and emotional consequences of male-to-female physical aggression appear to be greater on the female partners[6] and on children in the home[7] than female-to-male violence. For example, women are six times more likely than men to require medical care for injuries due to domestic violence.[8]

We also are not saying that a woman's violence justifies or makes her to blame for male violence. BCT strongly emphasizes that each person is responsible for controlling his or her own emotions and actions. Blaming the other person's actions for making one violent is not accepted in BCT. We are saying that female-to-male violence in couples starting BCT is not well understood currently. We need to get a better handle on IPV by female partners in their relationships: How much of it is in self-defense, how much of it is one-sided versus involving both partners, and so forth. Hopefully, studies currently in progress will answer these questions.

Table 10.2 summarizes key points about IPV among substance-abusing couples starting BCT.

Beliefs about Use of Couples Therapy with IPV

As noted, one professional view contends that couples therapy should not be used when there is partner violence. Much literature on IPV, including many practice guidelines, describe couples therapy for IPV as inappropriate, ineffective, and dangerous.[9] This strong opposition to couples therapy arises from a few key concerns. First, opponents believe that couples therapy implicitly or explicitly highlights participants' shared responsibility for IPV, which can lead to the victim assuming that she is at least partially responsible for her partner's violence and the abuser concluding that he is not fully responsible for his own aggressive behavior. Second, couples counseling encourages honest and open disclosure, with the risk that conflict in therapy sessions could escalate to violence outside the confines of therapy. Third, a victim of IPV may not be comfortable expressing her concerns honestly in the presence of her partner about such issues as the level of violence, her level of fear, and her thoughts about ending the relationship.

We agree that couples therapy should not be used with couples in whom very severe violence occurs. We think that opponents' concerns are valid for such couples. However, for the majority of substance-abusing couples that do not engage in very severe IPV, we believe that couples therapy (particularly BCT) may have certain advantages. First, BCT takes a strong

---

TABLE 10.2. IPV among Substance-Abusing Couples Starting BCT

- In male alcoholics starting BCT, over 60% were violent toward their female partner in the past year. Female-to-male violence was just as high.
- Nearly identical high violence rates are found among female alcoholic patients starting BCT.
- Most couples starting BCT engage in violence in the low to moderate severity range, akin to common couple violence, not patriarchal terrorism.
- The small number (< 2%) with very severe violence are excluded from BCT.
- If all couples with IPV were excluded from BCT, most patients would not be allowed to receive the benefits of this treatment.

stand against violence and in favor of individual responsibility. BCT stresses nonviolence by both partners and self-responsibility for violent acts. Second, we can get a more complete evaluation of the level and severity of the IPV because both partners provide information. Third, couples therapy provides a safe place in which to discuss emotionally charged topics, so that the couple can postpone talking about such topics at home until they learn the skills needed to do so constructively. Fourth, IPV most often occurs in the context of angry arguments between partners. BCT teaches anger management skills (e.g., recognition of anger, use of time-outs) and communication skills (e.g., active listening, use of "I" messages) that can reduce IPV by reducing the escalating arguments that often precede violence.

Opponents of couples therapy developed their beliefs mainly through treating and studying men entering domestic violence treatment programs and women seeking help and refuge at shelters. We developed our beliefs in favor of using BCT with substance-abusing couples by treating and studying this population. We think that opponents have overgeneralized the prohibition on couples therapy when they apply it to all couples who experience violence in their relationships. Given these conflicting beliefs, what does the research show? Is BCT safe and effective to use with substance abuse patients when there is IPV? Only very recently has sufficient evidence accumulated to answer this question with confidence.

Table 10.3 summarizes key points against using couples therapy with IPV.

Outcome Data on Use of BCT with IPV among Substance-Abusing Couples

Research shows that BCT with alcoholic and drug-abusing couples substantially reduces IPV, and reduces IPV more than standard individual counseling. Studies also suggest that BCT reduces IPV because it reduces the substance use and relationship problems that are risk factors for IPV and teaches specific skills to prevent violence. These conclusions run contrary to what opponents of couples therapy for IPV might have predicted. Notably, these conclusions come from studies that replicate similar findings across multiple reasonably sized samples. As we briefly consider this body of research, keep in mind that the studies excluded less than 2% of couples seeking BCT due to the woman's fear or very severe violence.

In two studies male-to-female partner violence was significantly reduced in the first and second years after BCT, and it was nearly eliminated with abstinence. O'Farrell and colleagues[3] examined partner violence before and after BCT for 303 married or cohabiting male alcoholic patients and used a demographically matched nonalcoholic comparison sample. In the year before BCT, 60% of alcoholic patients had been violent toward their female

---

TABLE 10.3. Beliefs against Using Couples Therapy with IPV

1. Many say you should not use couples therapy when there is partner violence.

2. Opponents believe that couples therapy implicitly highlights partners' shared responsibility for IPV and obscures individual responsibility for it.

3. Conflict in therapy sessions could escalate to violence outside of therapy.

4. A female victim of IPV may fear being honest in the presence of her partner.

5. We agree that BCT should not be used with very severe IPV, but BCT should not be banned for most substance-abusing couples that have less severe IPV.

partner—five times the comparison sample rate of 12%. In the year after BCT, violence had decreased significantly to 24% of the alcoholic sample but remained higher than the comparison group. Among remitted alcoholics after BCT, violence prevalence of 12% was identical to the comparison sample and less than half the rate among relapsed patients (30%). Results for the second year following BCT yielded similar findings to those found for the first-year outcomes. Thus, partner violence decreased after BCT, and clinically significant violence reductions occurred for patients who ceased drinking after BCT. An earlier study of 88 male alcoholics found nearly identical results.[10]

In four randomized studies conducted by Fals-Stewart and colleagues, BCT reduced partner violence more than individual substance abuse counseling. The design and results of each study were very similar. Only the patient population examined differed. All patients were scheduled to receive the same number of outpatient counseling sessions, and patients were randomized to receive all individual counseling sessions or half BCT and half individual sessions. When we talk about results for BCT in these studies, we are referring to the latter group who received half BCT and half individual sessions. All four studies found high levels of male-to-female violence in the year before treatment. Outcomes after BCT consistently showed significantly reduced violence in the year after BCT, and greater violence reductions among patients who received BCT than among those who got only individual counseling. BCT also showed more abstinence and greater relationship satisfaction than individual counseling. These nearly identical results occurred in four studies of (1) 80 mixed male drug-abusing patients (mostly with cocaine and heroin problems),[11] (2) 195 male alcoholic patients,[12] (3) 105 female alcoholic patients,[13] and (4) 215 cocaine-dependent patients.[14]

Reasons Why BCT Reduces IPV

Why does BCT reduce IPV more than standard individual substance abuse counseling? Some of the studies just reviewed examined this question. The answer is, as noted, that BCT reduces IPV because it reduces the substance use and relationship problems that are general risk factors for IPV, and it also teaches specific skills to prevent violence. In terms of general risk factors, the study of 80 mixed male drug-abusing patients[11] found that BCT reduced violence better than individual treatment because BCT reduced drug use, drinking, and relationship problems to a greater extent than individual treatment. The study of 303 male alcoholic patients[3] found that attending more scheduled BCT sessions and using BCT-targeted behaviors more during and after treatment were related to less drinking and less violence after BCT, suggesting that skills couples learn in BCT may promote both sobriety and violence reductions.

What specific skills taught in BCT may prevent violence? BCT teaches communication skills to reduce hostile conflicts that may escalate to violence. In the study of 195 male alcoholic patients,[12] those who participated in BCT reported less frequent hostile conflicts (e.g., yelling, name calling, threatening to hit, hitting) during treatment than those who received individual treatment. These results show that couples who take part in BCT do learn to handle their conflicts with less hostility and aggression. Most important, reduced hostile conflicts during treatment explained the lower violence for BCT than for individual treatment in the year after treatment, presumably because couples continued to use the conflict management skills they had learned during BCT. In addition to conflict management skills, less drinking and happier relationships among those in BCT also explained the lower violence for BCT.

Learning skills to reduce conflict when the patient relapses, which is part of the spouse's action plan to stay safe if relapse occurs (see Chapter 8), also may prevent violence. We know that there is a strong link between relapse and violence in the year after treatment; conversely, there is a strong link between abstinence and nonviolence. However, relying only on abstinence to reduce the risk of violence has limitations, given the high relapse rate among patients in alcoholism and drug-abuse treatment. BCT teaches the non-substance-abusing partner certain coping skills (e.g., leaving the situation, avoiding conflict-inducing and emotionally laden discussion topics with an intoxicated partner) designed to reduce the likelihood of aggression when the male partner is intoxicated. These skills are designed to reduce partner violence even when relapse occurs (i.e., BCT does not rely exclusively on abstinence as the way to avoid violence). Thus, we would expect to find differences in the likelihood of IPV on days of drinking or drug use among patients with a history of IPV who receive individual treatment for substance abuse versus those patients who receive BCT. A recent pilot study provided initial support for this hypothesis. Fals-Stewart[15] randomly assigned couples with an alcoholic male partner and recent history of IPV to BCT or to individual-based alcoholism treatment for the male partner only. During the year after treatment, the likelihood of IPV on days of substance use were compared for the two groups. As expected, on days when the male partner drank, the likelihood of male-to-female violence was lower for couples who had received BCT compared to couples in which the male partner got only individual alcoholism counseling.

Table 10.4 summarizes key points about outcome data that support using BCT for substance-abusing couples with a history of IPV.

Conclusions about Using BCT with Substance-Abusing Couples Who Have a History of IPV

We advocate using BCT with substance-abusing couples who have a history of IPV, unless the violence is very severe. Although nearly two-thirds of couples seeking BCT have experienced IPV in the past year, most of this violence is low to moderate in severity. For the most part, these couples do not engage in the very severe violence seen in men entering court-mandated batterer intervention programs and women seeking help at shelters, for which we agree that couples therapy is not indicated. Research clearly shows that BCT with alcoholic and drug-

---

TABLE 10.4. Outcome Data Support Using BCT for Substance-Abusing Couples with IPV

1. Research shows that BCT with alcoholic and drug-abusing couples
   a. Substantially reduces IPV, and
   b. Reduces IPV more than standard individual substance abuse counseling.
2. A series of studies has replicated these findings across multiple reasonably sized samples.
3. Studies also suggest that BCT reduces IPV because BCT
   a. Reduces substance use and relationship problems that are risk factors for IPV, and
   b. Teaches specific skills to prevent violence; namely, communication skills to reduce hostile conflicts and coping skills to minimize conflict when the substance abuser relapses.

---

abusing couples substantially reduces IPV, and reduces IPV more than standard individual counseling. If we eliminated couples who had experienced recent IPV from BCT, it would prevent most patients and their families from receiving the benefits of this treatment.

EXCLUDING COUPLES
WITH VERY SEVERE VIOLENCE FROM BCT

Specific Violence Exclusion Criteria for BCT

Most partner violence among substance abuse patients is not so severe that it precludes BCT. Unless the violence has been so severe that there remains an acute risk of violence that could cause serious injury or be potentially life-threatening, BCT generally can be used. However, it is important to identify and exclude from BCT the few couples that have a risk for very severe violence.

As described in Chapter 2, the first step is to find out if the couple has a history of partner violence. A history of partner violence is defined as pushing, grabbing, shoving, hitting, slapping, kicking, biting, choking, using weapons, or other violent or threatening acts by either the male or female partner. In separate interviews, we collect information from partners in couples with a history of violence to determine the degree, severity, and impact of the violence on the relationship. Our goal is to exclude couples who present an acute risk of very severe violence or are otherwise unsuitable for BCT due to partner violence. We use the specific exclusion criteria for BCT shown in Table 10.5 to guide our risk assessment. It is important to stress that these criteria are guidelines, not hard and fast rules. The decision to exclude a couple from BCT due to partner violence concerns should be based on an overall clinical assessment of the risk of harm that could occur from pursuing BCT. However, we rarely exclude couples on these grounds. As noted earlier, less than 2% of couples who have participated in our research or clinical programs have been excluded from BCT for these reasons.

Next we present two case examples to illustrate the process of violence risk assessment in BCT. The first case is one of the few couples that we excluded from BCT due to very severe violence. The second case is a more typical couple with a partner violence history that was treated in BCT.

TABLE 10.5. BCT for Substance-Abusing Couples with Partner Violence: Exclusion Criteria

- One or both partners report fear of injury, death, or significant physical reprisal from the other.
- Very severe violence (defined as resulting in injury requiring medical attention or hospitalization) has occurred in past 2 years.
- One or both partners have been threatened or harmed by the significant other using a knife, gun, or other weapon.
- One or both partners are fearful of participating in couples treatment.
- One or both partners want to leave the relationship due, in whole or in part, to the degree and severity of partner aggression.

From "Addressing Intimate Partner Violence in Substance-Abuse Treatment," by W. Fals-Stewart and C. Kennedy, 2005, *Journal of Substance Abuse Treatment*, 29, p. 13. Copyright 2005 by Elsevier Inc. Adapted with permission.

Case Example of a Couple Excluded from BCT
Due to Very Severe Violence

Max and Jen were a couple in their mid-30s. They had been living together, on and off, for 4 years in Jen's government-subsidized apartment. Jen received disability payments for being mentally disabled due to bipolar disorder. Max was unemployed and receiving public assistance income. Together they could afford to keep Jen's apartment and pay other expenses.

A week before their BCT intake session, Max had been drinking when he saw his probation officer, who told him that drinking violated his probation. The judge would likely send him to jail when he appeared for an upcoming court date for assault charges from a bar fight. The probation officer said that if he sought help for his drinking and stayed sober, he might be able to avoid jail. In addition, Jen was questioning whether to let Max continue to live with her if he continued drinking. Max scheduled an intake with the BCT program (rather than for individual counseling) because he wanted Jen to know that he was getting help so she would let him continue to live with her.

At the BCT intake session, when questioned about violence, Max reported that he had been released 2 months ago after 90 days in jail for domestic assault on Jen. The incident occurred when Max was drunk and they were arguing. He hit her and threw her to the floor; her ribs were broken when she fell against a table. Jen had been hospitalized overnight and still had pain from the rib injury. Both agreed that there had been a number of other violent arguments, including a few in which the police had been called by neighbors, but it had never been this bad before. The counselor also noticed that Max had obviously been drinking, and Jen was in an anxious, agitated state. They reported arguing that day, including on the way to the BCT session. Jen reported that she had stopped taking her lithium and attending her mental health counseling over a month ago. It was clear that this couple was a high-risk case and apparently in crisis.

After initial information gathering, the counselor met with each of them alone to get more details about the violence history and to formulate a plan. She met with Jen first. Jen was scared that there might be violence if they went home together. Max was drinking, they had been arguing, and he had threatened her on the way to the session. Jen also described additional violent incidents not revealed in the conjoint session. On occasion, this violence had caused red marks or bruises for which medical attention was not sought. It also led to an earlier restraining order—which he had violated, been jailed for, and was still on probation for.

Then the counselor met with Max, who admitted he had been drinking heavily for the past 3 weeks. Based on the probation officer's comments, he was afraid he might land back in jail. The counselor asked if he wanted to enter detox and consider a 30-day residential program. It would help him stop drinking and look good to his probation officer. Max agreed, and the counselor walked him to admitting for detox. Then she helped Jen call a friend to take her home. She also had Jen phone her therapist and psychiatrist and leave a message asking for appointments. When the counselor saw her 2 days later, Jen had talked with the psychiatrist by phone and restarted her lithium. She was going to see her therapist for a crisis appointment that afternoon and planned to restart weekly counseling.

At a follow-up appointment 2 weeks later, Jen was feeling a little better after restarting her medication and seeing her therapist. She was undecided about her relationship with Max and was discussing this issue with her therapist. The BCT counselor also followed up with Max. He had completed detox and was now in the first week of a 4-week residential program. At this point 2 weeks after the BCT intake session, the immediate crisis was over. Both Max and Jen had therapy commitments to address their individual needs. Therefore, the BCT counselor did not plan any further contact.

Case Example of a Couple with Partner Violence That Was Treated in BCT

Craig and Joan were a couple in their late 30s who had been married for 8 years and had lived together for 6 years before that. They were referred for evaluation for BCT by staff in a detox center when Craig was admitted for treatment of his problems with cocaine and alcohol. In the early years of their relationship, Joan had drunk and used cocaine together with Craig, but she had stopped cocaine and reduced her drinking soon after they married. In the past few years she had used alcohol only occasionally.

At the BCT intake session, when questioned about violence, they reported four incidents during their relationship. The first two incidents occurred in the early years of their relationship, on occasions when both of them had been drinking heavily and using cocaine. They would begin to argue verbally, then escalate to Joan's pushing and punching Craig, and Craig's slapping Joan. They denied that either of them sustained injury or required medical attention. They said that police intervened on one occasion, but no charges were filed. Both denied ever using a weapon against the other or threatening to hurt the other. There had been no restraining orders.

The other two episodes happened in the last year when Craig had been drinking or using coke. The most recent had occurred about 2 months ago. Both incidents had happened when Craig returned home intoxicated and high, after being out at a local bar, having told Joan that he had to work late. Craig would insist he wasn't intoxicated and had been at work, despite appearances to the contrary. Joan would get very angry at Craig's lying and repeated broken promises to stop cocaine and cut down on his drinking. Then both of them would begin yelling, which quickly escalated to pushing and shoving from both. No physical harm or legal involvement was reported in response to these violent incidents. In addition, they both reported fairly frequent intense arguments that did not end in violence, but did involve harsh criticism, name calling, yelling, and threatening to end the relationship.

Craig and Joan saw their violent actions in the past year as an integral part of their arguments over Craig's substance abuse problem and other relationship concerns. They were surprised when the counselor labeled their more recent actions of mutual pushing and shoving as "violence." However, they did consider the incidents in the earlier years of their relationship as violent in character. Both denied fear of violence currently and were not afraid that couples therapy sessions would lead to violence. Based on this violence history, the BCT counselor concluded that Craig and Joan were not currently at high risk for very severe violence. She therefore decided to proceed with BCT.

Craig and Joan were similar to many other couples with a violence history that we have treated in BCT. Both had been violent at times. There was no recent very severe violence. The few recent violent incidents that occurred were substance related, either when Craig was drinking or using drugs or Joan was feeling angry and helpless about his substance abuse. They readily agreed to the promise of nonviolence at the start of BCT and did not have much difficulty keeping their word. They still struggled with anger and, at times, intense verbal conflict about relationship problems, but they did not become violent. Once they had made a commitment to nonviolence, removed substance abuse from the picture, and started to work on improving their relationship, they were unlikely to experience violence. The BCT work on communication skills helped them discuss relationship problems more constructively. They also got better at handling conflicts and reduced their angry flare-ups. Finally, near the end of weekly BCT sessions, when planning how to handle a possible relapse, they agreed to avoid confrontation and thereby prevent violence between them.

ASPECTS OF BCT THAT AIM TO PREVENT VIOLENCE

The general goals of BCT are to promote abstinence and improve relationship functioning. BCT reduces violence by reducing the substance use and relationship problems that are general risk factors for IPV. In addition, a number of specific aspects of BCT aim to prevent violence. Beginning with the initial assessment and continuing to the point of planning for relapse prevention, specific BCT procedures focus directly on preventing violence. This section briefly reviews these five aspects of BCT, which have been covered in earlier chapters.

Assessment of Violence History and Exclusion of Couples with Very Severe Violence

The clinical assessment that starts during the initial couple session includes an assessment for partner violence for each couple who seeks BCT. For couples with a history of partner violence, in-depth questioning of the male and female partner determines the extent of current risk for very severe violence. If the assessment shows an active and acute risk for very severe violence that could cause serious injury or be potentially life-threatening, the couple is excluded from BCT. In such cases, it is better to treat the substance abuser and the partner separately rather than together. Although substance abuse patients seeking BCT frequently have a history of partner violence, most of this violence is not so severe that it precludes BCT. Chapter 2 and the preceding section provide more details.

Commitment to Nonviolence and Ongoing Monitoring

Each member of the couple agrees to refrain from violence or threats of violence as part of the promises made at the start of BCT. The therapist closely monitors compliance with this promise at each BCT session. Nearly all couples, even those with a history of IPV, successfully keep their promise of nonviolence while attending weekly BCT sessions. For the rare couple that experiences minor violence more than once or any incidents of more serious violence while attending BCT, we recommend terminating the couples therapy and providing separate treatment for each partner. The therapist also reviews situations when either person was concerned that anger might escalate to threats or violence. This helps identify factors that could trigger violence. It also provides an opportunity to teach the couple that each person is responsible for controlling his or her own emotions and actions. Blaming the other person's actions for making one violent is not accepted in BCT.

Teaching General Communication Skills

BCT teaches the general communication skills of listening, expressing feelings directly, and the use of planned, structured communication sessions. These general communication skills can reduce hostile conflicts that have the potential to escalate to violence. Applying these skills slows down couple interactions and reduces angry flare-ups that may lead to violence. The goal of these skills is to convey respect and understanding to each person even when there is disagreement. In addition, BCT teaches problem-solving skills to deal with external stressors and negotiation skills to resolve requests for change. Both can reduce stress, hostility, and potential for violence. Chapters 6 and 7 provide more details.

Teaching Specific Conflict Resolution Skills

BCT also teaches specific conflict resolution skills, beginning with the principle that conflict is inevitable when two people address emotionally charged issues and disagreements, and that how they handle the conflict is key. Couples learn about ineffective methods of dealing with conflict (e.g., verbal and physical aggression) and how to address conflict effectively with respect, understanding, and fairness. BCT provides couples with extensive coaching on general communication skills as partners apply them to high-conflict issues in their relationship. BCT also teaches couples to use a time-out agreement as a way to contain conflict: If either party feels uncomfortable that a discussion may be escalating, he or she says, "I'm getting uncomfortable and want a 5-minute time-out." Each partner goes to a separate room or location and uses slow, deep breathing or some other relaxation method to calm him- or herself. Afterward, the couple may restart the discussion if both desire it. Chapter 7 provides more details.

Action Plan to Stay Safe If Relapse Occurs

Near the end of weekly BCT sessions, the couple formulates an action plan for what to do if drinking or drug use occurs. Staying safe by preventing violence is an important part of the plan. Many couples tend to argue when the substance abuser drinks or uses drugs. It is only natural that the spouse becomes angry if the substance abuser relapses. However, arguing with an intoxicated person can lead to conflict and possible violence. Therefore, we ask the spouse to *avoid* confronting the substance abuser when he or she is under the influence of alcohol or drugs or hungover. In addition, for couples with a history of partner violence, we ask the spouse to leave the situation if warning signs of aggression occur and to call the police if violence or threats of violence erupt. This plan is one way to keep both members of the couple safe and protected from unwanted conflict that they could regret later. Chapter 8 provides more details.

Table 10.6 summarizes key points about aspects of BCT that aim to prevent violence.

OTHER CHALLENGES

This section considers a variety of other common clinical problems encountered in the course of BCT. We covered a few of these challenges, to some degree, in earlier chapters, and we present them here for easy reference.

TABLE 10.6. Aspects of BCT That Aim to Prevent Violence

- Assessment of violence history
  - Assess violence history during initial session.
  - Assess risk for couples with violence history.
  - Exclude couple if risk of very severe violence.
- Commitment to nonviolence
  - Ask couple to promise not to be violent.
  - Monitor nonviolence promise at each session.
  - Use close calls as teaching opportunity.
  - Stop BCT if two occasions of minor violence or any severe violence occurs.
- Teaching general communication skills
  - Teach listening skills and how to express feelings directly.
  - Explain and model planned, structured communication sessions.
  - Teach how to reduce hostile conflicts that can escalate to violence.
- Teaching specific conflict resolution skills
  - Explain that conflict is inevitable, how they handle it is key.
  - Explain that verbal and physical aggression are ineffective.
  - Coach communication about high-conflict issues.
  - Teach time-out agreement to contain conflict.
- Formulation of action plan to keep partner safe if relapse occurs
  - Do not argue with substance abuser who is drinking, using drugs, or hungover.
  - Leave situation if warning signs of violence occur.
  - Call police if violence or threats of violence erupt.

Resistance and Noncompliance

Frequently, each member of the couple will want the other person to change first, loving feelings to precede loving action, and to solve their most difficult problems first before committing further to therapy or the relationship. Often these attitudes and feelings are understandable, given the couple's history. Unfortunately, however, these attitudes do not fit well with BCT. BCT asks each person to voluntarily make changes that will improve the relationship, to act more positively toward the partner in hopes that doing so will lead to more positive feelings, and to start with small changes before attempting to tackle major issues. The therapist can point out that the couple's approach has not been working and that a new approach is needed if the relationship is to improve. The therapist needs to stress that the partners have neither the skill nor the goodwill and positive feeling needed for the negotiation and compromise that could help them resolve their major problems and differences. Changing how they act with each other and giving their relationship a good chance to improve will require risk and vulnerability. Repeating this rationale often helps partners initially decide to engage fully in the therapy and later to recommit themselves to the effort after backsliding or noncompliance.

Resistance to Behavioral Rehearsal

Most couples have some initial resistance to engaging in behavioral rehearsal ("role playing"), an important method used in BCT to help couples make positive behavior changes. Usually this resistance is overcome fairly easily if the therapist gives clear instructions and rationale for the role playing so that partners know what to do and why it is important. The therapist also must model the desired behavior. To get the person started in the role play, the therapist can prompt responses by providing the first words, if necessary. After the person role-plays his or her response, the therapist gives positive feedback first, followed by suggestions for improvement. Although reluctance to role-play generally decreases in later sessions, some resistance often remains and requires skillful effort to overcome it.

The therapist also might be reluctant to engage in behavioral rehearsal, especially a therapist who is new to this approach. The therapist and couple may talk a lot about the new skills but spend very little time actually participating in behavioral rehearsal. One way to deal with this problem is to record the amount of time spent role playing during each session; this tactic generally prompts increased time spent on rehearsal during the sessions. Additionally, sessions can be videotaped and used for review by the therapist and for supervision purposes.

Resistance to Home Practice

Weekly home practice assignments, which are designed to transfer new behaviors learned in the session to the couple's day-to-day life at home, require specific procedures to gain compliance. The therapist explains the reasons for weekly assignments and asks for a verbal commitment from the partners to do the home practice. When discussing a possible assignment for the coming week, stress that partners have a choice whether or not to accept the assignment. Indicate that you would rather they refused an assignment or agreed to do less than suggested than to agree and then not follow through. A midweek phone call between sessions can prompt and reinforce performance of the assignments. Such prompting phone calls can be done every session, only for the first few weeks, or only when a couple is having trouble completing assignments.

What do you do when the couple shows up in your office without having completed the assignment? This happens frequently despite therapists' best efforts to explain the assignment carefully and get explicit pledges to follow through. A few simple suggestions may help. First, respond matter-of-factly without blame, disappointment, or criticism. Do not question partners' commitment to the therapy or lecture them about the need for assignments or that they promised to do their assignments. Do not look for the deeper reasons behind their noncompliance (at least, not the first few times). Although some noncompliance does reflect a deeper anger or fear about the relationship, missing or incomplete assignments are so common that we expect them and do not infer underlying reasons. Therapists should reinforce and work with whatever the couple did manage to do, because compliance is often partial.

Second, have them do in session what they were supposed to do at home. This response emphasizes that in BCT they need to complete prior steps before going on to later steps. It is important to set this expectation right from the beginning. For example, as described in Chapter 3, a couple may fail to complete and discuss a worksheet meant to prepare them for signing the Recovery Contract. When this happens, explain that you will need the worksheet later in the session and ask them to complete and discuss it now. Leave the office for a few minutes to give them privacy while they complete the assignment. Do this matter-of-factly, without expressing disappointment or blame, and you will have sent a powerful message about the need for compliance with agreed-to assignments.

Another common example is when one or both partners bring in totally or partly blank Catch Your Partner Doing Something Nice sheets. In the daily review of the previous week, the person who failed to write down anything their partner did nice can be asked to remember at least something from the most recent days and provide the missing answers in session. Or consider the couple in which both partners brought blank sheets because they "had a bad week" and were not getting along very well. After processing the bad week and hopefully reaching some common ground (possibly just that the therapist heard and understood their conflicting view points), you can return to the assignment. You can ask each person to think back over the past week, unhappy as it may have been, and share the two most positive things the partner did. By having the couple do all or part of the missed assignment during the BCT session, you are reinforcing successive approximations to the desired goal of completing the assignments, as agreed.

Finally, if one or both members of the couple consistently fail to complete agreed-to assignments over several sessions, then the reasons for the noncompliance should be explored. The solution will depend on the cause of the problem. For couples who have very hectic lives with little time for BCT assignments, it may be best to limit assignments to the most critical elements (e.g., Recovery Contract) and work on other elements mainly during the couple sessions, with less required preparation or practice at home. This approach may slow progress but it may be a pragmatic solution. For other couples, consistent noncompliance may be due to underlying anger or uncertain commitment to the relationship by one of the partners. In such cases, one or more individual sessions may help to clarify whether the problem can be overcome (see the next section).

Clinical Impasse

If one or both partners are unable to move past their anger or other significant obstacles to progressing in treatment, an individual session for one or both partners between couple meetings may be necessary. This session (more than one, if necessary) allows for exploration of past hurt, pain, and anger. The therapist focuses on the individual with the goal of showing that the therapist understands and empathizes with the person's feelings. The session(s) also focuses on how the person might move past the feelings or how his or her partner could help the person to do so, in order to work on the relationship. When using individual sessions, it is vital that both partners understand that the therapist is not siding with one or the other. This point can be made explicit before and after the individual session with a summary of the goal of the individual sessions and the progress made toward that goal.

Couples Who Are Angry When They Come to Session

A common problem occurs when a couple comes to a session with one or both members feeling quite angry and upset over a conflict they had in the past week. Try to defer a full discussion of the conflict until assignments have been reviewed. At least review compliance with the Recovery Contract and whether there has been any substance use. If the anger and upset relate to substance use that happened in the past week, then use the guidelines for such situations discussed in Chapter 4.

When faced with an angry couple, your goal is to reduce anger and tension and prevent negativity from continuing at home after the couple leaves the session. (If feelings were particularly intense, you may want to call the couple 24–48 hours after the session to see how things are going.) If possible, you also would like each person to feel that their point of view was understood by the therapist and by the partner. Ideally, you also would help partners find common ground and at least a temporary resolution to the issue that provoked the conflict.

We suggest three main methods to use to achieve these goals when you encounter an angry couple. First, you can coach the couple to use the listener and speaker skills described in Chapter 6 to discuss the conflict. However, this option works only if both members of the couple have some mastery of these skills. Even with couples who have developed the skills, this approach will not work if negative emotions are too intense.

Second, you can coach the couple to talk out the problem using you, the therapist, as a "listening post." Have each person explain his or her feelings to you, and show your understanding of the person's message by using listening and understanding responses ("What I heard you saying was. . . . Did I get that right?"). Repeat this process with both partners until each person affirms that you have understood his or her point of view. This method slows down the conversation and defuses anger because each person feels understood. It may help the couple find common ground or a partial resolution. This is the method we use most often, and it is a good place to start. You can move back to the first option and let the couple take over if this seems like it would work, or you can move up to the next option if the couple is too upset to use this "listening post" method.

Finally, you can speak with each member of the couple alone while the other sits in the waiting area. We generally speak first with the person who seems the most upset. Usually meeting alone with each person once is sufficient, but occasionally you will have to do this more than once. When talking separately, empathize with each person's point of view and also try to help them see the partner's point of view. Then bring them back together as a couple. Based on what you learned from each individual, actively guide the couple to defuse the conflict and possibly find a partial resolution.

Psychiatric Comorbidity

In a number of couples who seek BCT, the substance abuser or the spouse has serious emotional problems that can present a challenge. However, often BCT can be effective with such cases when it is used along with appropriate individual therapy and psychotropic medication. In such cases, medications for psychiatric problems can be taken during the daily trust discussion. In addition, individual therapy appointments can be added to the couple's Recovery Contract and marked on the calendar the same way attendance at AA meetings is marked. Including such elements strengthens the Recovery Contract as a sign of a couple's joint commitment to improve their lives together. In addition, the BCT counselor should get a signed release to contact the person's individual therapist. The BCT counselor and the individual therapist should have ongoing periodic contacts to share information and monitor progress. It is important to ask the individual therapist to encourage his or her patient to discuss concerns about the couple's relationship in BCT sessions. Otherwise, a split often occurs wherein the patient complains about relationship problems to the individual therapist but does not share these fully in BCT sessions, where they could be addressed. Finally, for couples with significant psychiatric comorbidity, BCT sessions may need to proceed more slowly than usual and be carefully tailored to the special needs of such couples.

Reading Level

You may encounter couples in which one member has difficulty reading or is unable to read at all. This deficit can affect the presentation of the Recovery Contract and other parts of BCT that typically rely on understanding written material. In such cases, the therapist may be able to rely on the partner with the better reading skills, who may be accustomed to helping his or her partner in a natural way. Other options for the Recovery Contract include the therapist reading the contract to the partners; altering the agreement by making it a verbal one; or using a simplified written version. These same options apply to other aspects of BCT. The main response to the challenge of low reading level is to simplify most aspects of BCT. More details on how to reduce reliance on reading for the BCT methods intended to increase positive activities are given at the end of Chapter 5. Most couples can understand and carry out basic aspects of BCT, even if one has a low reading level.

Issues Related to Sexual Intimacy

Throughout the assessment and therapy process in BCT, issues related to sexual intimacy may become apparent. Although it is beyond the scope of BCT to address sexual issues in detail, therapists can encourage couples to use the skills they learn in BCT to address them. For example, the therapist might encourage the partners to plan a special evening together ("sex date") as their shared rewarding activity or to use "I" messages and positive specific requests to communicate what they would like from each other. If sexual concerns are long-standing, it may be better to address them during extended maintenance and relapse prevention sessions, after a period of stable abstinence and improved relationship functioning has been achieved.

Either Partner Discloses Infidelity or High-Risk Behavior for HIV

If either partner discloses infidelity to the therapist but the affair is in the past, we do not require disclosure to the other partner. If it is not an issue now and does not appear to be an issue going forward, we encourage disclosure for health reasons, but do not make it a requirement for continued BCT treatment. However, if a person reports being actively involved in an affair or has a competing love interest, we will not treat him or her in BCT. In that case, either the person has to end the affair immediately or tell the partner immediately, or we discontinue BCT. If the affair is terminated, we strongly encourage disclosure but do not make it a requirement. Early in our experience doing BCT, we tried disclosing past extramarital sex during couples therapy in a few cases, but all of the couples discontinued therapy.

If it is possible that there has been exposure to HIV through infidelity or risky drug-use practices, as described in more detail in Chapter 11, the partners should be strongly encouraged to do the following:

1. Immediately begin, or return to, using condoms in their relationship.
2. Get tested for HIV.
3. Partners will have to wait at least 3 months after the possible exposure before being tested, and they must use condoms during that time to protect from HIV infection.
4. If the partners test negative, they need to continue to follow the HIV risk-reduction plan, which involves avoiding risky behaviors in the future (see Chapter 11).

Either Partner Discloses HIV-Positive Status That Is Unknown to the Other

If either partner discloses HIV-positive status that is unknown to the other, the therapist might feel conflicted by individual moral obligations, professional ethical obligations, and the law. State laws vary on mandated partner notification, and partners are generally not notified without the HIV-positive patient's permission. Under the American Psychological Association (APA) Ethics Code Standard 1.14, psychologists have a duty to minimize harm when it is foreseeable and avoidable.[16] This standard would seem to dictate the necessity of disclosing the patient's HIV-positive status. However, state law might say otherwise. Current New York State law, for example, prohibits disclosure of a patient's HIV status without written permission from the patient. Given conflicting standards, counselors should become informed about their state laws and then act accordingly.

The National Institute on Drug Abuse (NIDA) suggests that HIV-positive patients should be counseled to inform their primary partner and other drug and sex partners, if possible, about potential risk of infection and the importance of getting tested and counseled for HIV and other blood-borne infections. Patients should be encouraged to seek medical treatment for HIV and to follow recommended practices with regard to obtaining and adhering to medications to slow or prevent the onset of HIV symptoms. They should also be advised to get off and stay off drugs and to maintain overall health through proper nutrition, rest, and exercise.

FREQUENTLY ASKED QUESTIONS

- *Question 1*: It seems as if you are at least partly blaming the woman for being physically abused by her husband or male partner. Toward the end of BCT, when planning for how to deal with relapse, you counsel the woman not to argue with the man if he relapses because he might get violent toward her. This advice seems to imply that you are making the woman responsible for the man's violence rather than holding him accountable for his own actions.

- *Answer*: We do not agree with this assessment for two reasons. First, the principle of individual responsibility that is integral to BCT certainly applies to partner violence. The woman is responsible for her own actions. In our opinion, if there are reasonable steps she can take to ensure her own safety, then she should take them. This does not mean that she is responsible for the man's behavior. In BCT the man is responsible and held accountable for his actions. For couples with a history of partner violence, we ask the spouse to leave the situation if warning signs of aggression occur when there is a relapse or a serious escalation of conflict and to call the police if violence or threats of violence erupt.

Second, Rychtarik and McGillicuddy[17] provide some support for the approach used in BCT of teaching women coping skills to deal with their partner's drinking in a way that protects them from being violently victimized. They compared coping skills training with Al-Anon facilitation therapy for women distressed by living with an actively drinking alcoholic husband or male partner. They taught women coping skills designed to reduce the likelihood of violence when the male partner was intoxicated (e.g., leaving the situation, not arguing with him). Coping skills training, as compared with Al-Anon facilitation therapy, resulted in less physical abuse from husbands, especially for women whose husbands drank greater amounts.

- *Question 2*: Although you do acknowledge challenges in BCT, you cite research studies and case examples that show positive outcomes for BCT. It seems as if you stress the positive outcomes of BCT too much. All couples cannot have good outcomes with BCT; some must have poor outcomes. What types of couples do not have positive outcomes with BCT?

• *Answer*: That is a really good question. We do not want to convey the idea that all patients benefit from BCT. What the research studies indicate is that patients who get BCT as part of their treatment, on average as a group, do better (on days abstinent, relationship happiness, violence reduction, child functioning) than patients who get only individual-based treatment (IBT). The fact that research shows that BCT does better does not mean that *all* patients benefit from this treatment. For example, among male drug abuse patients in the year after treatment, more of those treated in BCT showed clinically significant improvement in substance use (83% for BCT vs. 60% for IBT) and in relationship adjustment (60% for BCT vs. 35% for IBT) than for those who got individual treatment only.[18] Thus, patients experience a range of outcomes after BCT, just as they do with any treatment.

Factors that predict less good outcomes after BCT include couples with younger age, less than high school education, cohabiting rather than married, and more violence. These couples are more likely to drop out of BCT and to have poorer outcomes over time. Also, greater problems during the first month of BCT are associated with poorer outcomes on a clinical basis. These problems include continuing substance use, missing scheduled appointments, not completing assignments, and hostility during sessions that does not get defused.

SUMMARY

• Violence experts describe two types of IPV. *Patriarchal terrorism* is very severe man-to-woman violence that is likely to injure the woman, make her fear the man, and serve the goal of male domination. *Common couple violence* is mild to moderate in severity, often inflicted by both the man and woman, less likely to cause fear in, or endanger, the woman, and less likely to be used as a form of control.

• This second, less severe form of violence characterizes most couples starting BCT. Couples with very severe violence are excluded from BCT, and guidelines for implementing this exclusion criteria were provided.

• Over 60% of couples starting BCT reported partner violence in the previous year. However, less than 2% of couples reported very severe violence, which precludes BCT. If all couples with IPV were excluded from BCT, most patients would not receive treatment.

• BCT aims to prevent partner violence by teaching commitment to nonviolence, communication skills to reduce hostile conflicts, and coping skills to minimize conflict if the substance abuser relapses. The use of BCT with substance-abusing couples substantially reduces partner violence, and reduces violence more than typical individual treatment.

• Advising the woman not to argue with the man if he relapses because he might get violent toward her does not mean that the woman is held responsible for the man's violence. In BCT the man is held accountable for his actions. For couples with a history of violence, we ask the spouse to leave the situation if warning signs of aggression occur when there is a relapse or a serious escalation of conflict and to call the police if violence or threats of violence happen.

• The final section of this chapter considered a variety of other common clinical problems encountered in the course of BCT. Challenges covered include resistance to role playing and home practice, angry couples, psychiatric comorbidity, low reading level, and issues related to sexuality and HIV status.

NOTES

1. The sections of this chapter on partner violence draw heavily from "Addressing Intimate Partner Violence in Substance-Abuse Treatment," by W. Fals-Stewart and C. Kennedy, 2005, *Journal of Substance Abuse Treatment*, 29, pp. 6, 11–12. Copyright 2005 by Elsevier Inc. Adapted with permission.
2. Johnson (1995).
3. O'Farrell, Murphy, Stephan, Fals-Stewart, and Murphy (2004).
4. Chase, O'Farrell, Murphy, Fals-Stewart, and Murphy (2003).
5. Schumacher, Fals-Stewart, and Leonard (2003).
6. Cascardi, Langhinrichsen, and Vivian (1992).
7. Margolin (1998).
8. Stets and Straus (1990).
9. Massachusetts Guidelines and Standards for Certification of Batterers' Treatment Program (1994, May revision); Zubretsky and Knights (2001).
10. O'Farrell, Van Hutton, and Murphy (1999).
11. Fals-Stewart, Kashdan, O'Farrell, and Birchler (2002).
12. Birchler and Fals-Stewart (2003).
13. Fals-Stewart, Birchler, and Kelley (in press).
14. Fals-Stewart, O'Farrell, and Birchler (2003b).
15. Fals-Stewart (2004).
16. American Psychological Association (1992).
17. Rychtarik and McGillicuddy (2005).
18. Fals-Stewart, O'Farrell, Feehan, et al. (2000).

11

Enhancements to BCT

Most of the research on BCT has focused on two *primary outcomes*, namely, substance use and relationship outcomes. This is understandable, given that BCT for substance abuse is designed primarily to have a direct effect on these areas of functioning. However, recent studies show that BCT has broader effects on important *secondary outcomes*, including improved adjustment for children of couples receiving BCT and reduced HIV risk behaviors among the partners in these relationships. We call these *secondary outcome domains* not to diminish their importance but to signify that these outcomes were not the primary targets of the standard BCT intervention.

Currently we are trying to enhance key secondary outcomes by adding components to BCT targeted specifically to address these domains. This chapter describes two such additions to standard BCT: (1) parent training to enhance improvements in children's adjustment, and (2) HIV-risk reduction for couples.

A third enhancement described in this chapter involves using methods and techniques of BCT with the patient and a family member other than a spouse. We call this behavioral family counseling (BFC). Use of BFC would expand considerably the pool of patients that could benefit from the general therapeutic elements of BCT.

COMBINING PARENT SKILLS TRAINING WITH BCT

Rationale for Adding Parent Skills Training to BCT

Children living with a parent or parents who abuse alcohol or other drugs often have significant emotional, behavioral, and social problems, which are as severe as those of children who enter treatment for mental health services.[1] Unfortunately, substantial numbers of children live with, and are raised by, a parent or parents who have problems with alcohol or other drugs. For example, nearly 30% of female and 18% of male adult problem drug users live with children.[2] In the United States, nearly 8 million children live in homes with an alcoholic parent[3] and between 6 and 12 million children live in homes with a drug-abusing parent.[2, 4]

Treatment providers have long recognized that interventions are needed to help these children, not only to address their current difficulties, but also to help prevent future emotional and behavioral problems that often emerge as these children enter adolescence and early adulthood. Echoing this sentiment, the U.S. Secretary of Health and Human Services recently called for substance abuse treatment programs to recognize and deal with the emotional and behavioral problems of children whose parents seek help for alcoholism or drug abuse. As the secretary stated, "We must not allow our children to become the forgotten victims of substance abuse. By providing appropriate services and programs, we have the power to reduce the fear and confusion that they experience and to provide the knowledge and skills that they need to rebound and succeed as they mature into adults."[5]

Some interventions to help children of substance-abusing parents directly involve the children in treatment. The success of some well-known family-based treatments for substance abuse (e.g., Focus on Families Project[6]; Strengthening Families Program[7]) suggests that it is possible to engage some parents in family treatments that include their children. Although directly involving these children in treatment may be optimal, in many cases it is neither practical nor realistic. Most parents who enter treatment for substance abuse who are raising children are unwilling to allow their children to be involved in any type of counseling, regardless of whether it is individual treatment or part of family therapy.[8] Furthermore, with the exception of certain extenuating circumstances, parents who enter substance abuse treatment programs cannot be coerced to have their children participate in any type of intervention, whether it is delivered in the substance abuse program or elsewhere. In turn, the only access we may have to most of these children is indirect, through a parent entering treatment. Thus, interventions for adult substance-abusing patients that do not directly involve children, but nonetheless serve to improve the family environment as a whole, may actually hold the most potential for helping the children who live in these homes.

Impact of BCT on the Couple's Children

WHY MIGHT BCT BE HELPFUL TO CHILDREN?

Parents who take part in BCT are not only improving their own relationship but also may be helping their children. Conceptually, BCT might have positive "trickle down" effects on children because it has a positive impact on factors often associated with poor functioning among children who live with substance-abusing parents (i.e., parental substance use, partner violence, relationship conflict). Additionally, BCT training to improve communication and reduce parental conflict, if effective, is likely to create a healthier home environment for children, ultimately leading to better child adjustment. Next we examine research (mentioned briefly in Chapter 1) that investigated BCT's impact on children.

DOES PARENTAL PARTICIPATION IN BCT IMPROVE CHILD FUNCTIONING?

Recent studies show that parental participation in BCT leads to marked improvements in their children. More specifically, we found that school-age children of couples who participated in BCT showed greater improvements in emotional adjustment than children whose parents received individual-based treatment that did not involve BCT.[9] These encouraging findings indicate that BCT has effects on the family that extended beyond the couple to their children, even though (1) the children themselves were not actively involved in treatment, (2) parent skills training was not a component of the treatment, and (3) parenting issues were not discussed during the course of BCT. Thus, participation in BCT may provide an entry point to the family system from which to improve the psychosocial adjustment of children living in the homes of substance-abusing parents who refuse to involve their children in treatment. Table 11.1 summarizes key points about the impact of BCT on children of substance-abusing couples.

ENHANCING A COUPLE'S PARENTING SKILLS MAY IMPROVE THEIR CHILDREN'S FUNCTIONING

It also seems likely that the positive effects of BCT on children could be enhanced if some time in BCT sessions was devoted to improving parenting behavior. Research suggests that the parenting behaviors of alcoholic and substance-abusing caregivers significantly contribute to the problems observed in their children. Reviews of parenting and substance abuse literatures[10] identify the types of parenting practices that have been closely associated with the development of child problems: inconsistent discipline; irritable, explosive discipline; low supervision and involvement; inflexible, rigid discipline; poor nurturance; low levels of parental monitoring; and poorly developed general parenting skills.[11, 12] We found that lower levels of parental monitoring and poorer parenting skills were related to poorer adjustment among preadolescent children (i.e., 8- to 12-year-olds) in families with drug-abusing fathers and non-substance-abusing mothers.[13]

Can we improve parenting skills of substance-abusing patients and their partners if the children are not active participants in treatment? As it turns out, child attendance is not a necessary component for many parent skills training approaches. Parent training is defined as a method of treating child behavior problems by using "procedures by which parents are trained to alter their child's behavior in the home. The parents meet with a therapist or trainer who teaches them to use specific procedures to alter interactions with their child, to promote prosocial behavior, and to decrease deviant behavior."[14] Perhaps Bowen's comment about including children in parent skills training is most telling: "Some of the best results have come when the symptomatic child was never seen by the therapist. . . . The child's symptoms subside faster when the child is not present in the therapy."[15]

METHODS AND RESULTS OF COMBINING PARENT SKILLS TRAINING WITH BCT

With this research as a backdrop, we have recently developed a hybrid intervention consisting of parent skills training and BCT, which is referred to as PSBCT. The children are not actively involved in the treatment, but every other scheduled couple session is devoted to parenting

---

TABLE 11.1. Impact of BCT on Couples' Children

- Children of substance abusers are at risk for problems.
- Most parents won't let their children get counseling.
- BCT may be an entry point for helping children.
- BCT may help children indirectly by reducing risk factors (e.g., parental substance abuse, conflict and violence).
- Studies show that BCT helps children more than individual treatment for parent's substance abuse.

issues and parent skill development. Other sessions are more focused on the couple's relationship issues. Broadly, the parent skills sessions are devoted to improving basic parenting behavior (e.g., parental monitoring, limit setting, delivering consequences). The counselor interweaves similar topics for the BCT and parent skills modules. For example, a communication skills session for the partners on a given week is followed by a parent training module on communication skills between parents and children the following week. If parents are assigned to do a shared rewarding activity with each other one week, they are asked to do one with their children the next. Thus, the activities for the couple-based and parenting-based sessions are conceptually and practically related.

Does participation in PSBCT result in greater improvements in children's adjustment than standard BCT for parents? Although this research is ongoing, early results are very promising.[16] Preliminary findings indicate that, compared to standard BCT, PSBCT results in higher levels of parental monitoring and improvements in disciplining approaches. Additionally, children whose parents participated in PSBCT had significantly lower anxiety and depressive symptoms than children whose parents received BCT, as rated by the parents, the children, and the children's teachers. It is also important to note that PSBCT and BCT had very similar and positive effects on the parents, in terms of reduced substance use, reductions in parental conflict, and improvements in relationship happiness. Taken together, these findings suggest that PSBCT may be a viable alternative to standard BCT for couples in which the partners are also custodial parents. Table 11.2 summarizes key points about adding parent skills training to BCT.

Case Example of Combining Parent Skills Training with BCT

Jackson was a 40-year-old African American man entering outpatient treatment for a 12-year history of cocaine and alcohol dependence. During his intake interview, Jackson described significant conflict with his wife Ann, to whom he had been married for 15 years. He also reported that he and Ann had a daughter, Kim, age 11, with whom he had a very poor relationship. He said he left all parenting responsibilities to Ann and had very little patience with Kim when she misbehaved. He described himself as being an "absentee father"—although he lived in the home, he spent little time with Kim. Jackson said he did not punish Kim physically, but he would "yell and scream" at her when she misbehaved, and, as a result, she had learned to avoid him. As part of his treatment, Jackson reported that he wanted to take care of his drug problem

---

TABLE 11.2. Adding Parent Skills Training to BCT

- Substance abuse impacts children by its negative effect on parenting.
- Parental substance abuse is associated with
  - Inconsistent discipline
  - Irritable, explosive discipline
  - Low supervision and involvement
  - Inflexible, rigid discipline
  - Poor nurturance
- Adding parent training to BCT may address the added risk factor of poor parenting practices.
- Study shows parent training plus BCT improves parenting and child adjustment better than BCT or individual treatment alone.

---

and also to improve his life at home. He agreed to allow the intake team to interview his wife and daughter.

Ann, a 42-year-old African American woman with no history of alcohol or drug abuse eagerly accepted the counselor's invitation to come to the clinic to share her views about Jackson's problems and their life together. She described her relationship with Jackson as "one big fight" (but reported no episodes of partner violence) and said he "hardly does anything with Kim." She said that Kim was a very quiet child who was afraid of her father. Ann believed that Kim was depressed and "would rather go to school than be at home." Ann also said she resented Jackson because, as result of him having little involvement with her or Kim, she had to "do it all" and had little time for herself. In her interview Kim said that she was worried about her father because her mother told her "he was sick." So she tended to "leave him alone so he can rest and not get mad." Although Jackson and Ann were reluctant to allow Kim to participate in family therapy, they both agreed to take part in couples therapy combined with parent skills training.

The general sequence of sessions alternated between couples therapy activities during a given week and thematically related parent skills training the next week. As an example, during one week, Jackson and Ann worked on planning and carrying out a shared rewarding activity with each other. During the next week, Jackson planned and carried out a shared recreational activity with his daughter. The counselor worked extensively with Jackson and Ann on conflict resolution skills. Using these skills as a starting point, the counselor worked with Jackson on developing effective discipline to use with Kim (e.g., avoid yelling, identify the misbehavior, set clear boundaries of unacceptable behavior, reward good behavior).

Although Jackson remained abstinent from alcohol and cocaine during treatment, the couple had several setbacks in the course of BCT. Kim at first was uneasy interacting with Jackson, and Ann would often intervene—and, by Jackson's account, "take over," not allowing Jackson one-on-one time with Kim. Ann admitted it was hard for her to shift from being the primary parent in the home to sharing parenting with Jackson. In the course of the transition to Jackson's assuming a more active and positive role as a parent, conflicts arose between him and Ann. Ann reported that it was very difficult for her to share parenting responsibilities with Jackson after so many years of filling that role herself, but she also realized it was something she needed to allow. Thus, Jackson was assigned activities with Kim that he would do away from home and without Ann. Over time, as Jackson stayed sober and got more involved with his daughter and trust grew between the partners, Ann got used to Jackson's involvement with Kim as he monitored, disciplined, and spent time with his daughter. According to both partners, conflict in the home was reduced considerably. With parenting responsibilities more evenly shared, Ann had more time "for herself." Jackson maintained abstinence during the year after completing treatment, and he, Ann, and Kim reported significant improvements in the home environment.

BCT AS A METHOD OF HIV RISK REDUCTION

In our experience, addressing and managing HIV risk behaviors among substance-abusing patients present complex clinical challenges. In turn, approaches to HIV risk reduction need to be considered from the perspective of the patient, his or her partner, and the couple. This section describes HIV risk behaviors associated with the sexual relationships of substance-abusing couples and HIV risk reduction strategies we have added to BCT recently.

The Problem: Epidemiological Trends in HIV

It has now been over 20 years since the first cases of AIDS were reported in the United States. Since that time, a global HIV epidemic has unfolded. Today, nearly 1 million people live with HIV infection, and 450,000 have died due to AIDS thus far.[17] Nearly a quarter of a million individuals living with HIV in the United States remain unaware of their seropositive status and therefore may unwittingly transmit HIV to others. Although the pace of HIV infection has slowed since the 1980s, roughly 40,000 Americans continue to contract HIV each year.[18]

Women are the fastest growing group infected by HIV in the United States; HIV/AIDS infection is the fifth leading cause of death among women ages 25–44 and the third leading cause of death among African American women in this age group.[19] Epidemiological data indicate that the rise in HIV infection among women in the United States is attributable largely to heterosexual transmission. Among women, roughly 40% of new AIDS cases and 75% of new infections are due to heterosexual transmission.[18, 20]

Intimate Relationships and HIV Risk Behaviors

Certain high-risk behaviors have long been known to increase the likelihood of HIV exposure and infection. Primary among these are (1) intravenous (IV) drug use and risky needle practices (e.g., sharing syringes with other drug users), and (2) having sexual intercourse without using a condom in the context of relationships that are not mutually monogamous. Clearly, the more sexual partners with whom a person is involved, the greater the likelihood of him or her encountering a partner who is infected with, and might transmit, HIV.

However, an individual who has only one partner can be placed at risk indirectly, through his or her partner's behaviors. For example, a sexually monogamous woman is placed at high risk for indirect exposure to HIV in circumstances in which her only partner has other sexual partners or engages in other high-risk behaviors. This type of indirect exposure leading to HIV infection is, unfortunately, a common phenomenon for women. Most women who acquire HIV, both in the United States[21] and internationally,[22] are infected by their primary male partner. The only risk factor that many women who are infected report is unprotected sexual intercourse with their primary (and only) male partner.[23]

Results from several studies have indicated that marital status was a significant predictor of whether or not a person had more than one sexual partner; unmarried and cohabiting people were more likely to have multiple sexual partnerships than married respondents.[24–26] Thus, being married can serve as a type of social protective factor against infection from HIV. However, the reliability of this factor is often less than is commonly assumed. Several surveys of adult sexual behavior indicated that 26–50% of married men and 21–38% of married women have at least one lifetime occurrence of extramarital sex.[27, 28] Roughly 2% of married individuals engage in extramarital sex each year, and less than 20% of these individuals use condoms consistently.[29] Because condoms are used only by a comparatively small proportion of married couples as their primary method of birth control,[30, 31] extramarital sexual relationships have the potential to be a significant public health problem. This concern is not only for the partners who engage in these unprotected extramarital sexual encounters. It also extends to their spouses, who may be exposed to HIV indirectly when they have unprotected sex with their (unfaithful) husbands or wives.

HIV Risk Behaviors among Alcoholic and Drug-Abusing Couples

In a study of 362 married drug-abusing men entering outpatient substance abuse treatment and their non-substance-abusing female partners, we found that roughly 40% of the husbands reported having engaged in risky sexual behavior (e.g., penetrative intercourse with a partner who was not their spouse) or risky drug use behaviors in the previous year.[32] The most common HIV risk behavior reported by husbands in this study was extramarital sexual relationships. We recently completed a study with alcoholic couples and obtained similar results.[33]

Over two-thirds of the wives whose husbands had engaged in a high-risk behavior reported that they were not aware of it *and* were also having unprotected sexual intercourse with their husbands, thus placing them at high (and unknowing) risk for indirect exposure to HIV. Poor relationship quality, severity of drug use by the husbands, and wives' lack of knowledge of their husbands' high-risk behaviors were significant predictors of an increased likelihood of wives being placed at high risk for indirect exposure to HIV.

Unfortunately, wives of substance-abusing men are difficult to reach in most clinical settings. The women typically do not view themselves as being at high risk for HIV infection, and they are not identified as a clinical target populations for most interventions. An important exception is in the context of BCT for substance abuse, where the wives and significant others of substance-abusing partners participate in treatment. Thus, providers and programs that use BCT have access to individuals who have an elevated risk of HIV infection (i.e., patients' partners). In the context of BCT, providers have a unique opportunity to educate these partners about HIV and risk reduction, even though the partners may not view themselves as being at risk.

BCT and HIV Risk

As we have shown throughout this book, BCT is a very effective intervention for reducing substance use and improving relationship quality, particularly in comparison to more traditional individual-based interventions. As noted above, substance use severity and relationship problems are related to increased HIV risk behaviors by the partners in these couples. Drinking and drug use tend to lower inhibitions, thereby increasing the likelihood of extramarital encounters. Moreover, many drug-abusing patients purchase and use drugs in contexts that increase the likelihood of extramarital relationships (e.g., exchanging sex for drugs). Relationship problems serve to increase the likelihood that spouses will seek to meet their intimacy needs outside of the primary relationship. Thus, we might expect that, compared to individual-based treatments for substance abuse, participation in BCT might reduce HIV risk behaviors because it has a positive impact on the very factors that seem to promote these risky behaviors.

Preliminary studies of the effect of BCT on HIV risk behaviors support this notion. For example, we found that participation in BCT significantly reduced the proportion of drug-abusing male partners ($N = 270$) who engaged in high-risk behaviors during the year after treatment.[34] BCT showed greater reductions in HIV risk behaviors than did individual-based treatment or a couples-based psychoeducational attention control condition. Furthermore, as expected, the greater reductions in substance use and relationship problems experienced by BCT patients directly contributed to their greater reductions in HIV risk behaviors. These results were obtained with standard BCT, which did not include specific HIV risk reduction strategies as part of the intervention.

HIV Risk Reduction Strategies in the Course of BCT

Although the effects of BCT on substance use and relationship functioning influence HIV risk behaviors, BCT was originally not designed, nor did it include components, to address HIV risk behaviors directly. Indeed, descriptions of interventions directed toward persons in steady or primary relationships with high-risk partners are, for the most part, missing from the literature.[35] In much of the HIV prevention work, a primary risk reduction outcome is consistent condom use. However, among couples in committed relationships (vs. casual relationships), regular condom use is far more the exception than the norm.[36]

More recently, in our clinical practice and our research settings, we have added an HIV risk reduction module to standard BCT that offers related components: (1) health-oriented psychoeducation plus HIV testing and (2) safety agreements. These components are designed to address HIV risk behaviors directly with partners who enter BCT. Early in the course of BCT, the patient and spouse each take part in a separate, individual, psychoeducational session devoted exclusively to general health issues. The content of the session emphasizes identification, prevention, and treatment of certain health risks that are elevated among substance-abusing patients and their partners. These include risks that are emotional (e.g., depression) and physical (e.g., high blood pressure). Included in the latter is a discussion of HIV risk for both patients and their partners. As part of this presentation, we provide each person with a list of local agencies in which he or she can obtain confidential HIV testing, as well as testing for other sexually transmitted infections. We also provide testing for HIV in some of the clinics where we conduct BCT. This is often the only venue where many of the non-substance-abusing partners will receive such information.

However, does the inclusion of a health-oriented psychoeducational session have any impact on the likelihood of obtaining HIV testing among those who receive BCT? Although the research on this particular outcome is in its infancy, preliminary findings are encouraging. In a recent trial, over twice as many female partners of drug-abusing men who participated in BCT reported being tested for HIV, compared to female partners who participated in a psychoeducational control treatment for female partners who did not receive any treatment (i.e., their male partners received individual-based treatment; no couple-based treatment was offered).[37]

The second part of the HIV risk reduction module involves what we refer to as a *safety agreement*, which is often introduced in the session following presentation of the health-related information described above. As part of this agreement, partners are encouraged to get tested for HIV. Additionally, each partner is asked to reduce or eliminate behaviors that place him or her at higher risk for HIV infection. Thus, partners are encouraged to commit to mutual monogamy and to avoid high-risk drug use behaviors (e.g., needle sharing). Although these are the ideals which we promote with partners who participate in BCT, we also recognize that partners may engage in high-risk behaviors despite these agreements. Thus, we ask the partners to use precautions to reduce risk if they happen to engage in a risky behavior. For example, partners agree to use a condom if they have sexual intercourse with another person. They are also asked to agree to clean their needles or to use their own syringe exclusively if they return to IV use. Lastly, partners agree to let each other know if they have engaged in a high-risk behavior, so that appropriate precautions or actions can be taken (e.g., HIV testing).

At present, we do not know if the safety agreement had an effect on the behavior of partners in these couples. Clearly, simply making agreements to avoid high-risk behaviors is not likely, in and of itself, to be a powerful deterrent. However, an important aspect of couples entering into these agreements is that individuals become more aware of how their high-risk behaviors (e.g., extramarital affairs) may place their significant other at risk for infection (via unprotected sexual intercourse).

Table 11.3 summarizes key points about BCT as a method for HIV risk reduction.

TABLE 11.3. Key Points about BCT as a Method of HIV Risk Reduction

---

Women and HIV

- Women are fastest growing group infected by HIV in the U.S.
- 75% of new infections are due to heterosexual transmission.
- 40% of new AIDS cases are due to heterosexual transmission.
- This is a 25% increase in last 20 years.

Infidelity and HIV risk

- Sexual intercourse with multiple partners increases risk of HIV infection.
- Monogamous spouses are also placed at risk by their partners' sexual behavior.
- Infidelity is fairly common: 25–50% lifetime for men, 20–40% for women.
- Most partners in committed relationships assume mutual monogamy.
- If assumption is false, partners are not aware of their indirect risk exposure.

HIV risk behaviors in study of 362 married male drug-abusing patients

- Roughly 40% of the men engaged in high-risk HIV behaviors.
- 78% of married couples did not use condoms.
- 71% of wives were not aware of their husbands' HIV risk behaviors.
- Factors associated with infidelity in this study were:
  - Greater substance use, which leads to reduced inhibition, involvement with prostitutes, "sex for drugs";
  - Poor quality of primary couple relationship with wife.
- BCT might reduce HIV risk behaviors because it reduces substance use and relationship problems.

Impact of BCT on HIV risk behaviors in randomized study

- Study compared BCT with individual treatment for 270 cocaine-abusing men.
- BCT reduced HIV risk behaviors more than individual treatment.
- As expected, this was due to BCT's producing greater reductions in substance use and relationship problems.
- BCT did not include specific HIV risk reduction strategies in this study.

Adding specific HIV risk reduction strategies to BCT

- Educate about secondary risk of HIV among substance-abusing couples.
- Encourage both partners in couple to get tested.
- Encourage disclosure of high-risk behaviors and use of protective measures.
- Preliminary data are promising; controlled studies are in progress to see if this intervention will further reduce HIV risk behaviors beyond that achieved by standard BCT.

Case Example of HIV Risk Reduction in BCT

Marcus was a 32-year-old married African American man referred to outpatient substance abuse treatment by his probation officer for a 6-year history of alcohol and cocaine dependence. During his intake interview, Marcus reported that his wife, Joanna, was very supportive of his entering treatment and addressing his drug problem. When describing his marriage, Marcus lamented that he had "treated Joanna very badly." When the intake interviewer probed this statement, Marcus noted that he and his wife were "distant" and that he had engaged in two extramarital relationships in the last 3 months. He reported having had unprotected vaginal intercourse with a woman with whom he used cocaine and another woman he had met at work. To the best of his knowledge, his wife did not know about these extramarital relationships, and he was also having unprotected sex with her on a fairly regular basis. Marcus agreed to allow Joanna to be interviewed under the condition that the counselor not inform Joanna about the affairs. Although the counselor strongly encouraged Marcus to disclose the affairs to Joanna, he adamantly refused.

Joanna was a 30-year-old African American woman with no reported history of alcohol or other drug abuse. She stated that she was "very happy and very relieved" that Marcus was entering treatment and that she wanted to do whatever was necessary to help him get sober. She said that Marcus was uncaring, neglectful, and spent lots of time away from the home, leaving her alone. Based on her responses to self-report measures Joanna completed as part of her intake, she was not aware of Marcus's extramarital relationships.

Marcus and Joanna agreed to participate in BCT. As part of the program, both partners participated in individual psychoeducational sessions about HIV and comprehensive risk reduction methods. As part of these sessions, both partners were tested for HIV. Joanna agreed to the testing even though she believed she was not at any risk. Test results for both partners were negative. In the course of BCT, the couple entered into an HIV risk reduction contract. When she introduced the contract, the counselor highlighted the theme of mutual risk (if one person engaged in a high-risk behavior, then he or she put the partner at risk as well) and, in turn, couple-based risk reduction. As part of the contract, Marcus and Joanna agreed to remain monogamous, but they also agreed to use a condom if they had extramarital sex. Also as part of the contract, they agreed to tell each other if they engaged in a risky behavior (e.g., sharing needles, having unprotected sex with another partner) and seek HIV testing. Marcus admitted that initially he did not realize his extramarital relationships could put Joanna at risk, but he became more aware of the danger after taking part in BCT. However, he refused to discuss these affairs with Joanna.

The couple completed BCT. Although Marcus initially had some difficulty staying abstinent, he eventually was able to maintain stable sobriety, starting roughly 4 months after he finished the program. He reported that he did not engage in sexual relationships with other women, or engage in other HIV high-risk behaviors, during the year following treatment completion.

BEHAVIORAL FAMILY COUNSELING: EXPANDING BCT TO FAMILY MEMBERS OTHER THAN SPOUSES

The methods and techniques we have described thus far have been used with patients and their intimate partners, hence the name "behavioral couples therapy." However, the general principles on which BCT is founded are more broadly applicable to families, in general. Therefore, some studies have used these methods with other patient–family couple types (e.g., patient and parent, patient and sibling). As an example, in a study of male opioid patients taking naltrexone (Trexan), those assigned to receive BCT, compared with their individually treated counterparts, had better naltrexone compliance, which led to greater abstinence and fewer substance-related problems.[38] In this study family members taking part were spouses or cohabiting partners (49%), parents (36%), and siblings (15%). About half the patients took part in BCT with a spouse, whereas the other half took part in BCT with a family member other than a spouse. Most important, BCT had the same positive outcomes, whether it was a spouse or other family member who took part in BCT with the patient.

The success of BCT with both spouses and other family members in this study got us thinking. Could we develop a flexible behavioral family counseling (BFC) method, based on BCT, for use with substance abuse patients living with an adult family member other than a spouse? Developing a BFC intervention for family members other than spouses would considerably expand the number of patients who might benefit from the methods and techniques used as part of BCT. Among alcoholic patients living with an adult family member, 50–60% live with a spouse and the remaining 40–50% live with another adult family member not typically included in BCT. Among drug abuse patients seeking treatment, the percentage living with family members other than spouses is even higher.[39] Thus, if BCT were broadened to include family members other than spouses, it would nearly double the number of patients who could benefit from this treatment.

Adapting BCT Methods for Use in BFC

We are conducting a clinical development project to adapt BCT for use with family members other than spouses. The project is developing a treatment manual for BFC that is based conceptually on a behavioral approach to family treatment with alcoholic and drug abuse patients. A behavioral approach assumes that family members can reward abstinence and that substance abuse patients from happier families with better communication have a lower risk of relapse. This approach works directly to increase relationship factors conducive to sobriety. (These same principles guided the development of BCT for couples.)

The BFC manual is based procedurally on the BCT approach presented in this book. This BCT approach has several key components: (1) a Recovery Contract, consisting of a daily trust discussion and the taking of recovery medication (if any), attendance at 12-step meetings, and taking urine screens, as needed; (2) use of two techniques—Catch Your Partner Doing Something Nice and caring days—to increase positive feelings; (3) the planning of shared rewarding activities; (4) learning communication, negotiation, and problem-solving skills; and (5) a Continuing Recovery Plan of activities to maintain sobriety and prevent relapse. In adapting BCT to produce a manual for BFC, we retained certain aspects and we dropped or deemphasized other aspects of BCT.

The BFC manual retains the daily Recovery Contract, an emphasis on acknowledging behavior that is appreciated and on decreasing negative communication, and the Continuing Recovery Plan. The BFC manual places less emphasis on daily expressions of affection and shared rewarding activities, which are better suited to couples than to other family relationships. BFC also involves less extensive at-home practice of communication skills. Instead we place more emphasis on helping family members communicate constructively about key issues during the BFC sessions. The BFC manual includes core sessions (e.g., formulating the Recovery Contract, decreasing negative communication, Continuing Recovery Plan) that all patient–

family dyads receive. It also offers elective sessions from which the therapist can choose (e.g., shared activities, negotiating changes) depending on the role of the family member, the nature of the family relationships, and specific needs of the patient and family member. Table 11.4 contains key points about expanding BCT to family members other than spouses.

Case Example of BFC

Alex was a 24-year-old male addicted to heroin. He had dropped out of community college 12 months earlier when he became a daily IV heroin user. He had "graduated" to daily IV heroin after using Oxycontin pills daily for over a year. His first detox admission followed an arrest for possession of heroin. Alex lived at home with his divorced mother Sally and his 17-year-old sister. There was a great deal of conflict at home about his drug addiction. Sally would try to convince him to change, tearfully pleading with him to stop before he got killed on the street or sent to jail. Alex would yell, call his mother names, curse at her, and eventually leave the house to use drugs.

The doctor at the detox recommended that Alex try buprenorphine[40] for 90 days as an opioid substitute while he took part in outpatient substance abuse counseling. This approach would give him time to decide if he wanted to try a drug-free recovery program. He entered an intensive outpatient program for 6 weeks, followed by weekly individual counseling for another 6 weeks. He and his mother also started weekly sessions with a BFC counselor.

The first step in BFC was to arrange a Recovery Contract. As part of the contract, Alex and his mother had a daily trust discussion in which he stated his intent not to use illicit drugs that day and took his buprenorphine, and Sally thanked Alex for his efforts to abstain from drugs. At each BFC session, Alex and Sally did the trust discussion complete with medication taking and expressions of mutual appreciation, in similar fashion to standard BCT. Taking weekly urine screens, keeping other counseling session appointments, staying away from certain people and places linked to prior drug use, and making regular reports to his probation officer also were part of Alex's Recovery Contract.

To increase positive communication, at each session Alex and Sally were asked to tell the two things they appreciated most about each other from the previous week. It was also sug-

---

TABLE 11.4. Expanding BCT to BFC

- Recent study showed same positive outcomes if spouse or other family member took part in BCT with patient.
- Including family members other than spouses would double patients who could benefit from BCT.
- BFC is based on same principles as BCT:
  - Family members can reward abstinence.
  - Patients from happier families with better communication relapse less.
- BFC retained certain aspects of BCT but not others.
- BFC has core elements for all patient–family dyads:
  - Daily Recovery Contract
  - Acknowledging pleasing behavior
  - Decreasing negative communication
  - Continuing recovery plan
- BFC also has elective elements for individual needs.

---

gested that they show more appreciation to each other at home, but no specific assignments were given to do so. In terms of negative communication, conflict at home decreased considerably once Alex started counseling. However, when Sally would criticize him about something (e.g., his sloppy room) or ask him about his plans for the future, Alex often reverted to yelling, name calling, or leaving the house. The counselor coached Alex and Sally on how to talk about some of these volatile issues in a more constructive manner. The counselor helped Alex be assertive but not aggressive. Over a number of sessions, mother and son talked through several issues. They also got better at discussing issues at home without Alex resorting to negative communication.

After 12 weeks of treatment, Alex graduated from the intensive outpatient and individual counseling programs and joined an aftercare group that met weekly. He also elected, with guidance from the physician, to wean himself off the buprenorphine. Instead, he started taking naltrexone,[41] which would block any "high" if he took heroin or another opiate drug. BFC continued weekly for 2 more months, with naltrexone taken daily during the trust discussion. The Continuing Recovery Plan included naltrexone as part of the daily contract for 18 months, during which time the BFC sessions became less frequent. Alex also completed a training program and got a job as a technician in the heating, ventilation, and air conditioning field. Eventually, he moved into an apartment with some friends.

FREQUENTLY ASKED QUESTIONS

- *Question 1*: What do you do when you discover, during the parent training sessions, that one of the parents has engaged in recent or ongoing child abuse toward one of the children living in the home?
- *Answer*: In most states you have little choice about what to do; most states legally mandate counselors and therapists to report child abuse to the local designated child protection agency. However, you have some choice about *how* you carry out the mandatory reporting. Our general commonsense suggestion is to try to maintain the therapeutic relationship with the couple, despite the need to report them to the child protection agency. They are attending couples counseling that includes parent training, so they are trying to improve themselves and their parenting. If you can file the child abuse report without them dropping out of therapy, then you can continue to help them improve as parents.

There are a number of steps you can take to preserve the therapeutic relationship. Mainly, try to handle the situation sensitively and assume that they do not want to hurt their children. Treat them with respect and try to involve them in a collaborative process. Talk to them about why you need to file a report. Ask them how they feel about the abusive behavior and about you reporting them. Give them the opportunity to call the child protection agency themselves in your presence. Often they will fear having their children removed from the home. Although this certainly is possible, you can suggest that very often the agency will take into account that they are seeking help for substance abuse and family problems. Find out if they have ever been involved with the child protection agency before and, if so, what happened.

- *Question 2*: Is there a conflict between the typical confidentiality rules you use and how you handle affairs disclosed by one partner? In the case example on HIV risk reduction, the counselor accepted the husband's desire not to reveal his past extramarital sexual relationships to his wife. This does not seem consistent with the "limited confidentiality" approach described in Chapter 2 (i.e., "If you tell me, it can become part of couple sessions").

- *Answer*: Yes, how we handle affairs is an exception to our general approach to limited confidentiality. (The other exception is very severe violence that puts the victim at serious risk of harm, as discussed in Chapters 2 and 10.) If a person reports being actively involved in an affair or has a competing love interest, we will not treat him or her in BCT. In that case, either the person has to end the affair immediately or tell the partner immediately, or we discontinue BCT. If the affair is terminated, we strongly encourage disclosure but do not make it a requirement.

- *Question 3*: What problems have you encountered in your efforts to apply methods and techniques from BCT for use in behavioral family counseling (BFC) with a patient and family member other than the spouse?

- *Answer*: Although the general principles and many methods of BCT can be applied to other patient–family pairs, not everything translates directly from BCT to BFC. For example, many of the patients we have seen in BFC are young men in their 20s who have both alcohol and drug problems and are taking part in BFC with their mothers. The mother frequently likes the daily trust discussion and the emphasis on more positive communication and showing appreciation. However, often the patient is less comfortable with these aspects. As one patient said, "It's a little strange talking to your mother like that." Another put it this way: "I don't usually talk too much to my mother, so this seemed a little weird."

Generally, despite some initial discomfort, we have been able to help the patient and mother find a way to do these parts of BCT. Usually this involves empathizing with the patient's discomfort, explaining the reason behind what we are asking him to do, and asking both of them to help us find something that will work. In one case, the patient, John, felt uncomfortable with the wording of the standard trust discussion used in BCT:

PATIENT: I have been sober for the last 24 hours and plan to stay sober for the next 24 hours. Thank you for listening and being supportive of my effort to be drug and alcohol free.

MOTHER: Thank you for staying sober for the last 24 hours. I appreciate the effort you are making to stay clean and sober.

After some discussion, we decided he would just say "Things are going fine, Mom" and his mother would say "Thanks, John."

SUMMARY

- To enhance BCT outcomes, we have added parent training to help the couple's children, included a module to reduce HIV risk behaviors, and expanded BCT to include family members other than spouses or partners.

- Children of substance abusers are at risk for a range of problems, but most patients won't let their children get counseling. BCT may be an entry point for helping children indirectly, and parent training may address common poor parenting practices. Initial studies show that

BCT plus parent training improved parenting and child adjustment better than BCT or individual treatment alone.

- You may discover definite or suspected child abuse during BCT. Most states require counselors to report child abuse to the authorities. If you can make the child abuse report without the couple dropping out of BCT, then you can continue to help them improve as parents.

- Many male substance abuse patients engage in high-risk HIV behaviors that put their wives at risk. Adding an HIV educational module to BCT reduces HIV risk behaviors and encourages both members of couple to get tested.

- Our BCT "limited confidentiality" approach (i.e., "If you tell me, it can become part of couple sessions") is described in Chapter 2. How we handle extramarital affairs is an exception to this general approach. If the affair is in the past, we do not require disclosure to the other partner because such disclosure almost always leads to the couple's immediate discontinuance of BCT.

- A recent study showed the same positive outcomes if a spouse or another family member (e.g., parent, sibling) took part in BCT with the substance-abusing patient. These results led us to adapt BCT to produce behavioral family counseling, which, if successful, would double the number of patients who could benefit from BCT.

NOTES

1. Cooke, Kelley, Fals-Stewart, and Golden (2004); Kelley and Fals-Stewart (2004).
2. U.S. Department of Health and Human Services (1994).
3. Grant (2000).
4. Mrazek and Haggerty (1994).
5. See "Help for Children of Addicted Parents" (2003, p. 1).
6. Catalano, Gainey, and Fleming (1999).
7. Kumpfer, Molgaard, and Spoth (1996).
8. Fals-Stewart, Kelley, Fincham, and Golden (2004).
9. Kelley and Fals-Stewart (2002).
10. For example, see the review by Mayes and Truman (2002).
11. Chamberlain, Reid, Ray, Capaldi, and Fisher (1997).
12. Fals-Stewart, Kelley, Fincham, Golden, and Logsdon (2004).
13. Fals-Stewart, Kelley, Cooke, and Golden (2003).
14. Kazdin (1995, p. 82).
15. Bowen (1985, p. 309).
16. Kelley and Fals-Stewart (2003).
17. Joint United Nations Programme on HIV/AIDS (2004).
18. Centers for Disease Control and Prevention (2002).
19. Hader, Smith, Moore, and Holmberg (2001).
20. Centers for Disease Control and Prevention (1999).
21. Carpenter et al. (1991).
22. Newman et al. (2000).
23. O'Leary (2000).
24. Catania et al. (1992).
25. Kost and Forrest (1992).
26. Laumann, Gagnon, Michael, and Michaels (1994).

27. Blumstein and Schwartz (1983).

28. Kinsey, Pomeroy, and Martin (1948).

29. Choi, Catania, and Dolcini (1994).

30. Kwiatkowski, Stober, Booth, and Zhang (1999).

31. McCoy and Inciardi (1993).

32. Fals-Stewart, Birchler, Hoebbel, et al. (2003).

33. Hall, Fals-Stewart, and Fincham (2004).

34. Fals-Stewart, O'Farrell, and Birchler (2003a).

35. Kelly and Kalichman (2002).

36. Ku, Sonnenstein, and Pleck (1994).

37. Hoebbel and Fals-Stewart (2003).

38. Fals-Stewart and O'Farrell (2003).

39. Data on family members of alcoholics come from an unpublished survey, conducted by O'Farrell, of six alcoholism treatment programs in Massachusetts. Information on family members of drug abuse patients comes from Stanton and Todd (1982).

40. Buprenorphine is a newer medication for use in treating opiate addiction. It can be administered by properly trained physicians in office-based practice for (1) long-term maintenance as an opiate substitute, similar to methadone maintenance, or (2) medically supervised tapering for detoxification. This medication has two formulations: buprenorphine alone or a combination tablet consisting of buprenorphine plus naloxone. The purpose of the combination tablet is to reduce the chance of drug diversion and potential for abuse; the naloxone precipitates withdrawal symptoms if the combination tablet is misused and injected. In the case described here, the patient took the combination tablet daily for an initial 90-day opioid maintenance period during which drug-seeking behaviors were extinguished and recovery counseling begun. Then the patient opted to discontinue the opioid substitute medication and remain abstinent from opiates and other illicit drugs. For more details about use of buprenorphine in the treatment of opioid addiction, see Clark (2003) and Fudala et al. (2003).

41. Naltrexone is an opioid antagonist medication with proven efficacy to block the subjective reinforcing effects of opioid-based drugs (Kleber & Kosten, 1984; O'Brien, 1994). If a patient who is taking naltrexone uses heroin or some other opiate drug, he or she does not get high, thus reducing the patient's motivation to use drugs. Problems with patient compliance have been the biggest clinical challenge when using naltrexone to treat opioid dependence. The daily observation by the family member of the patient's medication ingestion, which is part of BCT/BFC, helps solve the compliance problem (Fals-Stewart & O'Farrell, 2003).

12

Implementing BCT in the Real World

In this closing chapter we consider the practical issues involved in the implementation of BCT in day-to-day practice in substance abuse treatment centers and other settings. After reviewing different settings and formats in which we have used BCT successfully, we consider lessons learned about possible barriers to establishing BCT as an ongoing program in community clinics. Based on these experiences, we provide suggestions for you to consider as you try to implement BCT "in the real world."

SETTINGS IN WHICH WE HAVE USED BCT

Starting in 1978 with O'Farrell's first BCT research project, over 2,400 alcohol- and drug-abusing couples have taken part in our BCT research projects and clinical programs. Of these couples, over 1,600 were treated in BCT (the rest comprised the control groups that received non-BCT treatments). We have implemented BCT in substance abuse treatment programs with typical patients presenting for help in those settings. With very few exceptions, we have not drawn patients from the pool of those who answer advertisements for research participants. Patients drawn from such ads tend to have less severe substance and relationship problems and are not typical of patients seeking help in community-based clinic settings. We have conducted our BCT research projects and clinical programs in over 20 substance abuse treatment programs and other settings. We have delivered BCT in the following types of settings:

- Part of outpatient services at a large VA substance abuse treatment program that also had inpatient detox, residential, and intensive outpatient programs.
- Part of outpatient services at a large, private, for-profit substance abuse treatment program that also had inpatient detox, residential, and intensive outpatient programs.
- Part of outpatient services at a private, nonprofit substance abuse treatment program that also had a detox unit and was part of a community hospital.

245

- Part of a small, private, nonprofit substance abuse treatment program that had a free-standing outpatient clinic only.
- Part-time private practice of clinical psychology.
- Methadone maintenance program.
- Outpatient substance abuse treatment program for gay and lesbian patients.
- Residential therapeutic community for drug abuse patients, for which BCT served as aftercare.
- Twenty-eight-day "Minnesota model" inpatient substance abuse program, for which BCT served as aftercare.

The settings in which we have implemented BCT have been quite varied and diverse. Some settings had many patients with complex comorbid nonpsychotic psychiatric and medical problems, whereas other settings did not. Patients' primary substance included alcohol, cocaine, heroin, and other opiates. Patients' income levels varied from those on public assistance to those solidly in the middle class. In some settings most patients paid for treatment with employment-based health insurance and out-of-pocket copayments. In other settings most patients' treatment was paid by a publicly funded government insurance program or other similar benefit. Many settings had a mix of payors. The proportion of minority group patients varied from settings in which there were almost none to settings in which over half were African American. Although most settings had mainly heterosexual couples, we did conduct two studies in a treatment program exclusively for gay and lesbian patients and their same-sex partners. Finally, location has varied with settings in greater Boston and other Massachusetts locations, in Buffalo and other New York state locations, in and around Norfolk, Virginia, and internationally in Calgary and Amsterdam.

As you can see, BCT has been successfully implemented in a range of practice settings. Many therapists in many different kinds of programs with different realities and obstacles have successfully implemented BCT. We hope that knowing this fact provides encouragement that you also can implement BCT successfully.

CONJOINT BCT FORMATS
DELIVERED TO ONE COUPLE AT A TIME

The formats we have used for BCT also have varied. We have delivered BCT to one couple at a time as well as in couples groups, in longer and briefer versions, and as a stand-alone intervention or combined with individual counseling. This section considers conjoint BCT formats delivered to one couple at a time. The next section covers BCT couples groups. Together, the two sections describe different versions of BCT that are available for counselors and programs to implement, according to their own structure and setting.

Twelve Weekly BCT Sessions for the Couple
plus Individual-Based Treatment for the Patient

A commonly used BCT format consists of 12 weekly, 60-minute, conjoint BCT sessions in which a couple receives the treatment we have described in the preceding chapters. Appendix A provides a therapist manual for this 12-session version of BCT. In our studies and clinical practice with this 12-session BCT format,[1] the patient has also attended individual-based treatment (IBT) sessions not attended by the partner. IBT means that the counseling is directed to the individual needs of the patient, and the partner is not involved. IBT can be delivered to one patient at a time or in a group of patients; both focus on the individual needs of the patient and do not include the spouse. So the substance abuse patient received a combination of BCT and individual-based counseling sessions.

TYPES OF SUBSTANCE ABUSE COUNSELING USED WITH 12-SESSION CONJOINT BCT

The types of IBT that we have successfully combined with BCT have varied. We have used manualized individual counseling[2] or group[3] counseling with a cognitive-behavioral approach. We also have used manualized individual counseling[4] or group[5] counseling with a 12-step approach. Finally, we have used treatment as usual for individual or group counseling delivered without a manual and guided by a largely 12-step disease model framework. This successful use of BCT with most major IBT methods is one of the reasons we like to say that BCT is a flexible treatment method that fits well with a variety of individual counseling approaches.

In much of our work, the same counselor conducted the BCT and IBT sessions for a given patient. Although at first glance this might sound problematic, a few steps minimized problems with this approach. First, the counselor had to make sure that "limited confidentiality" was well understood by both members of the couple. (As described in Chapter 2, this term means that the therapist would not keep secrets except in the case of very severe violence that puts the victim at serious risk of harm or in the case of a past affair.) Second, the counselor made a clear division of labor between individual and couple sessions so that couple issues mainly were dealt with in BCT, not in IBT. Third, the counselor had to carefully balance his or her alliance with the patient and the partner so as to not favor one partner over the other or be perceived as doing so. Finally, at weekly clinical supervision sessions, the counselor reviewed any problems that had arisen in managing both the BCT and IBT sessions.

TREATMENT PROGRAMS IN WHICH 12-SESSION CONJOINT BCT HAS BEEN USED

This 12-session weekly BCT format has been used as part of two main treatment programs. The first program was used in drug abuse outpatient clinics that treat mostly court-referred patients. These patients were scheduled to receive 56 counseling sessions over a 24-week (6-month) period. In the first 4 weeks of the program, the orientation phase, demographic, medical, and psychosocial information was collected. Patients had counseling sessions with their group (90 minutes, once weekly) and individual counselor (60 minutes, twice weekly). In the next 12 weeks, the primary treatment phase, patients attended 60-minute conjoint BCT sessions with their partners once weekly, in addition to one group and one individual session each week. For the final 8 weeks, the discharge phase, patients had one 60-minute individual counseling session each week.

The second treatment program was used in a number of alcoholism and drug abuse outpatient clinics treating a wide mix of patients. It had fewer sessions and lasted half as long as the first program, due mainly to changes over time in policies and in reimbursement practices that favored shorter and less intensive treatment programs. Patients were scheduled to receive 24 counseling sessions over a 12-week (3-month) period. They attended two counseling sessions each week for 12 weeks, a 60-minute conjoint BCT session with their partner and an IBT session. The IBT session varied, depending on the study and the clinic. IBT was either 60-minute individual counseling sessions or 90-minute group counseling sessions based on either a 12-step or a cognitive-behavioral approach.

Brief BCT Consisting of Six BCT Sessions

To address requests of treatment agencies for a briefer BCT model, we developed a six-session version of BCT.[6] This brief BCT version emphasizes support for abstinence and the Recovery Contract in a similar fashion as the 12-session BCT version, but less time is devoted to relationship-focused BCT components of positive activities and communication. Although our work with this manual is limited so far, we have used it as part of two treatment programs.

In the first program, patients were scheduled to receive 18 counseling sessions over a 12-week (3-month) period. They attended 12 weekly, 90-minute group counseling sessions based on a 12-step approach plus six 60-minute conjoint BCT sessions with their partners on alternating weeks. *In the second program*, patients received 12 counseling sessions over a 12-week (3-month) period. They attended six 60-minute individual counseling sessions and six 60-minute conjoint BCT sessions with their partners on alternating weeks.

Initial outcomes for this brief BCT version are quite encouraging.[7] However, these outcomes have not been examined in relation to the severity of patients' substance abuse and relationship problems. It seems likely that patients with more severe problems would need more than six sessions of BCT to achieve and maintain clinically significant benefits.

Flexible-Length Individualized BCT Program

Most of our experience with the conjoint BCT formats we just described (and with the group formats below) occurred while we were conducting research-funded outcome studies. Many believe that results from research studies do not hold up when new treatments are applied to routine clinical practice because research studies use carefully selected patients and have ideal conditions. However, this has not been our experience. BCT works well under routine clinical conditions when it is applied flexibly to meet any special needs of the patients or circumstances of the clinical setting.

For a number of years, O'Farrell has run a nonresearch BCT clinic in a VA substance abuse program in the Boston area. This BCT program follows the approach described in the preceding chapters. The number of BCT sessions and the duration of treatment are determined flexibly, based on the needs of each patient and couple. Typically patients attend from 12 to 20 weekly conjoint BCT sessions, followed by periodic checkups or more extended relapse prevention sessions for as long as deemed clinically needed. It is not uncommon for patients with more severe problems to attend BCT and couples-based aftercare for a number of years. Many (but by no means all) patients also attend individual substance abuse or mental health counseling, usually delivered on a treatment as usual basis by counselors other than the person providing BCT. A sizeable minority of patients include Antabuse or naltrexone as part of their Recovery Contract. Psychotropic medications for comorbid mental health problems also are commonly used, because many patients in this setting have complex comorbid psychiatric and medical problems.[8]

Table 12.1 lists key points about conjoint BCT formats delivered to one couple at a time that we have used in our studies and clinics.

TABLE 12.1. Conjoint BCT Formats Delivered to One Couple at a Time

1. 12 weekly BCT sessions plus individual-based treatment (IBT) for patient

   - Weekly 60-minute BCT sessions based on manual outline in Appendix A.
   - This BCT format has been combined with various types of IBT:
     - Manualized individual or group cognitive-behavioral or 12-step counseling
     - Nonmanualized treatment as usual based mainly on 12-step concepts
   - Twelve-session BCT has been studied in two treatment programs.
   - First combined BCT plus IBT program:
     - Fifty-six sessions over a 24-week period
     - Three times per week for first 4 weeks: 60-minute individual twice a week and 90-minute group once a week
     - Three time per week next 12 weeks: 60-minute BCT, 60-minute individual, 90-minute group
     - Once a week last 8 weeks: 60-minute individual
   - Second combined BCT plus IBT program:
     - Twenty-four twice-weekly sessions over 12 weeks
     - Twelve BCT and 12 IBT sessions with BCT and IBT alternating
     - IBT was 60-minute individual or 90-minute group sessions

2. Brief six-session BCT plus IBT program

   - Emphasized support for abstinence, less time on communication
   - Brief BCT has been studied in two treatment programs.
   - First combined brief BCT plus IBT program:
     - Eighteen sessions over a 12-week period
     - Twelve weekly 90-minute group sessions based on 12-step approach
     - Six 60-minute BCT sessions on alternating weeks
   - Second combined brief BCT plus IBT program:
     - Twelve sessions over 12 weeks
     - Six 60-minute BCT and six 60-minute IBT sessions on alternating weeks
   - Initial promising results, but more severe patients may need more sessions.

3. Flexible-length individualized BCT program

   - Number and duration of BCT sessions based on needs of each patient.
   - Typically 12–20 weekly BCT sessions over 3–6 months, followed by periodic checkups or relapse prevention sessions, as long as needed.
   - Optional IBT is treatment as usual, typically not delivered by BCT counselor.
   - Recovery and psychotropic medications commonly used.
   - Many patients have health care benefits for long-term outpatient care.

COUPLES GROUP BCT FORMATS
FOR THREE TO FIVE COUPLES

Ten Weekly BCT Group Sessions

This 10-session BCT group format[9] was developed for alcoholic patients in O'Farrell's first grant. After two initial 60-minute conjoint sessions to engage and assess each couple, it provided 10 weekly 2-hour BCT group sessions. In addition to the BCT group sessions, patients had weekly individual counseling with a 12-step orientation, delivered on a treatment as usual (TAU) basis by paraprofessional alcoholism counselors. This BCT group used a somewhat simpler version of the BCT methods described in this book. The alcoholic patients started Antabuse before they joined the group, and each couple negotiated the daily Antabuse contract during the first and second group sessions.

Each group had three to five couples, a male and female cotherapist team, and a group observer (usually an intern or therapist in training). The observer phoned each couple midweek to prompt homework completion, monitor progress, and confirm attendance for the next session. It was a closed group that, once begun, did not add additional members. Couples reported on the previous week's homework in the first half of each session, beginning with the Antabuse contract and any thoughts to drink or use drugs. New skills training and practice occurred in the second half, and each session ended with assignments for the coming week and each couple's statement of commitment to complete them.

The group format had a number of advantages. Social reinforcement from group members encouraged completion of homework assignments and attendance at group sessions. Feedback from fellow group members often made a greater impression than opinions from therapists. The group format provided extensive modeling and role playing of communication. This BCT group format was found to be more effective than TAU individual counseling.[10] It also was transported successfully to a clinic in Calgary, Canada, with similar favorable outcomes.[11]

Initial Conjoint Sessions Combined with a BCT Group

Despite its positive outcomes, the 10-session BCT group program did not provide sufficient time to deal with all the problems that these couples have. In addition, the group format made it difficult to individualize the treatment to the desired extent and to deal with sensitive issues a couple was unwilling to reveal to a group. We also found that negotiating the Recovery Contract in the group format made it difficult to give each couple the attention needed to be sure the daily contract was implemented correctly and consistently. To overcome some of these limitations, we designed a longer BCT program that combined conjoint BCT sessions with a BCT group.

The combined BCT program[12] consisted of 20–22 weekly BCT sessions over a 5–6 month period: 10–12 weekly 1-hour initial conjoint sessions with each couple followed by 10 weekly 2-hour couples group sessions (like the ones just described). In our studies of this program, patients did not get individual counseling; the BCT program was the patient's only source of substance abuse counseling. Most patients did attend at least some self-help group meetings, however. Many patients started this BCT program after an inpatient detox, residential rehab program, or intensive outpatient program.

The initial conjoint sessions set up and monitored the daily Recovery Contract and helped the couple solve immediate life problems. In these conjoint sessions the therapist also developed an individualized understanding of the substance abuse and relationship problems of each couple. The therapist who saw the couple in initial conjoint sessions was one of the cotherapists in the couples group. So each group therapist already had a strong rapport with some of the couples in the group. BCT group sessions focused on increasing positive couple activities, teaching communication skills, and monitoring the ongoing Recovery Contract. This conjoint and group BCT program provided an excellent combination of individual attention to each couple in the conjoint sessions with the added social reinforcement of a cohesive group. In short, both therapists and couples really liked this combined program.

Couple Relapse Prevention Sessions after Conjoint plus BCT Group Program

We developed and tested an extended BCT program that lasted for about 18 months to provide ongoing support for long term recovery. This program consisted of the 5- to 6-month conjoint plus couples group program just described, followed by 15 couples relapse prevention (RP) sessions (described in Chapter 8) over the next 12 months.[13] The couples RP sessions were scheduled at gradually increasing intervals and conducted conjointly with one couple at a time by one of the therapists who had led the couple's BCT group. The RP sessions aimed to (1) maintain gains achieved during weekly BCT, (2) deal with problems that were still unresolved or that emerged later, and (3) prevent or minimize relapse. Therapists liked this program because they believed it helped produce longer-lasting changes and more sustained recovery.

Study results showed that the therapists were correct. Over a 3-year period, patients who got the additional RP continued the daily Recovery Contract longer and had more abstinence and happier relationships than those who did not. Patients with more severe drinking and relationship problems got the most benefit from the extended program.[14] In our flexible-length BCT program in a VA setting, we still use this extended program for patients who have more severe problems or who have had trouble during the weekly BCT sessions.

Ongoing BCT Group with Rotating Content and Rolling Admissions

A very recent development is a 10-session BCT group program that allows "rolling admissions" of couples to the group, which is ongoing with rotating content.[15] This new program has similar content to the 10-session BCT group described above, which was a closed group that, once begun, did not admit additional members. A problem with the closed group format is that some couples inevitably have to wait many weeks to join a group. This waiting period increases the chance that they will drop out and no longer be interested by the time a new group begins. In this newly developed BCT group, new couples can periodically join an ongoing group, which has a rotating content that, once completed, begins again. A major advantage of the ongoing group format for BCT is that it fits with the way other types of groups generally are run in substance abuse treatment programs.

After an introductory conjoint session to prepare the couple to join the group, each couple attends nine 90-minute weekly group sessions divided into three modules, each lasting 3 weeks. At any time, three to five couples participate in the group. New couples can join the group at the end of each module (i.e., every 3 weeks). Completion of all three modules constitutes graduation from the group.

Initial feasibility testing and preliminary outcome data for this rotating BCT group format show promising results. This program may work best with couples in which the patient has achieved some initial abstinence and a track record of faithful attendance at other counseling sessions. Some settings may require more than one introductory session to prepare the couple for group, to test attendance and abstinence, and possibly to start the Recovery Contract. The point is that couples who drink or use, miss sessions, or drop out during the group sessions have a demoralizing effect on other couples in the group. Conversely, couples who faithfully attend sessions and mainly stay abstinent can serve as an uplifting example that inspires everyone to do better.

Table 12.2 summarizes key points about couples group formats for BCT that we have used in our studies and clinics.

TABLE 12.2. Couples Group BCT Formats for Three to Five Couples

1. 10-week BCT couples group

   - Two initial conjoint sessions to assess and prepare couple for group
   - Ten weekly 2-hour group sessions with 15-minute refreshment break
   - Male and female cotherapist team
   - Closed group that, once begun, did not add new members
   - Group cohesion encouraged attendance and assignments
   - BCT group combined with IBT delivered on treatment-as-usual basis
   - More effective than IBT alone
   - Transported internationally with favorable outcomes

2. Combined initial conjoint sessions with 10-week BCT couples group

   - Added 10–12 initial conjoint sessions before BCT group in #1 (above)
   - Combined program had 20–22 weekly BCT sessions over a 5- to 6-month period
     - Ten to twelve weekly 60-minute conjoint sessions
     - Ten weekly BCT groups, as in #1 (above)
     - Same therapist for conjoint and group session
   - Conjoint sessions set up Recovery Contract and gave individual attention
   - BCT was patient's only counseling (no IBT), but many patients came to BCT after initial detox or other treatment and attended 12-step meetings

3. Conjoint plus BCT group program with conjoint relapse prevention (RP) sessions

   - Added couples RP sessions after combined program in #2 (above)
   - Entire program lasted about 18 months
     - Weekly conjoint and group BCT sessions for first 5–6 months
     - Fifteen RP sessions at gradually increasing intervals for next 12 months
   - RP aimed to maintain gains, deal with problems, and prevent or minimize relapse
   - RP brought longer-lasting change and more sustained recovery
   - Patients with more severe problems got most benefit from extended program

4. Ongoing BCT group with rotating content and rolling admissions

   - Ongoing group repeats same content every 9 weeks
   - Initial conjoint session prepares couple to join weekly group
   - Each couple attends nine 90-minute sessions with three modules
   - After doing all three modules, couple graduates from group
   - New couples join group at each module (every 3 weeks)
   - Can be used with a wide variety of other treatment
   - Has only been tested in preliminary studies

LESSONS LEARNED ABOUT BARRIERS TO MAKING BCT AN ONGOING PROGRAM IN COMMUNITY-BASED CLINICS

We learned about practical barriers in implementing BCT from our experiences with the community-based treatment programs in which we have conducted research or training projects on BCT.[16] In these projects, we trained counselors employed in these settings to deliver BCT using a manualized protocol. Counselors gained considerable experience over the course of treating many couples with BCT. However, in each case, eventually the research or training project with its specialized grant funding ended. Then BCT was left to fend for itself, to either survive or perish.

What happened? This section provides an answer to that question by reporting a qualitative analysis of BCT's introduction in seven treatment programs. Six programs conducted BCT as part of a research project, and one program started a BCT program after on-site training followed by periodic phone consultation. We recently returned, 3–5 years later, to learn the status of BCT in these seven programs. We sought to find out whether BCT was still being used or, if not, when it was terminated and why. We recorded comments from medical-chart reviews and from interviews with counselors, supervisors, and administrators in these programs. We wanted to gain insight into why the seed we planted either sprouted and thrived or failed to take root.

Currently, four of the seven programs no longer offer BCT and stopped providing the service some time ago. BCT has flourished in three programs. In this qualitative summary, quotations from individuals in different organizational levels of these programs reveal some of the barriers to sustaining BCT implementation and, in the case of three programs, how these barriers were overcome.

Patient-Level Barriers

EXAMPLES OF PATIENT-LEVEL BARRIERS TO BCT

"Why would I want my wife involved? It's my problem, not hers." In the programs where BCT failed to survive, the choice of BCT participation was left almost completely in the hands of the patients themselves and was presented as one of several competing treatment options. Moreover, it was offered very early in treatment, typically in the first intake session. Other comments from patients' medical records included, "I don't want her here. My wife and my counselor would just gang up on me" and "I don't want her involved because I don't know what she might say behind my back." These comments reflect patients' distrust of the counselor and of couples therapy, which is common early in treatment before a therapeutic alliance has had a chance to form and solidify. The charts revealed no cases where the use of BCT was later revisited; once it was not chosen, BCT was not offered again.

EXAMPLES OF HOW PATIENT-LEVEL BARRIERS TO BCT WERE OVERCOME

"We did the assessment interviews together and it wasn't *too* bad, so we just kept going." Conversely, in a clinic in which BCT is thriving, patients are told that, as part of clinic policy, assessment with a spouse or other family member is "strongly suggested." Counselors are encouraged by their supervisor, barring some compelling reason to the contrary, to conduct assessment interviews with patients and their intimate partners together as part of the psychosocial intake assessment. BCT as a treatment choice is offered to both partners only after the psychosocial intake assessment is completed. This process enables the counselor and the partners to develop an alliance before the option of BCT is raised. This "stepped engagement approach" has resulted in excellent engagement rates of couples in BCT.

"We met with Mrs. Jones when I was in detox. She seemed to understand both of us. So we met with her when I got out and just kept going after that." This comment came from a patient in another program where BCT succeeded. This program set up routine family meetings when the patient was in detox. A counselor trained in BCT met with the patient and a family member with whom the patient lived to review aftercare plans for the patient postdetox. The meeting was with the spouse or partner for married or cohabiting patients. This was often a time of some anxiety for the spouse, who wanted the patient to continue in treatment and not return to using. For the patient undergoing detox, it was a time of heightened readiness to change, so both were receptive to the counselor's suggestions. Thus the couple was likely to agree to an initial outpatient couples session with the counselor they had met in detox, and if that went well, to continue in BCT.

The lesson is that delivery and timing are critical. As the experiences of these programs attest, couples therapy can be anxiety provoking for many patients. Routinely including the spouse in assessment and treatment planning with the patient reduces the anxiety. These meetings are not "couples therapy." They allow the couple to meet the counselor, with no obligation for continued couples involvement. Without a nonthreatening introduction and the opportunity for some trust in the counselor to develop, couples therapy is likely to be avoided.

Counselor-Level Barriers

EXAMPLES OF COUNSELOR-LEVEL BARRIERS TO BCT

"Never heard of it. What does BCT stand for, anyway?" A very significant counselor-level barrier we identified was the extensive staff turnover that has plagued many of these programs since the departure of the funded BCT projects. In one clinic, from which we had departed only 3 years ago, none of the primary treatment providers (including those who were trained in BCT) remained on staff. As a consequence of what is typically low pay, long working hours, and general burnout from treating difficult patients, turnover rates for substance abuse treatment providers hover around 50% annually.[17] Although several counselors in these clinics had been thoroughly trained in BCT, many were no longer in the programs to provide the specialized service. Importantly, none of the replacement counselors was subsequently trained in BCT and, in fact, most were not even aware of BCT when we interviewed them.

Another very interesting and recurring counselor barrier was captured by the comment of a former counselor on one of our BCT clinical trials who had remained on staff at the treatment program after we left: "We continued to use BCT for a short time with patients who seemed to really need it, but it just didn't seem to work anymore, so we eventually dropped it." Our review showed that counselors were applying BCT almost exclusively to very highly distressed, difficult couples. This was not done by design; rather, it evolved from consideration of BCT only for cases in which the need for a relationship intervention, because of extreme relationship problems, was simply too extensive and overt to ignore. For example, these were couples with very frequent arguments, partner violence, and serious threats to end the relationship. In sharp contrast, in our BCT trials the intervention is not reserved only for highly distressed couples; most married or cohabiting patients, with a range of relationship distress levels, are eligible and recruited. The selection of only extremely difficult cases that were less likely to respond to BCT appeared to leave the counselors discouraged about its effectiveness. Consequently, BCT eventually was discarded from the program's services.

EXAMPLES OF HOW COUNSELOR-LEVEL BARRIERS TO BCT WERE OVERCOME

"BCT works and, honestly, it is interesting to do something other than 12-step all day long." Counselors in the programs that continued to use BCT reported that they found it to be generally effective, that it increased client retention and attendance and added variety to their work routine. These program had low counselor turnover in the time since our departure (perhaps due to substantially higher pay compared to counselors in the programs no longer using BCT). As part of program policy, newly hired counselors were trained in BCT by those on staff who had experience with it. Finally, programs in which BCT prospered made it a routine part of their services, available to most married or cohabiting patients, and did not limit BCT to a small number of very severely distressed couples.

Supervisor-Level Barriers

EXAMPLES OF SUPERVISOR-LEVEL BARRIERS TO BCT

"I think relationship work should only be initiated after 1 year of complete sobriety. Then BCT might be appropriate." Strongly related to the high staff turnover problem was the fact that in two of the four programs that had discontinued BCT, there were clinical supervisors who were not working in the agencies when the funded BCT projects were conducted. In both cases, the supervisors held somewhat traditional philosophical views about addiction treatment. They believed that alcoholism and drug abuse are individual problems best treated on an individual basis. This position has its roots in the early alcoholism treatment literature.[18] The quotation at the start of this section reflects a commonly held belief recited by many in the addiction field today. Ironically, if the counselor waits for a year of abstinence before initiating BCT, in many treatment programs patients with such extended sobriety would no longer meet criteria for a current substance-use disorder and thus would not be eligible for program admission!

EXAMPLES OF HOW SUPERVISOR-LEVEL BARRIERS TO BCT WERE OVERCOME

"I am trained in the model and find that it helps with attendance and retention. I require everyone to be trained in BCT and to use it. It is a unique service only we provide in town, which helps us in the market." In contrast to the programs in which BCT failed, clinical supervisors in the agencies that still use BCT continued to work in these agencies and now both provide and supervise BCT. For example, the clinical supervisor just quoted did couples therapy in a BCT research project and got promoted after the research project ended. The demands of her new position include not only clinical success but also patient recruitment, keeping a high patient census, and maintenance of high attendance rates for scheduled (and billable) sessions. BCT appears to work on all of these fronts. Not only is BCT clinically effective, but our review of medical records showed that most patients involved with BCT attended their scheduled appointments at a higher rate than individual or group therapy sessions.

Anecdotally, often non-substance-abusing partners will encourage the substance-abusing patients to attend scheduled BCT appointments, even when the patients themselves may be less motivated to participate. Conversely, factors influencing attendance at scheduled individual and group appointments (e.g., counselor pressure) are usually not going to be as powerful as a spouse or intimate partner.

Administration-Level Barriers

EXAMPLES OF ADMINISTRATION-LEVEL BARRIERS TO BCT

"We stopped using BCT because we couldn't find a way to bill for it. Simple." Proving that BCT is effective in no way requires third-party payers to reimburse providers for the service. In programs that stopped using BCT, administrators found that most third-party payers were not familiar with BCT, were generally unwilling to reimburse for couples therapy, or were only willing to pay for one or two family sessions. During the course of the BCT projects we conducted, grant funding paid to deliver BCT, making the issue of reimbursement moot. After the grant funds ended, these programs found that they could not bill most third-party payers for the couples sessions. Most substance abuse treatment programs are notoriously underfunded and are appropriately concerned about their economic stability. The unwillingness of payers to reimburse for BCT sessions was a fatal blow to the viability of the intervention in these programs.

EXAMPLES OF HOW ADMINISTRATION-LEVEL BARRIERS TO BCT WERE OVERCOME

"We educated our third-party payers about BCT before you left and now get reimbursement for these sessions. In fact, because the BCT sessions are so well attended compared to our other services, it's a money-maker for us. We successfully bill for all, or nearly all, the sessions." For one of the programs in which it is actively used, BCT is strongly supported by the administration—largely on economic grounds! The executive director and the clinical supervisor made significant efforts to educate third-party payers prior to, and early after, our departure to establish that BCT sessions would be reimbursable. They also met with a local politician about the issue, who wrote a letter of support for the use of BCT in the program to several of the local and regional managed care companies.

For the other two programs in which BCT continued, government health funding paid for services to patients deemed eligible for these services. In these programs, reimbursement for services was not the major concern. Rather, administrators needed to be sure that their annual budgets had ongoing funding for staff to deliver BCT. For example, in the program that brought us in to train their staff in BCT, the administrator already had committed a part-time counselor to deliver BCT for at least a year before we started the training. After we helped them establish a BCT program that was well-regarded by staff and patients, the administrator arranged to continue funding the counselor who was doing BCT.

A second example was a program where we conducted a research project in which a grant provided the funding to add therapists to deliver BCT. When the grant ended, the specially funded staff left. However, the administrator used psychology and social work trainees as couples therapists to keep a small BCT program going, until he was able to obtain government-funded staff to expand BCT services. Both administrators strongly supported BCT because they had read about research verifying its effectiveness. In addition, they had personally observed high attendance rates and excellent patient satisfaction for BCT in their programs. These administrators had a commitment to providing evidence-based services. They took pride that their program was the only one providing BCT in their area. They saw it as a way of marking their program as unique to their patients, government superiors, and local community stakeholders.

The Dynamic Interplay of These Different Barriers

For convenience and clarity, we have described the barriers to BCT we observed at different organizational levels. However, we recognize that these barriers are not really so separate and do not operate in isolation from one another. There is considerable overlap among, and a dynamic interplay between, barriers at different levels. Trying to overcome a barrier at one level, without at the same time dealing with, or at least understanding, the interrelated barriers at other levels, may be doomed to fail.

For example, we reported that many counselors in these programs were not even aware of BCT, let alone trained to use it. That is a counselor-level barrier, to be sure, but it is also an important reflection of a supervisor-level and administrative-level barrier. Supervisors who do not believe in couples therapy for substance-abusing patients, on philosophical grounds, are not going to promote training in BCT. Moreover, administrators who cannot bill for BCT sessions will also not encourage counselors to participate in, or pay for, training in a technique that is ultimately not going to boost the agency's bottom line. Similarly, the philosophical patient-level barrier of viewing substance abuse as an individual problem that should be addressed by the alcoholic or addict without involving family members also reflects, to some extent, a community-level barrier. This idea that substance abusers and their family members each should address their problems separately on an individual basis (vs. in a couples or family therapy context) is a fairly commonly held view expressed by members of the 12-step community. We saw in Chapter 1 that, despite their different philosophical beliefs, BCT and 12-step actually are quite compatible in practice. A major barrier to BCT arises when these differing beliefs cause counselors, supervisors, and others to reject BCT without giving it a try.

We learned a great deal about barriers to implementing BCT from our qualitative analysis of organizations in which BCT prospered versus those where it did not. For BCT to become an ongoing part of a program's services, the "buy-in" needs to occur at multiple levels of the treatment community, in general, and within a given treatment agency, ranging from the patient to policymakers. Attempts to implement BCT in the real world must be multifaceted and multilevel to have the best chance to succeed. Table 12.3 summarizes key points about overcoming barriers to implementing BCT as an ongoing service in a substance abuse treatment program or other setting.

SUGGESTIONS FOR IMPLEMENTING BCT

This section provides some commonsense suggestions for implementing BCT as well as some ideas that might not be obvious at first. It includes guidance for initially trying out BCT and for establishing an ongoing BCT program.

TABLE 12.3. Barriers to Implementing BCT as an Ongoing Program

1. Patient-level barriers

   - Patients' distrust and fear of couples counseling
   - Patients asked to take part in BCT at initial intake session, where most refused

   Solutions to patient-level barriers:
   - Routinely include spouse in assessment and treatment planning interviews with patient to gradually overcome fear of spouse involvement
   - Delay invitation to BCT until counselor has developed rapport with patient

2. Counselor-level barriers

   - High staff turnover: Staff trained in BCT left, replacements not trained in BCT
   - Targeting BCT only to couples with severe relationship problems led to poorer outcomes and loss of faith in BCT's effectiveness

   Solutions to counselor-level barriers:
   - Low staff turnover; new counselors trained in BCT
   - Use BCT with all couples, not just those with severe relationship problems

3. Supervisor-level barriers

   - Supervisor turnover
   - New supervisor with anti-couples-therapy philosophy

   Solutions to supervisor-level barriers:
   - Low supervisor turnover
   - Hire new supervisors who value BCT

4. Administration-level barriers

   - Difficulty finding third party or other resources to pay for BCT

   Solutions to administration-level barriers:
   - Proactive steps to gain financial support for BCT sessions and staff
   - Commitment to providing BCT because it contributes to key program values (e.g., evidence-based services, high patient satisfaction)

Suggestions for Getting Started with BCT

For the counselor or program just getting started with BCT, we suggest you implement it under conditions where it is most likely to succeed. This approach will allow you to build skill and confidence in BCT under less challenging conditions before moving on to more difficult situations. Applying the following suggestions will maximize your chance of success as you learn BCT.

First, BCT counselors typically have a master's degree and a few years of experience in substance abuse treatment. Although experienced substance abuse counselors with a bachelor's degree performed successfully in one study, they received very extensive supervision and monitoring from BCT experts that would not be available in most settings.[19]

Second, a counselor who is going to try out BCT should receive specific training in it, preferably followed by ongoing consultation from a BCT expert.

Third, choose a BCT format that is relatively simple and user-friendly. We suggest the 12-session conjoint BCT format, delivered to one couple at a time, while the patient receives concurrent group or individual substance abuse counseling. (Appendix A provides a therapist manual for this BCT format.) You may be tempted to start with a BCT group, especially the rotating group format because it fits with group formats used for patients in so many agencies. However, a great deal of skill is needed to handle multiple couples, deal with group dynamics, *and* remain focused on behavioral rehearsal of new skills and completion of home assignments. A BCT group led by a novice therapist can easily deteriorate into just another psychoeducational group without providing the active ingredients of BCT: a strong, skillful focus on behavior change *in group* and *at home*.

Fourth, and probably most important when beginning to implement BCT in your program, choose your patients carefully. We suggest you choose couples according to the following criteria:

- Married or cohabiting for at least a year
- Living together and not planning separation
- Only one person has a current substance problem
- Absence of psychosis, major mental illness, or severe violence

In addition, learning BCT is easier with patients who recognize that they have a problem, have stopped using for a short time, and enter BCT after detox, rehab, or some court involvement. Finally, avoid couples who have very severe relationship problems until you gain more BCT experience. You can expand to more challenging couples later, after you have mastered the basics of BCT in these less complicated cases.

Suggestions for Establishing an Ongoing BCT Program

After trying out BCT on some initial cases, a counselor or treatment program director may want to make BCT an ongoing part of their services. Establishing an ongoing BCT program requires (1) deciding the target group for the BCT program, (2) engaging patients and spouses, and (3) getting "buy in" from key individuals. Each of these points is considered next.

DECIDING THE TARGET GROUP FOR THE BCT PROGRAM

We recommend that you use BCT for most married or cohabiting patients seeking substance abuse treatment, not just those with serious relationship problems. (Of course, you should exclude couples who report very severe violence and probably dual-problem couples in which only one person wants to change.) Years ago, when we started our BCT work, we thought that BCT was most useful for patients with serious relationship problems or with spouses who enabled patients' use. Now, based on many studies and years of clinical experience, we have changed our thinking. BCT should not be reserved for patients who have serious relationship problems secondary to, preceding, or coexisting with the substance problem. Couples with less serious problems often are better able to work together in BCT to support patients' sobriety and enrich their relationships. Furthermore, even when relationship factors do not trigger or maintain substance use, daily spouse support in BCT may help the patient stay abstinent by strengthening alternative behaviors to substance use.

ENGAGING PATIENTS AND SPOUSES

To run a BCT program, you need to engage patients and spouses in BCT, despite some patients' fear and distrust of spouse contact, as described above. We recommend that you routinely include the spouse or other family member with whom the patient lives in family assessment and treatment planning interviews in your treatment program. Most patients will consent to their families being contacted if you describe this contact as routine and present it in a positive manner. After the patient agrees, contact the family member yourself to invite him or her to meet with you and the patient to share insights about the substance problem and give input into the patient's treatment plan.

After completing the family assessment interview, you can offer an initial BCT session to the patient and partner as a treatment option. The family interview is an opportunity to cultivate trust in the counselor, so that couples sessions do not seem so threatening. If the family interview goes well, the couple is likely to agree to an initial BCT session. This approach works best when the counselor who does the family assessment interview with the patient and spouse is the same person the couple will see if they choose to schedule an initial BCT session. (Chapter 2 provides more details on the process of engaging couples in BCT.)

The practice of routine family involvement in family assessment interviews has a number of advantages beyond engaging couples for BCT. First, it meets the requirement by the Joint Commission on Accreditation of Healthcare Organizations (JCAHO) that a family member who lives with the patient be included in the assessment process for patients in substance abuse programs.[20] Second, it increases aftercare participation postdetox[21] and reduces readmission rates in inpatient or residential programs.[22] Finally, it also contributes to favorable satisfaction ratings from patients and family members.

GETTING "BUY-IN" FOR A BCT PROGRAM FROM KEY INDIVIDUALS

Establishing BCT as an ongoing service requires a program champion who will take the lead to start and sustain the program. The program champion is a counselor, supervisor, or (more rarely) an administrator who persuades key individuals in the treatment program to embrace BCT and the principle of family involvement. Persuading key individuals of BCT's value is challenging because individuals vary in which aspect of BCT they might find appealing.

For those with a commitment to providing evidence-based services, the research supporting BCT can be important and persuasive. You will have to overcome the belief that recent research shows that different types of counseling are equally effective. For example, results from Project MATCH showed that 12-step and cognitive-behavioral counseling were equally effective for alcoholism.[23] The NIDA Collaborative Cocaine Treatment Study showed that 12-step-oriented drug counseling was more effective than professional psychotherapy.[24] However, neither MATCH nor the NIDA cocaine study examined family or couples counseling. In fact, family-involved treatments, especially BCT, are one of the few types of counseling that have better outcomes than 12-step or cognitive-behavioral counseling. The fact that BCT also has a more positive impact on children, spouses, social costs, and other socially relevant outcomes (partner violence, marital stability, HIV risk behaviors) is important to emphasize. This evidence for BCT and family counseling is summarized in Chapter 1 and in recent literature reviews.[25]

For others, realizing that a sizable subgroup of patients could benefit from BCT may be persuasive. About 30% of adult patients entering substance abuse treatment live with a spouse or partner, and an additional 20–25% live with a parent or other adult family member.[26] Staff and administrators in many treatment programs do not see the value of BCT because "most of our patients don't have a partner." Although this is true, how big does a subgroup of patients need to be to get specialized services to fit its unique needs? On the one hand, some program administrators like "one-size-fits-all" programming because it is easier and cheaper. On the other hand, specialized programming is accepted for other subgroups of patients that are no larger than our subgroup. For example, most programs have ongoing groups or other programs for women patients separate from men patients. Women typically comprise about 25–35% of patients in substance abuse programs—very similar in size to the subgroup of patients living with partners and smaller than those living with all family members combined. Women patients get specialized programming because we believe it improves their comfort and retention in treatment and ultimately their chances of staying abstinent. Thus, subgroup size and beliefs about the beneficial impact of specialized services both influence the decision to provide such services. Following this logic, BCT is well justified because the size of the subgroup needing it is significant and the evidence that it improves patient outcomes and helps family members is strong.

Although published research and appeals to logic may influence some, patients' positive responses to BCT may carry more weight with many key individuals. We suggest that you use positive results from initial BCT cases to highlight the value of the treatment. Patients' testimonials about their satisfaction with BCT, responses to satisfaction questionnaires from patients and spouses, and comments patients make about BCT to other program staff all increase acceptance of BCT. Once they try BCT, many program staff like it due to better retention of patients in treatment and high levels of patient and family satisfaction.

Finally, a program may value BCT for its appeal to patients. We have noted that many patients view substance abuse as an exclusively individual problem and have some anxiety about couples sessions. Nonetheless, increasingly we see patients initiating requests for couples sessions when they know that these services are available. This is especially true for spouses. Thus a BCT program can be a marketing tool to attract patients to a program— something that gets the attention of many program supervisors and administrators.

Table 12.4 summarizes key points about practical suggestions for implementing BCT.

CONCLUDING COMMENTS

BCT aims to build support for abstinence and to improve relationship functioning among married or cohabiting individuals seeking help for alcoholism or drug abuse. This volume has provided detailed clinical guidelines for counselors who want to use BCT with their patients. After briefly reviewing the extensive research support for BCT, we described the BCT Recovery Contract to support abstinence and the BCT methods used to increase positive activities, improve communication, and prevent or minimize relapse. To round out this clinical guide, Appendix A provides a 12-session BCT treatment manual that includes a checklist for each session that a counselor can use to guide the session. Remaining appendices contain handouts and other forms used in BCT.

TABLE 12.4. Practical Suggestions for Implementing BCT

1. Getting started with BCT

- Try out BCT under favorable conditions, build skill and confidence, then move to more difficult situations.
- Be a master's-level counselor with training in BCT plus ongoing consultation.
- Use 12-session BCT conjoint format plus substance abuse counseling.
- Carefully choose couples for initial trial of BCT.
  - Married or cohabiting for at least a year
  - Living together and not planning separation
  - Only one person has a current substance problem
  - Absence of psychosis, major mental illness, or severe violence
  - Patients who admit they have a problem, have stopped using for a short time

2. Establishing an ongoing BCT program

- Decide the target group for the BCT program.
  - All patients with partners, not just those with relationship problems
  - BCT provides support for abstinence, something all patients can use
- Engage patients and spouses in the program.
  - Routinely include spouse in family assessment interviews.
  - Offer initial couple session as an option at end of assessment.
- Get "buy in" from key program staff (counselors, supervisor, administration).
  - Research support for BCT will convince those who value evidence-based care.
  - Realizing that a sizable subgroup of patients could benefit from BCT may persuade others.
  - Use positive response of initial BCT cases to sell program.
  - BCT's appeal to patients and spouses can help attract new patients.

We also described solutions to challenges faced in BCT and enhancements to extend the impact of BCT. Solutions to challenges such as dual-problem couples and enhancements such as parent training were developed only very recently as the findings of new BCT studies were reported. Future developments will continue to refine and reevaluate BCT. We hope that this volume will lead to increased use of BCT to benefit substance abuse patients and their families. Insights gained from widespread clinical application of BCT and new research findings will make what is already a very effective intervention even more so.

SUMMARY

- This closing chapter considers pragmatic issues in implementing BCT in day-to-day practice in substance abuse treatment centers and other settings.

- Over 2,400 couples have taken part in our BCT projects in over 20 different substance abuse treatment programs. Patients varied considerably in their primary substance, psychiatric comorbidity, ethnicity, income level, payor (private or public) for services, and the BCT format (conjoint or group) received.

- Conjoint BCT formats delivered to one couple at a time have included 12 weekly BCT sessions, brief BCT with six BCT sessions, and a flexible-length individualized BCT program. These conjoint BCT formats were combined with individual-based treatment (IBT) for the patient. IBT included 12-step counseling, cognitive-behavioral sessions, or treatment as usual, provided in individual or group counseling.

- Couples group BCT formats for three to five couples include a 10-week closed group delivered alone or with conjoint sessions added before to prepare couples and afterward to prevent relapse. A newly developed ongoing BCT group format has rotating content and rolling admissions in which couples join the group, complete the nine group sessions, and "graduate."

- A number of suggestions flow from lessons we have learned about practical barriers to implementing BCT in substance abuse treatment programs.

- To get started with BCT, use the 12-session conjoint BCT format with couples who are likely to benefit before moving on to more difficult situations. To establish an ongoing BCT program, use BCT with most couples, not just those with serious relationship problems; make family assessment interviews a routine part of your program; and get "buy-in" for BCT from key individuals.

- This volume has provided detailed clinical guidelines for counselors who want to use BCT. Future developments will continue to refine and reevaluate BCT and to make what is already a very effective intervention even more so.

NOTES

1. Appendix A of this book, which contains this 12-session BCT manual, draws heavily from Fals-Stewart, O'Farrell, Birchler, and Gorman (2004a).
2. For this manual, see Kadden et al. (1992).
3. For this manual, see Daley and Marlatt (1997).
4. For this manual, see Mercer and Woody (1999).
5. For this manual, see Daley, Mercer, and Carpenter (2002).
6. For this manual, see Fals-Stewart, O'Farrell, Birchler, and Gorman (2004b).
7. Fals-Stewart, Klosterman, Yates, O'Farrell, and Birchler (2005).
8. For more details on BCT for patients with comorbid mental health problems, see Rotunda, Alter, and O'Farrell (2001).
9. For a detailed description of this BCT program, see O'Farrell and Cutter (1984b).
10. O'Farrell, Choquette, Cutter, Floyd, et al. (1996); O'Farrell, Cutter, Choquette, Floyd, and Bayog (1992).
11. el-Guebaly, Richard, Currie, and Hudson (2004).
12. For a detailed description of this BCT program, see O'Farrell (1993a).
13. For a detailed description of this BCT program, see O'Farrell (1993b).
14. For study results, see O'Farrell, Choquette, Cutter, Brown, and McCourt (1993), and O'Farrell, Choquette, and Cutter (1998).
15. For this BCT manual on the rotating group format, see Fals-Stewart, O'Farrell, Golden, and Birchler (2004).
16. The section on barriers to BCT and the following section on suggestions for implementing BCT draw heavily from "Dissemination of Empirically Supported Treatments for Substance Abuse: An Organizational Autopsy of Technology Transfer Success and Failure," by W. Fals-Stewart, T.

Logsdon, and G. R. Birchler, 2004, *Clinical Psychology: Science and Practice*, *11*, pp. 179–181. Copyright 2004 by Oxford University Press. Adapted with permission.

17. Carise, McLellan, Gifford, and Kleber (1999).
18. Jellinek (1960).
19. Fals-Stewart and Birchler (2002).
20. Brown, O'Farrell, Maisto, Boies, and Suchinsky (1997).
21. O'Farrell, Fals-Stewart, et al. (2004).
22. Peterson, Swindle, Phibbs, Recine, and Moos (1994).
23. Project MATCH Research Group (1997).
24. Crits-Christoph et al. (1999).
25. O'Farrell and Fals-Stewart (2003); Stanton and Shadish (1997).
26. These data on percent of patients living with family members are based on Tracy, Kelly, and Moos (2005) and an unpublished survey of six substance abuse treatment programs in Massachusetts conducted by O'Farrell.

APPENDICES

Appendix A contains a 12-session BCT treatment manual. Each session has a therapist checklist and an outline for the session. Once familiar with BCT, a counselor can use the checklist to guide their conduct of the session.

Appendix B contains posters that are often used to convey key points to couples getting BCT. These posters can be enlarged and kept in the counselor's office for use in BCT sessions. Appendix C contains forms used in BCT. Appendices A, B, and C are adapted from an unpublished manual by Fals-Stewart, O'Farrell, Birchler, and Gorman (2004a), and use of this material is gratefully acknowledged.

The checklist for each session provided in Appendix A lists posters and forms needed for the first time in that session. Some posters and forms also may be needed for later sessions, but they are only mentioned once when first introduced. For example, the Catch Your Partner Doing Something Nice form is listed in the Session 1 checklist because it is introduced for the first time in this session. This form also is needed in some later sessions, but it is not listed in these later sessions to keep repetition to a minimum.

Appendix D contains a list of materials for training in BCT and other related resources.

A 12-Session BCT Treatment Manual

Checklist for BCT Session 1:
Introduction, Recovery Contract, Catch Your Partner Doing Something Nice

Posters Needed	Forms Needed
B.1. Why BCT?	C.1. Recovery Contract
B.2. Promises	C.2. Recovery Contract Calendar
B.3. Typical Sequence of Sessions	C.3. Catch Your Partner Doing Something Nice Worksheet
B.4. Daily Trust Discussion Formula	C.4. Home Practice Session 1
B.5. Sample Recovery Contract Calendar	
B.6. Sample Caring Behaviors	
B.7. Catch Your Partner Doing Something Nice	

Note: B.1 refers to Poster B.1 in Appendix B, C.1 to Form C.1 in Appendix C.

Cover the following material as completely as possible. Place a checkmark next to each completed section.

1. Introduction and Welcome

___ Reaffirm couple's interest in starting BCT.

___ Discuss "limited" confidentiality or "No Secrets Policy."

2. Explanation of BCT and Why It Is Important

___ Explain rationale for BCT.
→(Show *Why BCT? Poster B.1.*)←

___ Give preview of future sessions.

___ Cover missed sessions policy.

3. Promises

___ Introduce concept of Promises.

___ Explain and discuss four Promises.
→(Show *Promises Poster B.2.*)←

___ Ask for verbal commitment to keep Promises in coming week.

(continued)

4. Overview of Sessions

___ Explain general structure of sessions.
→(Show *Typical Sessions Poster B.3.*)←

___ Explain drug urine tests if patient has drug problem.

___ Explain review of urges or actual substance use in past week.

___ Explain review of relationship problems or concerns from the past week.

___ Explain home practice assignments.

5. Trust Discussion and Recovery Contract

___ Introduce Trust Discussion concept.

___ Explain and discuss Trust Discussion format.
→(Show *Trust Discussion Poster B.4.*)←

___ Couple practices Trust Discussion with coaching from therapist.

___ Explain and discuss Recovery Contract, including possible use of recovery medication.
→(Show *Recovery Contract Poster B.5.*)←

___ Have each person verbally commit to Recovery Contract.

___ Assign home practice: Trust Discussion and completion of contract.
→(Hand out *Recovery Contract and Calendar Forms C.1 and C.2.*)←

6. Catch Your Partner Doing Something Nice

→(Show *Sample Caring Behaviors Poster B.6.*)←

___ Discuss rationale for "Catch Your Partner Doing Something Nice" exercise.

___ Ask each person to name one Caring Behavior partner did in past week.
→(Show *Catch Your Partner Poster B.7.*)←

___ Solicit questions or concerns about Catch Your Partner exercise.

___ Assign home practice.
→(Hand out *Catch Your Partner Form C.3.*)←

7. Assign Home Practice

→(Hand out *Home Practice Session 1 Form C.4.*)←

___ Recovery Contract

___ Do Trust Discussion (with medication, if taking it) and mark on calendar.

___ Complete self-help and other parts of contract.

___ Catch Your Partner (write down one nice thing partner does each day).

8. Session Closing

___ Answer questions about home practice assignments.

___ Get commitment from each person to do home practice assignments.

270

BCT SESSION 1 OUTLINE
INTRODUCTION, RECOVERY CONTRACT,
CATCH YOUR PARTNER DOING SOMETHING NICE

This session introduces behavioral couples therapy (BCT) and explains what will be covered in the counseling. This session occurs after one or more initial couple sessions to engage the couple and explore their interest and suitability for BCT. It begins the segments on the Recovery Contract and Catch Your Partner Doing Something Nice.

1. Introduction and Welcome:

Generally this session comes after an initial couple meeting in which basic clinical information has been gathered, a very brief orientation to BCT and to the local clinic or program has been provided, and the couple has expressed an interest in starting BCT.

1A. Welcome Back: The therapist asks about reactions to the first couple session and finds out if they are still interested in starting BCT. If the answer is "yes," then proceed to the issue of confidentiality.

1B. Limited Confidentiality or "No Secrets Policy": Educating the couple about the "No Secrets Policy" and the limits to confidentiality associated with this policy, as well as soliciting and answering their questions, is critically important.

SUGGESTED THERAPIST SCRIPT

Along with couple sessions, I may meet with each of you separately to talk about our work here. Therefore, I would like to talk about something that we call our "No Secrets Policy." This means that if one of you tells me something that I believe is important to your relationship, I retain the option of whether, when, and to what extent I will discuss this in a couple's session. Also, if appropriate, I will first allow the partner who shared the information the chance to bring the issue up in a couple's session.

Holding information that one of you shares with me can be interpreted as taking sides, and that goes against what we are trying to do here.

This may seem strange and may lead you to keep certain information to yourself. Although I don't want to encourage that, I also want to make our time together most effective, and holding "secrets" may hurt that process.

Also, I will not disclose any information to someone else unless required by law or with your written consent. The law mandates reporting when a person discloses an intent to harm him- or herself or someone else, or if there is abuse against a child or an elderly or disabled person.

What questions do you have about this?

---

2. Explanation of BCT and Why It Is Important:

2A. Why BCT?: →(Show *Why BCT? Poster B.1*.)←
Use the poster to show why BCT can help maintain abstinence and improve the relationship.

(continued)

2B. Preview of Future Sessions:

SUGGESTED THERAPIST SCRIPT

I want you to know what to expect in counseling. Here are specific things we will be covering:

1. **Recovery Contract:** You will both do the daily Trust Discussion together. There also may be AA or NA meetings, urine drug screens, and recovery medication.
2. **Catch and Tell:** Each of you is asked to notice and acknowledge one nice thing each day that your partner does for you.
3. **Shared Rewarding Activity:** This activity is designed to put fun back into your relationship. You will be asked to do something special together each week.
4. **Caring Day:** A Caring Day is when you take the time and energy to plan something special for your partner, as a way of putting caring back into your relationship.
5. **Communication Skills:** Learning to listen and express feelings directly will improve communication with your partner so that you can resolve disagreements and problems.
6. **Conflict Resolution:** You will learn different ways to reduce and resolve conflicts.
7. **Problem Solving:** You will learn a five-step process that will help you effectively address a variety of problems that may exist in your relationship, with the children, finances, etc.
8. **Continuing Recovery Plan:** This tool will help you identify activities and skills you have learned during BCT and that you can continue to use after weekly BCT ends.
9. **Action Plan:** This tool will help you prevent or minimize relapse when faced with high-risk situations for drinking or using drugs.

2C. Missing Sessions: Partners need to attend sessions faithfully and only cancel when necessary.

3. Promises:

→(Show *Promises Poster B.2.*)←

SUGGESTED THERAPIST SCRIPT

There are four Promises that can start making your relationship better. They are:

1. No threats of divorce or separation: Such threats interfere with making things better. If you need to discuss the possibility of divorce or separation, I ask that you do so during a session, so that we can discuss it together. *(Ask each person, "Will you make this promise for the coming week?" Repeat this question after you describe each remaining promise below.)*

2. No violence or threats of violence: I want you to learn how to communicate without resorting to violence. So pushing, shoving, hitting, and so forth, are unacceptable. So are threats. Using violence to address conflict is ineffective and can be dangerous.

3. Focus on the present and future: I ask that both of you focus on the present and future and avoid negative arguments about past problems and resentments. In sessions with me, we will talk about things that happened in the past and how your relationship was affected.

4. Attendance and active participation: I ask that both of you promise to attend scheduled sessions, to participate actively in sessions, and to complete home practice assignments. This counseling is based on you changing actions with each other. It only works if you work it.

I will ask about your success in keeping these Promises at our next session.

(continued)

4. Overview of Sessions:

→(Show *Typical Sequence of Sessions Poster B.3.*)←

It helps to educate the couple so that they are not "put off" by the highly structured nature of BCT.

SUGGESTED THERAPIST SCRIPT

Our sessions together will be fairly structured. Some things we will be doing every week are:

- *Urine screen*: If you have a drug problem, a negative screen can help to rebuild trust by verifying your progress. A positive screen can alert us to problems we need to deal with.
- *Review of use or urges to use in the last week*: Most people have urges to use in recovery. Reviewing urges can help you identify potential triggers and successful coping methods. Use of alcohol or drugs also happens, although less often. You need to be honest if there has been use, so we can address it and help you get back on track.
- *Review of relationship issues in the last week*: Reviewing how things went in the past week will alert us to problems you may be having as well as progress you're making.
- *Review of Promises*: Reviewing the four Promises will help you keep these important commitments.
- *Review of home practice in last week*: We will review assignments from last session and may practice some more in session. We will practice the Trust Discussion at each session.
- *Cover new material*: Each session you will learn a new skill. I will explain each skill, show you how to do it, and coach you as you practice the new skill in session.
- *Assign home practice for next week*: You'll have the chance to take on assignments each week, such as planning fun activities together or practicing how to communicate.

As you can see, there are a lot of things we cover each session. I also want you to know that I will be as flexible as possible as personal needs or any crisis situations arise.
   Do you have any questions or concerns about the structure of the sessions?

---

5. The Recovery Contract:

Rationale: Regaining lost trust after a substance problem can be difficult. The Recovery Contract helps build trust, reward abstinence, and minimize arguments about alcohol and drugs.

→(I hand out the *Recovery Contract Form C.1.*)←

5A. Components of the Recovery Contract:

SUGGESTED THERAPIST SCRIPT

The Recovery Contract has five parts:

1. The Trust Discussion, a brief daily ritual that may include recovery medication;
2. Agreement not to bring up past use or fears about future use of drugs or alcohol;
3. Self-help commitments (e.g., AA, Al-Anon);
4. Urine drug screens, if there is a problem with drugs; and
5. Other regular actions to support recovery.

   We'll begin by filling in your names at the top of the contract. Then we'll review each part.

(continued)

5A.1. The Trust Discussion:

5A.1.A. Decide on a Time and Place:

> **SUGGESTED THERAPIST SCRIPT**
>
> The Trust Discussion is a tool that can help to ease tension and rebuild trust in a relationship that has been affected by drugs and alcohol. It is important to have a set time when you can give your undivided attention to each other. Try to do the discussion at an already established event that occurs each day, such as during a meal or when you go to bed. This will help make it part of your daily routine. When would be a good time to do your Trust Discussion?

→(Show *Trust Discussion Formula Poster B.4.*)←

5A.1.B. Substance User's Statement:

> **SUGGESTED THERAPIST SCRIPT**
>
> The substance user should make a statement to his or her partner about his or her recovery for the last 24 hours and his or her intentions for the next 24 hours. An example sounds like:
> "I have been drug and alcohol free for the last 24 hours and plan to remain drug and alcohol free for the next 24 hours. I want to thank you for listening and being supportive of my effort to be drug and alcohol free."
> Do you think you can make this statement to your partner?

5A.1.C. Non-Substance-Abusing Partner's Statement:

> **SUGGESTED THERAPIST SCRIPT**
>
> The non-substance-user should thank his or her partner for remaining abstinent for the last 24 hours and offer support for the next 24 hours. An example may sound like:
> "Thank you for staying drug and alcohol free for the last 24 hours, and let me know how I can help during the next 24 hours."
> Do you think you can make this statement to your partner?

Partners can come up with their own version of the above statements. If they add their own words, be sure to check for negative statements. If medication is included, add "I'm taking this medication to help my recovery" to the patient's statement and "Thanks for taking the medication to help your recovery" to the spouse's statement.

5A.1.D. In-Session Practice of the Trust Discussion:

> **SUGGESTED THERAPIST SCRIPT**
>
> Now, I'd like you to practice the Trust Discussion. This will help you learn how you would like to have the discussion. It also gives me a chance to make sure you fully understand your roles in the discussion. This may feel awkward at first, but you'll get more comfortable with it over time. I may jump in to give you feedback or let you know if you are getting off track.
> I'll start by modeling the Trust Discussion with one of you. Then you'll practice together.

This is the couple's first time practicing in front of a therapist, so try to make them as comfortable as possible. Validate any concerns. Emphasize the need to practice skills in session to show that they understand the task. Give feedback and guidance they can use to be effective.

(continued)

5A.1.E. Get Verbal Commitment from the Partners:

Have the partners commit to doing the Trust Discussion each day this week.

5A.2. Not a Time to Bring Up the Past:

SUGGESTED THERAPIST SCRIPT
The Trust Discussion is not a time to bring up past substance use or fears about future use. It should be a positive discussion. Introducing a negative into the discussion may sound like this: "Thank you for staying drug and alcohol free, but I know this is only the calm before the storm because I have seen this before."

5A.3. Self-Help Involvement:

Both partners may also agree to attend self-help meetings as part of the Recovery Contract (e.g., AA three times a week for the substance user; Al-Anon weekly for the non-user) and record the times and dates for these meetings in the space provided on the contract and calendar.

5A.4. Urine Drug Screens:

At each BCT session, those with a current drug problem submit a urine screen. Positive (e.g., drugs in the urine) or negative (e.g., drug free) results are marked on the calendar.

5A.5. Other Recovery Activities:

SUGGESTED THERAPIST SCRIPT
This part of the contract covers other activities such as engaging in daily meditation, contacting your sponsor, reading the Big Book, or attending individual sessions.

5B. Early Warning System:

If the Trust Discussion does not take place for 2 days in a row, the partners should contact the therapist. There is a space on the Recovery Contract for the therapist's name and phone number.

5C. Length of Contract:

The Recovery Contract covers the time from the day it is signed until the end of weekly BCT sessions. Changes must be discussed in a face-to-face meeting of couple and therapist.

5D. The Recovery Calendar:

(Show *Sample Recovery Contract Calendar Poster B.5*; hand out *Recovery Contract Calendar Form C.2.*)

The Recovery Calendar provides an ongoing record of progress that is reviewed at each session.

Recovery Contract Home Practice:
- Do Trust Discussion (with medication, if taking it) every day at specified time.
- Mark on the calendar when discussion is done, self-help meeting attended, and urine screen results.
- Review Recovery Contract and bring it to the next session to be signed.

(continued)

6. Catch Your Partner Doing Something Nice Exercise:

→(Show *Sample Caring Behaviors Poster B.6*; show *Catch Your Partner Poster B.7*.)←

6A. Rationale: Couples often say that substance use has interfered with their expressions of caring. Catch Your Partner Doing Something Nice can help put caring back into the relationship.

SUGGESTED THERAPIST SCRIPT
Caring behaviors show that you respect and appreciate one another. Too often we take these behaviors for granted. The first step in learning to give and receive caring behaviors is learning to notice them. That is the purpose of Catch Your Partner Doing Something Nice. Keep in mind that these don't have to be out-of-the-ordinary things. They can be everyday actions that show caring or affection. For example, it could be something as simple as your partner bringing you a cup of coffee in the morning or telling you that you look nice. Do either of you have any questions or concerns?

6B. In-Session Practice of Catch Your Partner:

Next, explain to partners how to identify and record caring behaviors on the *Catch Your Partner Worksheet (Form C.3)*. Ask each partner to give an example of one caring behavior he or she noticed in the previous week. Give examples of caring behaviors if the partners appear to be struggling.

6C. Catch Your Partner Home Practice:

→(Hand out *Catch Your Partner Form C.3*.)←
- Each partner is asked to identify one caring behavior that his or her partner does each day. They should look for ordinary, "everyday" behaviors that express caring and affection. This exercise may seem awkward at first, but it will become second nature with practice.

7. Assign Home Practice:

→(Hand out *Home Practice Session 1 Form C.4*.)←

7A. Recovery Contract:
- Do Trust Discussion (with medication, if taking it) every day at specified time.
- Mark on the calendar each time the Trust Discussion is completed.
- Review Recovery Contract and bring it to next session to be signed.

7B. Catch Your Partner Doing Something Nice:
- Notice one nice thing your partner does each day and write it on the *Catch Your Partner Worksheet* (*Form C.3*), but do not tell each other what you wrote down.
- Bring the completed worksheet to the next session.

8. Session Closing:

8A. Answer Questions: Answer any questions about the home practice assignments.

8B. Commit to Home Practice: Get verbal commitment to do the home practice. Stress that they have a choice whether or not to accept an assignment. It is better if they refuse an assignment or agree to do less than suggested, than to agree and then not follow through.

Checklist for BCT Session 2:
Catch Your Partner Doing Something Nice and Tell Him or Her

Posters Needed:	Forms Needed:
B.8. Acknowledging Caring Behaviors	C.5. Catch and Tell
	C.6. Home Practice Session 2

Note: B.8 refers to Poster B.8 in Appendix B, C.5 to Form C.5 in Appendix C

Cover the following material as completely as possible. Place a checkmark next to each completed section.

1. Welcome Back

___ Review typical sequence of sessions.

___ Collect urine screen, if patient has drug problem.

___ Review urges or actual substance use in past week.

___ Review relationship problems or other concerns from past week; defer details until after review of home practice.

___ See if Promises were kept past week; commit to Promises for coming week.

2. Review Home Practice from Past Week

___ Recovery Contract

   ___ Review daily Trust Discussion (with medication, if taking it) and calendar of past week.

   ___ Couple practices Trust Discussion (with medication, if taking it) with therapist feedback.

   ___ Review self-help and other parts of Recovery Contract.

   ___ Sign Recovery Contract as ongoing commitment.

___ Catch Your Partner Doing Something Nice

   ___ Partners take turns reading caring behaviors they noticed in past week.

   ___ Go slowly, with therapist stressing positive impact of noticed behaviors.

3. Deal with Current Problems/Other Support for Abstinence

___ Explain that stress from life problems (e.g., job, financial problems) can trigger relapse.

___ Address past week or other problems directly or by referral to another source of help.

(continued)

4. Catch Your Partner Doing Something Nice and Tell Him or Her

___ Explain importance of telling partner about (acknowledging) caring behaviors. →(Show *Acknowledging Caring Behaviors Poster B.8.*)←

___ Therapist models how to acknowledge caring behaviors.

___ Couple practices acknowledging caring behaviors with therapist coaching.

___ Assign home practice. →(Hand out *Catch and Tell Form C.5.*)←

5. Assign Home Practice

→(Hand out *Home Practice Session 2 Form C.6.*)←

___ Recovery Contract

   ___ Do Trust Discussion (with medication, if taking it) and mark on calendar.

   ___ Do self-help and other parts of contract and mark on calendar.

___ Catch and Tell (acknowledge one nice thing partner does each day).

6. Session Closing

___ Answer questions about assignments.

___ Get commitment from each person to do home practice assignments.

BCT SESSION 2 OUTLINE
CATCH YOUR PARTNER DOING SOMETHING NICE AND TELL HIM OR HER

This session increases support for abstinence by using the Recovery Contract and increases positive activities by using the exercise Catch Your Partner Doing Something Nice and Tell Him or Her.

1. Welcome Back:

BCT sessions tend to be moderately structured and follow a specific agenda. A typical session starts by welcoming the partners back to BCT.

1A. Review Sequence of Sessions:
A general overview of the session offers an outline of what the couple can expect in a session.

SUGGESTED THERAPIST SCRIPT
As you can see, we will be covering quite a bit today. If, at any time, either one of you is thinking about stopping our couples sessions, I ask that you talk with me before stopping. With that said, is each of you willing to continue with today's session?

1B. Collect Urine Screen if Patient Has Drug Problem:
Administer the urine screen to the substance-using patient.

1C. Review Urges or Actual Substance Use in Past Week:
Ask: "Could you tell me about times since we last met when you drank or used drugs or had an urge or temptation to do so?"

1D. Review Relationship Problems or Other Concerns from Past Week:
Ask: "How did things go between the two of you in the past week? Any arguments? Positive times? Other important issues?" This segment should provide a brief overview of how the past week went. Defer any extensive discussion until after review of the home practice.

1E. Review Promises:

SUGGESTED THERAPIST SCRIPT
Each week we will review the Promises made in the last session.
1. No threats of divorce or separation.
2. No violence or threats of violence.
3. Focus on the present and future.
4. Attendance and active participation.
Review each Promise, asking each person "Have you been able to keep these Promises since last week? Can you commit to these Promises for the upcoming week?"

(continued)

2. Review Home Practice from Last Week:

Home practice helps couples change how they act in their day-to-day lives—a key goal of BCT. Reviewing home practice let's the counselor see how well the couple carried through with the assignment, reinforce that skills and activities build on each other, and discuss any problems with the assignment. Much of this session is spent reviewing the couple's first week using the Recovery Contract and doing the Catch Your Partner Doing Something Nice exercise.

2A. Recovery Contract:

1. **Repeat Assignment:** The patient and partner were to practice the Trust Discussion daily and record on the calendar each day it was done. They also were to review the Recovery Contract to see what other elements to add, and bring it to the session. Most couples will have other parts to their contract, including self-help meetings, urine screens, and recovery medication. These other elements can be added or changed at this or future sessions. For example, a patient might start or increase AA attendance or add medication.
2. **Rationale for Assignment:** To rebuild trust in the relationship and help the substance abuse patient stay abstinent.
3. **Review Assignment:** Ask the partners if they practiced the Trust Discussion and reviewed the Recovery Contract. Review the calendar to see how often they did the Trust Discussion and other elements of their contract.
4. **In-Session Practice:** The partners practice the Trust Discussion (with medication, if taking it) in session, allowing for feedback and correction if necessary. Address any difficulties they report or you observe during practice. Stress the importance of doing all parts of the Recovery Contract.
5. **Sign Recovery Contract:** Therapist and couple sign the Recovery Contract to reinforce the couple's commitment to follow it on a daily basis. If they did the Trust Discussion less than 5 of the past 7 days, let them practice another week before signing contract.

2B. Catch Your Partner Doing Something Nice:

1. **Repeat Assignment:** Each person was to notice one nice thing that his or her partner did each day and record it on the *Catch Your Partner Worksheet*.
2. **Rationale for Assignment:** To help each person notice pleasing things their partner is already doing rather than take them for granted.
3. **Review Assignment:** Have each person take turns reading caring behaviors recorded in past week. Start with the woman, because she is more likely to have done it completely. Ask her to read what she wrote for the day after the last session. Then ask the man to read what he wrote for that same day. Proceed in this manner through the week, day by day, alternating partner reports for each day. After each person reads a behavior, you can note the possible underlying meaning behind what the person is saying. For example, the husband's checking the tire pressure on his wife's car shows he is concerned about her safety.
4. **Compliance Problems:** When a partner did not write anything positive on the sheet, try to find out what kept him or her from doing so. Being too busy, feeling angry, or thinking it had to be something major or out of the ordinary are the most common reasons. Clarify and ask the person to think back over the week and pick one or two things he or she could have written down.
5. **Refine Statements:** With prompting and feedback, help the couple be more specific and explicit in describing caring behaviors they noticed, as well as how those behaviors made them feel.

(continued)

3. Deal with Current Problems/Other Support for Abstinence:

3A. Current Problems:

Rationale: Stress caused by life problems (e.g., medical, job, legal, financial, psychiatric, or other problems) can trigger relapse. Resolving stressful life problems reduces relapse risk.

- *Choose problem wisely*: A problem from past week noted earlier in session or an ongoing concern. Start with problem that may show quick progress. Defer complex, contentious, nonurgent problems until gains in abstinence and communication have been made.
- *Find solutions*: Help partners discuss solutions. Invite them to take action to resolve a problem and report back at next session on their progress. Actions to deal with life problems can be part of Recovery Contract: (1) take medications for medical or psychiatric problems during Trust Discussion; (2) mark attendance at other counseling or probation sessions on the calendar. Even if no solution can be found, a shared problem may be easier to bear.
- *Refer to other providers*: Refer to other help, as needed. Link with other providers who are helping patient with life problems to encourage patient's problem solving and abstinence.

4. Catch Your Partner Doing Something Nice and Tell Him or Her:

Rationale: People tend to focus more on negative than on positive aspects of their relationships, especially when they are not getting along. Catch Your Partner Doing Something Nice and Tell Him or Her, or Catch and Tell for short, helps build positive communication.

4A. Explain Importance of Telling Partner about (Acknowledging) Caring Behaviors:
→(Show *Acknowledging Caring Behaviors Poster B.8.*)←

SUGGESTED THERAPIST SCRIPT

We already talked about how to notice caring behaviors your partner does for you. Now we are going to talk about how to acknowledge caring behaviors by letting your partner know how you felt when they did something nice. We call this Catch Your Partner Doing Something Nice and Tell Him or Her, or Catch and Tell for short.

Acknowledging caring behaviors can increase positive feelings in your relationship. It lets your partner know what you appreciate, so they are more likely to continue these actions. Finally, by sharing your positive feelings, you can start opening your hearts to each other.

Catch and Tell begins our work together on your communication skills, starting with communicating positive feelings. Let's start by reviewing the chart on "what to say" and "how to say it" when acknowledging caring behaviors.

Review *Poster B.8* on effective ways to acknowledge caring behaviors. Elicit the couple's comments and questions to be sure they understand the basic concept.

4B. Therapist Models How to Acknowledge Caring Behaviors:

SUGGESTED THERAPIST SCRIPT

You are going to practice acknowledging caring behaviors by telling your partner what you liked that he or she did for you or said to you. Although this may feel awkward at first, remember that sometimes behavior change comes first and is followed by a change in feelings.

I'll start by showing you some examples.

(continued)

4.B.1. Therapist Models Correctly:

The therapist models how to acknowledge caring behaviors correctly, first using an actual example from his or her own day.

SUGGESTED THERAPIST SCRIPT

It may be helpful to both of you if I give you an example of how to do this correctly:
 "Thank you for coming on time to the session. It shows that you have a real commitment to your relationship and to your recovery."

In modeling, be sure to use positive nonverbal components (e.g., pleasant tone of voice, smile). Ask the couple to point out which of the elements listed on *Poster B.8* were part of your demonstration. Point out elements that they miss and be sure they understand your feedback.

4.B.2. Therapist Models Incorrectly:

The therapist models an ineffective example so that the couple can see the difference between correct and incorrect ways of acknowledging caring behaviors.

SUGGESTED THERAPIST SCRIPT

Now, what might an ineffective example of acknowledging caring behaviors look like?
 Perhaps: "I liked it when you did the laundry yesterday, but you should try doing it every day. Besides, you don't thank me when I do YOUR laundry."

If you do this modeling in a low tone of voice, without smiling or looking at the partner, it will also show incorrect nonverbal communication.

- Solicit feedback on your modeling in relation to the elements on *Poster B.8*. Ask them first to say which aspects were done well (e.g., it started off positive), then what needed improvement (e.g., had a lot of negative content, and nonverbal aspects were all wrong).
- The therapist reenacts the scenario correctly, based on feedback provided by the couple.

4C. In-Session Practice of Catch and Tell:

Each person takes a turn acknowledging caring behaviors, using the most pleasing example from the Catch Your Partner form completed the previous week.

SUGGESTED THERAPIST SCRIPT

Now I would like each of you to look at the Catch Your Partner form. Pick the caring behavior that was most pleasing to you, and then tell your partner what you liked about the behavior and how it made you feel. Try to follow the guidelines on the Acknowledging Caring Behaviors chart (*Poster B.8*). You can start with:
 "I liked it when you . . . " or "Thank you for . . . " or "It made me feel . . . "

- When the first person has stated his or her acknowledgment, identify positive aspects of the performance first and then move on to any constructive suggestions. You can model, if necessary, to demonstrate improvements.
- The person tries the acknowledgment again. You give positive feedback, noting even small improvements. Usually one, or at most two, "replays" are needed for the person to get it right.

(continued)

- Repeat this process with the second member of the couple.
- Practice, not perfection, is the goal, especially when doing this exercise for the first time. Try to get a convincing, sincere statement of appreciation within the current limits of the couple's relationship and each partner's background and skill level.

4D. Catch and Tell Home Practice: →(Hand out *Catch and Tell Form C.5.*)←

- Each person is asked to notice and acknowledge one nice thing that the partner does each day.
- Ask partners to write down the behavior noticed on the Catch and Tell form and to check off that they acknowledged it.
- Many couples share the most pleasing thing they have noticed in their partners' behavior in the last 24 hours after the Trust Discussion that is part of the Recovery Contract.

5. Assign Home Practice:

→(Hand out *Home Practice Session 2 Form C.6.*)←

5A. Recovery Contract:

- Do Trust Discussion (with medication, if taking it) every day at specified time.
- Do self-help and other parts of contract.
- Mark on calendar each time Trust Discussion and other parts of contract are done.

5B. Catch and Tell:

- Notice and acknowledge one nice thing your partner does each day and write it on the *Catch and Tell Worksheet (Form C.5)*.
- Bring the completed worksheet to the next session.

6. Session Closing:

6A. Answer Questions: Answer any questions about the home practice assignments.

6B. Commit to Home Practice: Get verbal commitment to do the home practice. Stress that they have a choice whether or not to accept an assignment. It is better if they refuse an assignment or agree to do less than suggested, than to agree and then not follow through.

Checklist for BCT Session 3: Shared Rewarding Activities and Caring Day

Posters Needed:	Forms Needed:
B.9. Possible Shared Activities B.10. Caring Day!	C.7. List of Possible Shared Activities C.8. Home Practice Session 3
Note: B.9 refers to Poster B.9 in Appendix B, C.7 to Form C.7 in Appendix C.	

Cover the following material as completely as possible. Place a checkmark next to each completed section.

1. Welcome Back

___ Review typical sequence of sessions.

___ Collect urine screen, if patient has drug problem.

___ Review urges or actual substance use in past week.

___ Review relationship problems or other concerns from past week; defer details until after review of home practice.

___ See if Promises were kept past week; commit to Promises for coming week.

2. Review Home Practice from Past Week

___ Recovery Contract

    ___ Review daily Trust Discussion (with medication, if taking it) and calendar of past week.

    ___ Couple practices Trust Discussion (with medication, if taking it) with therapist feedback.

    ___ Review self-help and other parts of Recovery Contract.

___ Catch Your Partner Doing Something Nice and Tell Him or Her

    ___ Review Catch and Tell (acknowledge one nice thing partner did each day).

    ___ Practice acknowledging caring behaviors of past week, with therapist coaching.

3. Deal with Current Problems/Other Support for Abstinence

___ *Problems:* Explain that stress from life problems (e.g., money problems) can trigger relapse.

    ___ Address past week or other problems directly or by referral to another source of help.

___ *Exposure:* Explain that exposure to alcohol or drugs is a high-risk situation for relapse.

    ___ Help partners decide how to deal with upcoming exposure situations.

(continued)

4. Shared Rewarding Activities

___ Explain importance and types of fun couple and family activities.
→(Show *Possible Shared Activities Poster B.9.*)←

___ Therapist models how to plan a Shared Rewarding Activity (SRA).

___ Couple practices planning an SRA for coming week, with therapist coaching.

___ Assign home practice (do planned SRA, complete list of possible SRAs).
→(Hand out *List of Possible SRAs Form C.7.*)←

5. Caring Day

___ Explain importance of doing special things to show caring to your partner.
→(Show *Caring Day Poster B.10.*)←

___ A Caring Day is when you plan ahead to do special things for your partner.

___ Couple gives examples of possible Caring Day actions.

___ Assign home practice (give your partner a Caring Day this week).

6. Assign Home Practice

→(Hand out *Home Practice Session 3 Form C.8.*)←

___ Recovery Contract

   ___ Do Trust Discussion (with medication, if taking it) and mark on calendar.

   ___ Do self-help and other parts of contract and mark on calendar.

___ Catch and Tell (acknowledge one nice thing partner does each day).

___ Shared Rewarding Activity (do planned SRA, list possible future SRAs).

___ Caring Day (give your partner a Caring Day this week).

7. Session Closing

___ Answer questions about assignments.

___ Get commitment from each person to do home practice assignments.

BCT SESSION 3 OUTLINE
SHARED REWARDING ACTIVITIES AND CARING DAY

This session introduces more ways to increase positive activities and feelings in the relationship by using Shared Rewarding Activities and Caring Day.

1. Welcome Back:

1A. Collect Urine Screen, If Patient Has Drug Problem.

1B. Review Urges or Actual Substance Use in Past Week:
Ask: "Could you tell me about times since we last met when you drank or used drugs or had an urge or temptation to do so?"

1C. Review Relationship Problems or Other Concerns from Past Week:
Ask: "How did things go between the two of you in the past week? Any arguments? Positive times? Other important issues?" This segment should give a brief overview of how the past week went. Defer any extensive discussion until after review of the home practice.

1D. Review Promises:
Review each Promise, asking each person: "Have you been able to keep these Promises since last week? Can you commit to these Promises for the upcoming week?"

2. Review Home Practice from Last Week:

2A. Recovery Contract:
1. **Repeat Assignment:** The patient and partner were to do all parts of their Recovery Contract.
2. **Rationale for Assignment:** To rebuild trust in the relationship and help the substance abuse patient stay abstinent.
3. **Review Assignment:** Review the calendar to see how often they did the Trust Discussion and other elements of their contract. Discuss obstacles and ways to get more benefits; for example, if going to AA, may consider getting a sponsor, joining a group.
4. **In-Session Practice of the Trust Discussion:** The partners practice the Trust Discussion (with medication, if taking it) in session, allowing for feedback and correction by therapist.

2B. Catch Your Partner Doing Something Nice and Tell Him or Her:
1. **Repeat Assignment:** Each person was to notice and acknowledge one nice thing their partner did each day and record it on the Catch and Tell Worksheet.
2. **Rationale for Assignment:** To help each person notice and acknowledge pleasing things their partner is already doing rather than take them for granted.
3. **Review Assignment:** Ask if they completed the assignment. Troubleshoot problems and encourage partners to do acknowledging ("daily compliment") after they do Trust Discussion.
4. **In-Session Practice of Catch and Tell:** Ask each person to practice acknowledging the two most pleasing, caring behaviors they noticed in the past week. With prompting and feedback, help the partners become more specific and explicit in describing caring behaviors they noticed, as well as how those behaviors made them feel.

(continued)

3. Deal with Current Problems/Other Support for Abstinence:

3A. Current Problems:

Rationale: Stress caused by life problems (e.g., medical, job, legal, financial, psychiatric, or other problems) can trigger relapse. Resolving stressful life problems reduces relapse risk.

- *Choose problem wisely*: A problem from past week noted earlier in session or an ongoing concern. Start with problem that may show quick progress. Defer complex, contentious, nonurgent problems until gains in abstinence and communication have been made.
- *Find solutions*: Help them discuss solutions. Invite them to take action to resolve a problem and report back at next session on their progress. Actions to deal with life problems can be part of Recovery Contract: (1) take medications for medical or psychiatric problems during Trust Discussion; (2) mark attendance at other counseling or probation sessions on the calendar. Even if no solution can be found, a shared problem may be easier to bear.
- *Refer to other providers*: Refer to other help, as needed. Link with other providers who are helping patient with life problems to encourage patient's problem solving and abstinence.

3B. Exposure to Situations Where Alcohol or Drugs Are Available:

Rationale: Patients' exposure to situations where alcohol or drugs are available or others are using such substances is a high-risk situation for relapse. Reducing exposure can reduce relapse.

The safest plan is for the patient to avoid situations where alcohol or drugs are available, especially in the early months of abstinence. However, many people are not willing or able to do this. You should help patients develop their own plan using the following common areas.

- Will alcohol be kept and served at home?
- Will the spouse drink in front of the patient?
- Will they attend social gatherings involving alcohol?
- Identify how to handle other exposure situations (work, friends, family).
- Identify exposure situations expected in coming week.

Pick one of these to discuss at a session. At each session ask what exposure situations they expect to face in the coming week, and discuss how they plan to deal with them. Pay special attention to seasonal events such as Thanksgiving, Christmas, and summer cookouts.

4. Shared Rewarding Activities:

Rationale: The upset that comes with a substance abuse problem can cause a couple to stop doing enjoyable things together. Participating in Shared Rewarding Activities puts fun back in the relationship.

4A. Explain Importance and Types of Fun Couple and Family Activities:
→(Show *Possible Shared Activities Poster B.9.*)←

SUGGESTED THERAPIST SCRIPT

Dealing with a substance abuse problem can cause a couple to stop doing enjoyable things together. Often a pattern develops in which the couple spends less time together, and the substance abuser spends more time isolating or using substances.

They no longer do activities they once enjoyed. The spouse often fears that the substance abuser will get intoxicated and embarrass the family. They may not enjoy each other's company anymore. Hobbies, sports, and other interests often take a back seat to trying to keep the family together, the bills paid, and the substance abuser out of trouble. As a result, it is not surprising that many couples have not done anything fun together or with the family in a long time.

(continued)

The goal of Shared Rewarding Activities is to begin to put fun back in your relationship. Fun activities together can bring you closer together as a couple and family. In addition, substance abusers who do activities with their spouse and children have better recovery rates.

In the Shared Rewarding Activity exercise, you will be asked to plan and do fun activities together each week. In planning, you can choose from three types of activities: (1) as a couple, (2) with the kids, or (3) with other couples or families. Activities can take place at home or out and they can be inexpensive (watch a TV movie together) or extensive (plan a weekend away). The activity should be something that both of you agree on and is mutually enjoyable. The ultimate goal is to spend more quality time together.

Please keep a few rules in mind while you do this exercise. First, make sure you compromise when choosing the activity, rather than having only one person decide. Second, make sure the activity you choose is feasible. The activity should be something that you can easily see yourself doing, meaning you can afford it, you have the time to do it, and you have a reasonable idea of how to do it. Finally, try to think of any obstacles (such as weather, babysitter, money) that may affect the activity and think of ways to handle those obstacles. For example, if you plan to go to the park for a walk and it starts to rain, what will you do instead?

Do you have any questions or concerns?

4B. Therapist Models How to Plan a Shared Rewarding Activity (SRA):

SUGGESTED THERAPIST SCRIPT

I will plan an activity using the rules we just talked about to show you how it works.

I want to be specific when choosing my activity. Therefore, I might say to my partner, "I would like to rent a movie this Saturday night." I stated what I want to do, not what I wouldn't want to do.

Next, I would check that my partner wants to do the same thing. Let's say that the movie idea is appealing to my partner, but then we realize that Saturday can't work because the kids will be home. Brainstorming on what we could do, we realize that it is high time the kids had a sleepover at Grandma's house. I will call my mom and make the arrangements for the kids, so that we can watch a movie and spend some time alone.

Now, that solution worked out. But in the event babysitting arrangements could not be made, we could consider a different night or decide that the activity could still be on Saturday but as a family night at home.

Are there any questions before you work together to plan an activity?

4C. In-Session Practice of Planning an SRA for Coming Week:

Following the therapist's model, the couple should plan the Shared Rewarding Activity that they will do in the coming week. If they cannot agree on an activity they both want to do, they can alternate week to week.

SUGGESTED THERAPIST SCRIPT

Following my example and using the rules we talked about, I would like for you to plan a Shared Rewarding Activity. Once you have chosen an activity, I want you to plan a day and time that you will do the activity during the upcoming week. Remember that the activity does not have to be expensive and should be something that you both want and are able to do. [You should guide the couple through the discussion, if necessary. Keep partners focused on the task and using the rules as a guideline when planning the activity.]

Great! Now that you have picked the activity, are there any obstacles to completing it? If so, what might you do differently?

(continued)

4D. Shared Rewarding Activity Home Practice:

→(Hand out *List of Possible Shared Activities Form C.7*.)←

- Partners do the Shared Rewarding Activity planned in this session in the upcoming week.
- Partners write down possible future activities on the *List of Possible Shared Activities Form C.7*.
- Remind couple that they don't need to feel that everything about their relationship is perfect in order to have a good time together. Usually, change in behavior comes first and then feelings will change. In other words, the couple may not be enthusiastic about doing an activity together, but planning and doing the activity may change their feelings about the situation.

5. Caring Day (Stuart, 1980):

→(Show *Caring Day Poster B.10*)←

5A. Explain Caring Day and Importance of Doing Special Things to Show Caring:

SUGGESTED THERAPIST SCRIPT
Now I will introduce a new way to bring more caring into your relationship, called Caring Day. Often, early in a relationship, we tend to do more "caring activities"—small demonstrations of affection and kindness shown to our partner. Later in a relationship, these behaviors may decrease. Our lives get busy, and we forget to take the time to show our partner that we care.
A Caring Day is when you plan ahead to surprise your partner with some special things to show you care. You can do a number of little things throughout the day or a bigger, special gesture of caring. The aim is to put more caring back into your relationship by taking the time and energy to plan special activities that you think will please your partner.
Does this make sense to you? What might be some examples you can think of that could be part of a Caring Day? Is this something you are willing to commit to?

5B. Caring Day Home Practice:
- Each person picks one day during the week to complete a Caring Day for their partner.

6. Assign Home Practice:

→(Hand out *Home Practice Session 3 Form C.8*.)←

6A. Recovery Contract:
- Do Trust Discussion (with medication, if taking it) every day at specified time.
- Do self-help and other parts of contract.
- Mark on calendar each time Trust Discussion and other parts of contract are done.

6B. Catch and Tell:
- Notice and acknowledge one nice thing your partner does each day and write it on the *Catch and Tell* (*Form C.5*). Bring the completed worksheet to the next session.

(continued)

6C. Shared Rewarding Activity
- Do the Shared Rewarding Activity planned in this session in the upcoming week.
- Write down possible future activities on the *List of Possible Shared Activities* (Form C.7).

6D. Caring Day
- Surprise your partner with a Caring Day on which you plan ahead to do some special things to show you care.

7. Session Closing:

7A. Answer Questions: Answer any questions about the home practice assignments.

7B. Commit to Home Practice: Get verbal commitment to do the home practice. Stress that they have a choice whether or not to accept an assignment. It is better if they refuse an assignment or agree to do less than suggested, than to agree and then not follow through.

Checklist for BCT Session 4:
Introduction to Communication Skills Training

Posters Needed:	Forms Needed:
B.11. Message Intended = Message Received B.12. Nonverbal Communication B.13. Barriers to Communication B.14. Direct and Indirect Communication B.15. Communication Session B.27. Enabling	C.9. Dos and Don'ts C.10. Communication Session C.11. Home Practice Session 4

Note: B.11 refers to Poster B.11 in Appendix B, C.9 to Form C.9 in Appendix C.

Cover the following material as completely as possible. Place a checkmark next to each completed section.

1. Welcome Back

___ Review typical sequence of sessions.

___ Collect urine screen, if patient has drug problem.

___ Review urges or actual substance use in past week.

___ Review relationship problems or other concerns from past week; defer details until after review of home practice.

___ See if Promises were kept past week; commit to Promises for coming week.

2. Review Home Practice from Past Week

___ Recovery Contract

   ___ Review daily Trust Discussion (with medication, if taking it) and calendar of past week.

   ___ Couple practices Trust Discussion (with medication, if taking it) with therapist feedback.

   ___ Review self-help and other parts of Recovery Contract.

___ Catch Your Partner Doing Something Nice and Tell Him or Her

   ___ Review Catch and Tell (acknowledge one nice thing partner did each day).

   ___ Practice acknowledging best caring behavior of past week, with therapist coaching.

___ Shared Rewarding Activity (SRA)

   ___ Did they do planned SRA? If yes, review experience. If not, troubleshoot.

   ___ Review each person's lists of possible SRAs to find common elements.

   ___ Plan SRA for coming week.

___ Caring Day: Did each do a Caring Day for partner? If yes, review. If not, troubleshoot.

(continued)

3. Deal with Current Problems/Other Support for Abstinence

___ *Problems:* Explain that stress from life problems (e.g., money problems) can trigger relapse.

___ Address past week or other problems directly or by referral to another source of help.

___ *Exposure:* Explain that exposure to alcohol or drugs is a high-risk situation for relapse.

___ Help partners decide how to deal with upcoming exposure situations.

(The following is optional, based on couple's needs.)

___ *Enabling:* Explain enabling behavior, like giving the user money to buy alcohol or drugs.

___ Help couple identify and stop enabling behaviors. →(Show *Enabling Poster B.27.*)←

4. Communication Skills Training: Introduction

___ Explain that good communication occurs when speaker's intended message matches message received by listener. →(Show *Message Intended = Message Received Poster B.11.*)←

___ Explain nonverbal communication. →(Show *Nonverbal Communication Poster B.12.*)←

___ Explain barriers to communication. →(Show *Barriers to Communication Poster B.13.*)←

___ Explain direct and indirect communication and "dos and don'ts" of communication.
→(Show *Direct and Indirect Communication Poster B.14.*)←
→(Hand out *"Dos and Don'ts" Form C.9.*)←

___ Elicit partners' reactions and examples of these aspects of communication.

5. Communication Session

___ Introduce Communication Session. →(Show *Communication Session Poster B.15.*)←

___ Therapist models a Communication Session about a positive or neutral topic.

___ Couple practices a Communication Session about a positive or neutral topic.

___ Assign home practice (have a 10- to 15-minute Communication Session at home).
→(Hand out *Communication Session Form C.10.*)←

6. Assign Home Practice →(Hand out *Home Practice Session 4 Form C.11.*)←

___ Recovery Contract

___ Do Trust Discussion (with medication, if taking it) and mark on calendar.

___ Do self-help and other parts of contract and mark on calendar

___ Catch and Tell (acknowledge one nice thing partner does each day).

___ Shared Rewarding Activity (do planned SRA; plan one for following week).

___ Caring Day (give your partner a Caring Day this week).

___ Communication Session (for 10–15 minutes on positive or neutral topic at home).

7. Session Closing

___ Answer questions about assignments.

___ Get commitment from each person to do home practice assignments.

BCT SESSION 4 OUTLINE
INTRODUCTION TO COMMUNICATION SKILLS TRAINING

So far, sessions have focused on supporting abstinence and increasing positive activities. This session introduces some basic concepts behind good communication.

1. Welcome Back:

1A. Collect Urine Screen If Patient Has Drug Problem.

1B. Review Urges or Actual Substance Use in Past Week:
Ask: "Could you tell me about times since we last met when you drank or used drugs or had an urge or temptation to do so?"

1C. Review Relationship Problems or Other Concerns from Past Week:
Ask: "How did things go between the two of you in the past week? Any arguments? Positive times? Other important issues?" This segment should give a brief overview of how the past week went. Defer any extensive discussion until after review of the home practice.

1D. Review Promises:
Review each Promise, asking each person: "Have you been able to keep these Promises since last week? Can you commit to these Promises for the upcoming week?"

2. Review Home Practice from Last Week:

2A. Recovery Contract:
1. **Repeat Assignment:** The patient and partner were to do all parts of their Recovery Contract.
2. **Rationale for Assignment:** Rebuild trust and help substance abuse patient stay abstinent.
3. **Review Assignment:** Review the calendar to see how often they did the Trust Discussion and other elements of their contract. Discuss obstacles and ways to get more benefits; for example, if going to AA, may consider getting a sponsor, joining a group.
4. **In-Session Practice of the Trust Discussion:** The partners practice the Trust Discussion (with medication, if taking it) in session, allowing for feedback and correction by therapist.

2B. Catch Your Partner Doing Something Nice and Tell Him or Her:
1. **Repeat Assignment:** Acknowledge one nice thing his or her partner did each day.
2. **Rationale for Assignment:** Acknowledge pleasing things rather than take them for granted.
3. **Review Assignment:** Troubleshoot problems. Encourage them to do acknowledging ("daily compliment") after they do Trust Discussion each day.
4. **In-Session Practice of Catch and Tell:** Ask each person to practice acknowledging the two most pleasing, caring behaviors they noticed in the past week. Give feedback.

(continued)

2C. Shared Rewarding Activity:
1. **Repeat Assignment:** Do planned activity and make list of possible future activities.
2. **Rationale for Assignment:** Put some fun back into their couple and family relationships.
3. **Review Assignment:** Did they do planned SRA? If yes, review experience. If not, troubleshoot. Assess for level of discomfort and for possible problem areas.
4. **In-Session Practice of Shared Rewarding Activity:** Review their lists of possible SRAs to find common elements. If list not done, have them do it now. Plan SRA for coming week.

2D. Caring Day:
1. **Repeat Assignment:** Give your partner a Caring Day on which you plan ahead to do some special things to show you care.
2. **Rationale for Assignment:** To increase the level of caring in the relationship.
3. **Review Assignment:** Did each person do a Caring Day for their partner? Did the partner notice? If yes, review. If not, troubleshoot.

3. Deal with Current Problems/Other Support for Abstinence:

3A. Current Problems:

Rationale: Stress caused by life problems (e.g., medical, job, legal, financial, psychiatric, or other problems) can trigger relapse. Resolving stressful life problems reduces relapse risk.
- *Choose problem wisely*: A problem from past week noted earlier in session or an ongoing concern. Start with problem that may show quick progress. Defer complex, contentious, nonurgent problems until gains in abstinence and communication have been made.
- *Find solutions*: Help them discuss solutions. Invite them to take action to resolve a problem and report back at next session on their progress. Actions to deal with life problems can be part of Recovery Contract: (1) take medications for medical or psychiatric problems during Trust Discussion; (2) mark attendance at other counseling or probation sessions on the calendar. Even if no solution can be found, a shared problem may be easier to bear.
- *Refer to other providers*: Refer to other help, as needed. Link with other providers who are helping patient with life problems to encourage patient's problem solving and abstinence.

3B. Exposure to Situations Where Alcohol or Drugs Are Available:

Rationale: Patients' exposure to situations where alcohol or drugs are available or others are using such substances is a high-risk situation for relapse. Reducing exposure can reduce relapse.

The safest plan is for the patient to avoid situations where alcohol or drugs are available, especially in the early months of abstinence. However, many people are not willing or able to do this. You should help patients develop their own plan using the following common areas.
- Will alcohol be kept and served at home?
- Will the spouse drink in front of the patient?
- Will they attend social gatherings involving alcohol?
- Identify how to handle other exposure situations (work, friends, family).
- Identify exposure situations expected in coming week.

Pick one of these to discuss at a session. At each session ask what exposure situations they expect to face in the coming week, and discuss how they plan to deal with them. Pay special attention to seasonal events such as Thanksgiving, Christmas, and summer cookouts.

(continued)

3C. Spouse Enabling *(optional, based on couple's needs)*: →(Show *Enabling Poster B.27.*)←

Rationale: Spouses try many ways to cope with a loved one's substance abuse. Unfortunately, some coping behaviors by the spouse unintentionally trigger or reward substance use.

- Review poster examples. Enabling often has short-term benefit (e.g., avoid couple conflict or protect family from legal or economic problems), but chance of future substance use increases.
- Help them identify enabling behaviors in their relationship and recognize the potential harm of such actions.
- Discuss how they plan to stop enabling in the future.

4. Communication Skills Training: Introduction:

4A. Explain That Good Communication Happens When Speaker's Intended Message Matches Message Received by Listener:
→(Show *Message Intended = Message Received Poster B.11.*)←

SUGGESTED THERAPIST SCRIPT

So far we have focused on your Recovery Contract and increasing positive activities and feelings in your relationship. Now we are going to start working on communication. Many things can get in the way of effective communication. Busy lifestyles often make it difficult to talk regularly. Also, conflict and disagreement may make us reluctant to communicate about certain topics. Regardless of the cause, a breakdown in communication is at the root of many problems.

   Good communication happens when the speaker's intended message matches the message received by the listener. The chances of the message intended matching the message received increases dramatically when the speaker clearly states what he or she wants, thinks, or feels instead of assuming the listener already knows. In turn, the listener should make every effort to understand the message without filling in gaps with his or her own assumptions.

   Effective communication is the result of a blend of listening and speaking. The speaker clearly states what he or she think, feels, or wants, and the listener checks with the speaker to make sure he or she heard the speaker's message correctly. The listener should not filter the message with his or her emotions or try to guess what the speaker means. Both speaker and listener work together to ensure that the message intended equals the message received.

   Do you have any questions or comments before we go on?

4B. Explain Nonverbal Components of Communication:
→(Show *Nonverbal Communication Poster B.12.*)←

Good body language and tone of voice help the intended message match the message received.

SUGGESTED THERAPIST SCRIPT

Making sure that the message sent equals the message received helps to decrease any conflict that comes from negative communication patterns. When a message is unclear and delivered with an angry tone, the chance of the person actually listening drastically decreases because he or she is focusing on the negative. The key here is to really listen to the words and avoid interpreting or assuming what the other person is going to say.

   One way to ensure that the message sent equals the message received is to make certain your body language matches your message. Some helpful hints are: (1) make eye contact, (2) face the person who is talking to you, and (3) make every effort to listen to what the speaker is saying.

(continued)

You also want to be aware of your tone of voice. For example, if you want to ask your partner whether a household task needs to be done, make sure your tone is neutral or pleasant. Your partner is more likely to really hear what you are trying to say. Matching voice tone to your intended message clarifies and increases understanding of the message.

Are there any questions before we move forward?

4C. Explain Barriers to Communication:
→(Show *Barriers to Communication Poster B.13.*)←

SUGGESTED THERAPIST SCRIPT

There are a number of barriers to effective communication. I think that as we go through them, you will see how they can interfere with making the message intended match the message received.

Filters are the first barrier we'll talk about. When we filter messages, we are putting our own spin on what is being said to us. Examples of filters are fatigue, being under the influence of substances, feeling unhappy or very happy, or particularly sensitive to a certain subject. These situations or feelings influence how you interpret messages. For example, one partner may present the other with a compliment, but if the recipient is feeling depressed or moody, the compliment might sound insincere because of the mood of the listener, not the actual message. However, if the listener is in better spirits, the compliment might be well received.

The **"all-talk-and-no-listen" syndrome** is another communication barrier. This occurs when both partners think they are right and are unwilling to listen to what the other has to say.

An example might look like this (note: SA = substance abuser; P = partner):

SA: Blah, blah.

P: Yak, yak.

SA: What I said was "blah, blah."

P: What I said was "yak, yak."

Does this sound familiar to either of you?

The "blah, blah" and "yak, yak" can be replaced with anything. The point is that each person continues to restate his or her position without hearing the other at all. All talk and no listening can seriously impair your ability to resolve disagreements and relationship issues.

Blaming and shaming is another communication no-no. This might sound like: "You did this! It's all your fault." Or "You decided to do that on your own—live with your own choices!" Or "You lied before; why should I believe you now?" These are examples of statements that blame and shame the other person. These types of statements prevent each person from taking responsibility for their own feelings and ideas.

Individual communication styles can also interfere with effective communication. Someone who has an *aggressive style* might use intimidation and insults to get their own way and be less concerned about the other person. The opposite is a *passive style.* This person often takes the back seat to others' needs, may do things they don't want in order to avoid confrontation, and often does not stick up for him- or herself. An *assertive style* is best because it allows for negotiation, fairness without intimidation or ridicule, and does not take advantage of others. This counseling should help each of you gain a more assertive communication style.

Does either of you recognize how some of these barriers may have existed, or still do exist, in your communication with each other?

(continued)

4D. Explain Direct and Indirect Communication:

→(Show *Direct and Indirect Communication Poster B.14*; show *Dos and Don'ts Form C.9*.)←

SUGGESTED THERAPIST SCRIPT

We are going to briefly describe the differences between direct and indirect communication.

Direct communication involves expressing a feeling, thought, or belief in a clear and direct manner. The speaker takes responsibility for his or her own feelings and doesn't blame the other person for how he or she feels. This reduces the listener's defensiveness and makes it easier to receive the intended message. Helpful hints in expressing yourself directly include:

DO:
Actively and assertively express yourself
Say what you think, feel, believe
Take personal responsibility for thoughts, feelings, and behaviors
Express yourself with words, not actions
Discuss one issue at a time

    Indirect communication is marked by use of barriers and defenses as the speaker tries to avoid responsibility and remove focus from the issue being discussed. It involves not taking personal responsibility for actions, avoiding the issue, and trying to redirect the conversation away from the topic at hand. Some helpful hints to avoid using indirect expressions include:

DON'T:

Accuse or blame the other person	Delay the conversation
Passively withdraw	Sulk or act aggressively
Mind read	Lecture
Say "you never"	Use angry gestures
Bring up the past	Try to "win" or "punish"

Do you see any of this in your relationship?

---

5. Communication Session:

→(Show *Communication Session Poster B.15*.)←

5A. Introduce Idea of a Communication Session

Rationale: A Communication Session is a time to practice effective communication skills and to deal with concerns and problems. Partners begin practicing active listening and direct communication slowly, starting with "safe" topics, and progressing toward more sensitive topics.

SUGGESTED THERAPIST SCRIPT

We have spent much of this session talking about things that help or hinder communication. To close out this session, I would like to introduce a helpful technique that we will use a lot in the rest of counseling—a Communication Session.

    A Communication Session is a planned conversation in which you practice communication skills. The two of you talk privately, face-to-face, without distractions. You take turns as speaker or listener, without interruptions. You use communication skills learned in counseling sessions. The goal is that the message intended by speaker matches the message received by listener.

    Now we will use a Communication Session as a time to practice communication skills. We'll start first with easier skills (simple communication about positive or neutral topics) and build up in future sessions to harder skills (more complex communication about charged issues in your relationship).

(continued)

5B. In-Session Practice of a Communication Session about a Positive or Neutral Topic:

In this section, you model a Communication Session with one person and then have the couple engage in their own Communication Session about a neutral or positive topic (examples below).
- Neutral topics: Where would your dream vacation be? What animal is your favorite pet? What would you do if you won $1,000? What is your favorite childhood memory?
- Positive topics: What is your fondest memory of your relationship with your partner? What do you love the most about your partner? Talk about when you first met each other.

SUGGESTED THERAPIST SCRIPT

The goal of this first Communication Session is for both of you to pay attention to your body language, your tone of voice, and how you are feeling. Try to really listen to each other.

First, I will role-play a Communication Session for you. [Patient/spouse name], you'll be the listener and I'll be the speaker. Let's try this out. (*Model the desired behaviors.*)

Now you'll both do a Communication Session. There are a few steps that will help guide your discussion. Let's choose a positive or neutral topic to talk about for your first session. (Therapist note: See topics listed above). Sit face-to-face and use brief statements (two or three sentences) to describe your topic. This makes it easier for the listener to hear and remember what you said. You will both get the chance to be the speaker and the listener. I will allow 2–5 minutes to talk. I may interrupt to help keep the conversation focused. (*Partners engage in Communication Session.*)

How did that feel? What are some of the things you noticed about yourself? Are there some Dos or Don'ts that you have used in the past? What did you do differently today?

Provide corrective and supportive feedback to each partner after both complete the *Communication Session*. Interrupt and redirect the partners if they go off topic.

5C. Communication Session Home Practice:
→(Hand out *Communication Session Form C.10.*)←
Have a Communication Session during the upcoming week using the following guidelines:
- Sit face-to-face.
- Choose a time/place where you will have privacy; no distractions such as TV, radio, etc.
- Schedule 2–5 minutes each.
- Choose a topic that is neutral or positive.
- Work together, taking turns; decide who will go first as the speaker.
- Speaker should be brief (two to three sentences).
- Listener should not respond to the speaker except to ask related questions.
- Pay specific attention to body language, tone of voice, filters, and avoid the "all-talk-and-no-listen" syndrome. Refer to the Dos and Don'ts sheet.

6. Assign Home Practice:

→(Hand out *Home Practice Session 4 Form C.11.*)←

6A. Recovery Contract:
- Do Trust Discussion (with medication, if taking it) every day at specified time.
- Do self-help and other parts of contract.
- Mark on calendar each time Trust Discussion and other parts of contract are completed.

(continued)

6B. Catch and Tell:

- Notice and acknowledge one nice thing your partner does each day and write it on the *Catch and Tell Worksheet (Form C.5)*. Bring the completed worksheet to the next session.

6C. Shared Rewarding Activity

- Do the *Shared Rewarding Activity* planned in this session in the upcoming week.
- Plan an activity for the following week.

6D. Caring Day

- Surprise your partner with a Caring Day on which you plan ahead to do some special things to show you care.

6E. Communication Session on Positive and Neutral Topics

- Have a Communication Session using guidelines listed above and on home practice sheet.

7. Session Closing:

7A. Answer Questions: Answer any questions about the home practice assignments.

7B. Commit to Home Practice: Get verbal commitment to do the home practice.

Checklist for BCT Session 5:
Communication Skills Training: Expressing Feelings Directly

Posters Needed:	Forms Needed:
B.16. Expressing Feelings Directly Using "I" Messages	C.12. Home Practice Session 5

Note: B.16 refers to Poster B.16 in Appendix B, C.12 to Form C.12 in Appendix C.

Cover the following material as completely as possible. Place a checkmark next to each completed section.

1. Welcome Back

___ Review typical sequence of sessions.

___ Collect urine screen, if patient has drug problem.

___ Review urges or actual substance use in past week.

___ Review relationship problems or other concerns from past week; defer details until after review of home practice.

___ See if Promises were kept past week; commit to Promises for coming week.

2. Review Home Practice from Past Week

___ Recovery Contract

   ___ Review daily Trust Discussion (with medication, if taking it) and calendar of past week.

   ___ Couple practices Trust Discussion (with medication, if taking it) with therapist feedback.

   ___ Review self-help and other parts of Recovery Contract.

___ Catch Your Partner Doing Something Nice and Tell Him or Her

   ___ Review Catch and Tell (acknowledge one nice thing partner did each day).

   ___ Practice acknowledging best caring behavior of past week, with therapist coaching.

___ Shared Rewarding Activity (SRA)

   ___ Did they do planned SRA? If yes, review experience. If not, troubleshoot.

   ___ What shared activity have they planned for coming week?

___ Caring Day

   ___ Did each do a Caring Day for partner? If yes, review. If not, troubleshoot.

___ Communication Session

   ___ Review how planned Communication Session at home went.

   ___ Practice a Communication Session with coaching from therapist.

(continued)

3. Deal with Current Problems/Other Support for Abstinence
(Each of the following is optional, based on couple's needs. Refer to Session 4 for details.)

___ *Problems:* Address past week or other problems directly or refer to another source of help.

___ *Exposure to substances:* Help partners decide how to deal with upcoming exposure situations.

___ *Enabling:* Help couple identify and stop enabling. →(Show *Enabling Poster B.27.*)←

4. Communication Skills Training: Expressing Feelings Directly

___ Explain use of "I" Messages to express feelings directly.
→(Show *"I" Messages Poster B.16.*)←

___ Have partners take turns role-playing the direct expression of feelings.

___ Assign home practice (practice expressing feelings directly).

5. Assign Home Practice
→(Hand out *Home Practice Session 5 Form C.12.*)←

___ Recovery Contract

   ___ Do Trust Discussion (with medication, if taking it) and mark on calendar.

   ___ Do self-help and other parts of contract and mark on calendar.

___ Positive activities—pick at least one of following to do:

   ___ Catch and Tell (acknowledge one nice thing partner does each day).

   ___ Shared Rewarding Activity (do planned SRA; plan one for following week).

   ___ Caring Day (give your partner a Caring Day this week).

___ Communication Session (for 10–15 minutes using "I" Messages to express feelings directly).

6. Session Closing

___ Answer questions about assignments.

___ Get commitment from each person to do home practice assignments.

BCT SESSION 5 OUTLINE
COMMUNICATION SKILLS TRAINING: EXPRESSING FEELINGS DIRECTLY

This session continues the work on improving communication, using "I" Messages to express feelings directly and make it more likely that the speaker's intended message will be received by listener.

1. Welcome Back:

1A. Collect Urine Screen If Patient Has Drug Problem.

1B. Review Urges or Actual Substance Use in Past Week:
Ask: "Could you tell me about times since we last met when you drank or used drugs or had an urge or temptation to do so?"

1C. Review Relationship Problems or Other Concerns from Past Week:
Ask: "How did things go between the two of you in the past week? Any arguments? Positive times? Other important issues?" This segment should give a brief overview of how the past week went. Defer any extensive discussion until after review of the home practice.

1D. Review Promises:
Review each Promise, asking each person: "Have you been able to keep these Promises since last week? Can you commit to these Promises for the upcoming week?"

2. Review Home Practice from Last Week:

2A. Recovery Contract:
1. **Repeat Assignment:** The patient and partner were to do all parts of their Recovery Contract.
2. **Rationale for Assignment:** Rebuild trust and help substance abuse patient stay abstinent.
3. **Review Assignment:** Review the calendar to see how often they did the Trust Discussion and other elements of their contract. Discuss obstacles and ways to get more benefits; for example, if going to AA, may consider getting a sponsor, joining a group.
4. **In-Session Practice of the Trust Discussion:** The partners practice the Trust Discussion (with medication, if taking it) in session, allowing for feedback and correction by therapist.

2B. Catch and Tell:
1. **Repeat Assignment:** Acknowledge one nice thing their partner did each day.
2. **Rationale for Assignment:** Acknowledge pleasing things rather than take them for granted.
3. **Review Assignment:** Troubleshoot problems. Encourage them to do acknowledging ("daily compliment") after they do Trust Discussion each day.
4. **In-Session Practice of Catch and Tell:** Ask each person to practice acknowledging the two most pleasing, caring behaviors they noticed in the past week. Give feedback.

2C. Shared Rewarding Activity:
1. **Repeat Assignment:** Do planned activity and make list of possible future activities.
2. **Rationale for Assignment:** Put some fun back into their couple and family relationships.
3. **Review Assignment:** Did they do planned SRA? If yes, review experience. If not, troubleshoot. Did they plan SRA for coming week? If not, plan it now.

(continued)

2D. Caring Day:
1. **Repeat Assignment:** Give partner a Caring Day on which you plan ahead to do some special things to show you care.
2. **Rationale for Assignment:** To increase the level of caring in the relationship.
3. **Review Assignment:** Did each person do a Caring Day for their partner? Did the partner notice? If yes, review. If not, troubleshoot.

2E. Communication Session:
1. **Repeat Assignment:** The partners were to have a Communication Session using general guidelines on *Communication Session Poster B.18.* Specific instructions were as follows.
   - They were to choose a topic that was neutral or positive. Speaker should be brief (two or three sentences). Listener should not respond to the speaker except to ask related questions.
   - Notice body language, tone of voice, filters; and avoid "all-talk-and-no-listen" syndrome.
2. **Rationale for Assignment:** Practicing new communication skills will help the couple learn how to resolve problems and concerns in their relationship.
3. **Review Assignment:** Ask if they completed the Communication Session following the guidelines provided. Ask for specific feedback regarding the assignment.
4. **In-Session Practice of Communication Session:** Have couple role-play a Communication Session, using skills learned up to this point. Provide feedback and correction, as necessary.

3. Deal with Current Problems/Other Support for Abstinence:

(*Each of following is optional, based on couple's needs. Refer to Session 4 for details.*)

3A. Current Problems:
   Address past week or other problems directly or by referral to another source of help.

3B. Exposure to Situations Where Alcohol or Drugs Are Available:
   Help couple decide how to deal with upcoming exposure situations.

3C. Spouse Enabling:
   Help couple identify and stop enabling behaviors. →(Show *Enabling Poster B.27.*)←

4. Communication Skills Training: Expressing Feelings Directly:

4A. Explain Use of "I" Messages to Express Feelings Directly
→(Show *"I" Messages Poster B.16.*)←

SUGGESTED THERAPIST SCRIPT

Learning to express feelings directly is an important communication skill. Expressing feelings directly can help the speaker send clear and direct messages that have a better chance of being received and understood by the listener.

   Becoming aware of feelings is an important part of the recovery process. Often when individuals begin recovery, they become aware of some feelings for the first time. It is important not only to become aware of these feelings, but also to learn how to express them.

   An important tool in expressing feelings directly is the use of "I" Messages. We will discuss and role-play the use of "I" Messages today.

   The "I" Message skill is the first of several communication skills you will learn over the next few weeks. "I" Messages can help you slow down and express yourself directly, without blaming your partner. It is an effective tool for expressing positive and negative feelings.

(continued)

You can use "I" Messages by making a statement using this simple formula:

"I feel _____ [emotion] when you _____ [behavior]."

Partners should consider using an "I" Message particularly when they want to share feelings or thoughts without blaming, any time there is an inordinate amount of stress in the relationship, and when both partners are upset.

Therapist note: These statements encourage the speaker to slow down his or her speech, to choose words carefully, and to speak directly using feelings.

4B. In-Session Practice of a Communication Session to Express Feelings Directly:

The couple should now have a Communication Session to practice speaking skills using "I" Messages. You may use the "I" Messages poster to help guide them through this exercise.

SUGGESTED THERAPIST SCRIPT

I would like each of you to come up with two "I" Messages. For this exercise, focus on a positive behavior or feeling. For example, your statement may be a general one: "I feel happy when I have a Saturday to relax." Or it may be more specific to the relationship: "I feel appreciated when you bring me breakfast in bed." You may want to use an example from Catch and Tell.

---

1. Allow the partners an opportunity to share each of their "I" Messages. Provide corrective feedback, as needed. Make sure the statements are positive in nature.
2. Once the partners become comfortable with this simple formula, other components can be added, such as adding the reason for the feeling. Below you will find the addition of "because . . . "

SUGGESTED THERAPIST SCRIPT

You both did great with the first formula. Now that you are comfortable using an "I" Message, I would like to tack on one more piece to the formula. Now you will say something positive using the following formula:

"I feel _____ [emotion] when you _____ [behavior] because _____ (specific reason)."

For example: "I feel excited when you plan a date for us because it shows me how much you care." The speaker says why they felt the way they did.

---

1. Ask them to build on their earlier statements or to create two more using the new formula. Give feedback, allowing each partner time to incorporate it and get the formula right.
2. **Therapist note:** At this point, the couple should not be responding to each other's statements. Once the couple appears comfortable with the use of "I" Messages, you can move on to the Listening Skills (discussed in the next session).

4C. Assign Communication Session Home Practice to Express Feelings Directly:

SUGGESTED THERAPIST SCRIPT

Up to now, we have discussed effective communication Dos and Don'ts, barriers, and now "I" Messages. At the end of last week's session, I introduced the Communication Session. I would like you to have another Communication Session at home, this time using the "I" Message skill and your awareness of Dos and Don'ts and barriers. This exercise may feel awkward at first, but the idea is to learn to use the skill until it becomes second nature.

(continued)

Remember, there are a few simple guidelines to help you through a Communication Session: Sit face-to-face, allow no distractions, take turns talking, and be brief (two or three sentences). We want you to use "I" Messages as you practice discussing a positive or neutral topic. Remember to pay attention to the Dos and Don'ts as well.

- Have the couple conduct a 5- to 10-minute Communication Session in the coming week to practice the "I" Message skill discussed in this session.

5. Assign Home Practice:

→(Hand out *Home Practice Session 5 Form C.12.*)←

5A. Recovery Contract:
- Do Trust Discussion (with medication, if taking it) every day at specified time.
- Do self-help and other parts of contract.
- Mark on calendar each time Trust Discussion and other parts of contract are completed.

5B. Positive Activities—pick at least one of following to do:
- "Catch and Tell"—acknowledge one nice thing about partner each day when doing Trust Discussion.
- Shared Rewarding Activity—do planned SRA; plan one for following week.
- Caring Day—give your partner a Caring Day this week.

5C. Communication Session
- Have a Communication Session to practice using "I" Messages to express feelings directly on positive and neutral topics using guidelines on home practice sheet.

6. Session Closing:

6A. Answer Questions: Answer any questions about the home practice assignments.

6B. Commit to Home Practice: Get verbal commitment to do the home practice.

Checklist for BCT Session 6:
Communication Skills Training: Listening and Understanding

Posters Needed:	Forms Needed:
B.17. Listening and Understanding	C.13. Home Practice Session 6

Note: B.17 refers to Poster B.17 in Appendix B, C.13 to Form C.13 in Appendix C.

Cover the following material as completely as possible. Place a checkmark next to each completed section.

1. Welcome Back

___ Review typical sequence of sessions.

___ Collect urine screen, if patient has drug problem.

___ Review urges or actual substance use in past week.

___ Review relationship problems or other concerns from past week; defer details until after review of home practice.

___ See if Promises were kept past week; commit to Promises for coming week.

2. Review Home Practice from Past Week

___ Recovery Contract

   ___ Review daily Trust Discussion (with medication, if taking it) and calendar of past week.

   ___ Couple practices Trust Discussion (with medication, if taking it) with therapist feedback.

   ___ Review self-help and other parts of Recovery Contract.

___ Positive Activities—review which of the following they chose to do:

   ___ Catch and Tell (acknowledge one nice thing partner does each day at home and best of past week in session).

   ___ Shared Rewarding Activity (do planned SRA; plan one for following week).

   ___ Caring Day (give your partner a Caring Day this week).

___ Communication Session

   ___ Review how planned Communication Session at home went.

   ___ Practice a Communication Session with coaching from therapist.

(continued)

3. Deal with Current Problems/Other Support for Abstinence

(Each of following is optional, based on couple's needs. Refer to Session 4 for details.)

___ *Problems:* Address past week or other problems directly or refer to another source of help.

___ *Exposure to substances:* Help partners decide how to deal with upcoming exposure situations.

___ *Enabling:* Help couple identify and stop enabling behaviors. →(Show *Enabling Poster B.27.*)←

4. Communication Skills Training: Listening and Understanding

→(Show *Listening and Understanding Poster B.17.*)←

___ Listening: Listener restates and checks accuracy of message received from speaker (*"What I heard you say was _____. Did I get that right?"*).

___ Therapist explains and models Listening.

___ Each person practices Listening while therapist coaches.

___ Understanding: Listener says speaker's ideas make sense (*"It makes sense that you feel _____ because . . . "*) and shows empathy (*"That must make you feel . . . "*).

___ Therapist explains and models Listening with Understanding.

___ Each person practices Listening with Understanding while therapist coaches.

___ Assign home practice (practice listening with understanding).

5. Assign Home Practice

→(Hand out *Home Practice Session 6 Form C.13.*)←

___ Recovery Contract

   ___ Do Trust Discussion (with medication, if taking it) and mark on calendar.

   ___ Do self-help and other parts of contract and mark on calendar.

___ Positive activities—pick at least one of following to do:

   ___ Catch and Tell (acknowledge one nice thing partner does each day).

   ___ Shared Rewarding Activity (do planned SRA; plan one for following week).

   ___ Caring Day (give your partner a Caring Day this week).

___ Communication Sessions (three times for 10–15 minutes to practice Listening with Understanding on everyday problems and events but not charged issues).

6. Session Closing

___ Answer questions about assignments.

___ Get commitment from each person to do home practice assignments.

BCT SESSION 6 OUTLINE
COMMUNICATION SKILLS TRAINING: LISTENING AND UNDERSTANDING

This session continues the work on improving communication, by using Listening and Understanding to make it more likely that the speaker's intended message will be received by listener.

1. Welcome Back:

1A. Collect Urine Screen If Patient Has Drug Problem.

1B. Review Urges or Actual Substance Use in Past Week:
Ask: "Could you tell me about times since we last met when you drank or used drugs or had an urge or temptation to do so?"

1C. Review Relationship Problems or Other Concerns from Past Week:
Ask: "How did things go between the two of you in the past week? Any arguments? Positive times? Other important issues?" This segment should give a brief overview of how the past week went. Defer any extensive discussion until after review of the home practice.

1D. Review Promises:
Review each Promise, asking each person: "Have you been able to keep these Promises since last week? Can you commit to these Promises for the upcoming week?"

2. Review Home Practice from Last Week:

2A. Recovery Contract:
1. **Repeat Assignment:** The patient and partner were to do all parts of their Recovery Contract.
2. **Rationale for Assignment:** Rebuild trust and help substance abuse patient stay abstinent.
3. **Review Assignment:** Review the calendar to see how often they did the Trust Discussion and other elements of their contract. Discuss obstacles and ways to get more benefits; for example, if going to AA, may consider getting a sponsor, joining a group.
4. **In-Session Practice of the Trust Discussion:** The partners practice the Trust Discussion (with medication, if taking it) in session, allowing for feedback and correction by therapist.

2B. Positive Activities:
1. **Repeat Assignment:** Pick at least one of following to do:
   - Catch and Tell: Acknowledge one nice thing each day when doing Trust Discussion.
   - Shared Rewarding Activity: Do planned SRA; plan one for following week.
   - Caring Day: Give your partner a Caring Day this week.
2. **Rationale for Assignment:** Increase positive activities and feelings in the relationship.
3. **Review Assignment:** Review chosen assignment(s) following instructions in Session 5.
4. **In-Session Practice:** Practice chosen assignment(s) following instructions in Session 5.

(continued)

2C. Communication Session:

1. **Repeat Assignment:** The partners were to have a Communication Session using general guidelines on *Communication Session Poster B.18.* Specific instructions follow:
   - They were to choose a topic that was neutral or positive. Speaker should be brief (two or three sentences) and practice expressing feelings directly using "I" Messages. Listener should not respond to the speaker except to ask related questions.
   - Notice body language, tone of voice, filters, and avoid "all-talk-and-no-listen" syndrome.
2. **Rationale for Assignment:** Practicing new communication skills will help the couple learn how to resolve problems and concerns in their relationship.
3. **Review Assignment:** Ask if they completed the Communication Session following the guidelines provided. Ask for specific feedback regarding the assignment.
4. **In-Session Practice of Communication Session:** Have couple role-play a Communication Session, using skills learned up to this point. Provide feedback and correction, as necessary.

3. Deal with Current Problems/Other Support for Abstinence:

(*Each of the following is optional, based on couple's needs. Refer to Session 4 for details.*)

3A. Current Problems:

Address past week or other problems directly or by referral to another source of help.

3B. Exposure to Situations Where Alcohol or Drugs Are Available:

Help couple decide how to deal with upcoming exposure situations.

3C. Spouse Enabling:

Help couple identify and stop enabling behaviors. →(Show *Enabling Poster B.27.*)←

4. Communication Skills Training: Listening and Understanding:

→(Show *Listening and Understanding Poster B.17.*)←

4A. Explain the Listening Response:

SUGGESTED THERAPIST SCRIPT

Listening may seem simple enough, but often it is not so easy, especially when you are discussing an important or sensitive topic from opposing viewpoints. When couples argue, the discussion often gets faster, louder, and more intense as emotions flare and both people try harder to make their point. Often people assume they know what message is being sent without really listening to what is being said. If you're thinking about what you want to say next, you are not listening to the speaker.

To listen better, we have to slow down the conversation. You don't have to agree with your partner to understand their point of view. I'm going to ask you to listen to your partner and then repeat what you believe you heard them say. You may not get it right the first time. That's OK. Just try to really listen without judging or adding your own thoughts. You'll get a chance to talk, after you have understood what your partner had to say.

Here's how this whole thing works. We are going to be doing what's called the Listening Response. Remember that good communication happens when the intended message of the speaker matches the message received by the listener. The Listening Response is a key tool of good communication. Using this tool, the listener restates the message received from the partner and then asks if they heard correctly. We do this in order to decrease the tension that comes with not feeling heard.

Now, I'll walk you through both parts of the Listening Response.

(continued)

First, you **restate the message received.** The listener should state what he or she heard the speaker say by using the following formula. In addition, the listener should refrain from adding their own point of view, thoughts, or anything other than the speaker's intended message.

After the speaker has finished speaking, the listener will say:

"What I heard you say was . . . "

Next, **ask if you heard correctly.** The idea behind this step is to make sure the message was received correctly.

After restating the message received, the listener will say:

"Is that right?" or *"Did I get that right?"*

If the message was not heard correctly, the speaker will simply state what the listener missed, and the listener will try to restate the message received again. When the speaker feels his or her message has been understood, then roles change and the listener gets to speak.

What questions do you have about the Listening Response before we practice it together?

4B. In-Session Practice of the Listening Response:

4B.1. Therapist Models How to Use the Listening Response:

SUGGESTED THERAPIST SCRIPT

Let's start with me showing you how to use the Listening Response. Would one of you like to volunteer to act this out with me? OK, great. Let me give you a brief recap so that we know what we are going to do.

We have two roles, the speaker and the listener. First, you'll be the speaker and I'll be the listener. Pick a positive or neutral topic, such as the weather or a local news event, to discuss. Keep your statements brief and clear so that I, as the listener, do not become overwhelmed. I will use the Listening Response formula—*"What I heard you say was. . . . Did I get that right?"*—to show I have received your message. (*Now the role play is enacted.*)

You said I heard your message correctly, so let's change roles and try it again. This time I'll be the speaker and you'll be the listener. (*Now the second role play is enacted.*)

[**Therapist's note:** If the listener does not fully understand the major parts of your intended message, try again to send your message until the listener gets it right. Gently correct the listener, as needed, if they interject their own opinion before checking the accuracy of the speaker's message, or if they fail to use the listening response formula.]

4B.2. Couple Practices How to Use the Listening Response:

Next, partners take turns using the Listening Response, while you offer supportive and corrective feedback. The listener should continue to restate and check the accuracy of the message received until the speaker feels they were heard. Then partners switch roles and continue the conversation.

SUGGESTED THERAPIST SCRIPT

I would like you to take turns being the speaker and listener, practicing the Listening Response together. The speaker should try to say something positive about the listener, such as an example from Catch and Tell, the thing you like best about your partner, or something similar. You should not talk about any issue that is "charged" or "heavy" at this time. There will be opportunities for that later. The listener will be

(continued)

doing most of the work because we focused on the speaker previously. You may feel awkward at first, but remember, behavior change comes first and feelings will follow.

Remember to stick with one issue. It's OK if you need to clarify a few times before getting the message correct. The listener should not feel bad for doing this and the speaker should try not to get mad. Listening is a process. With practice, you will find your own way of doing this, and it will feel more natural and "real."

Are you ready to give this a try? (*Now the role-play is enacted.*) How did that feel? What did you like best about this exercise?

Therapist note: We add two components to the basic Listening Response. First, we try to move beyond very brief, often stilted exchanges to a more complete consideration of the speaker's topic. To do this, once the speaker has told the listener that they heard the message correctly, the listener should ask

"Is there more?"

The speaker may want to talk more about the topic now that they feel heard by the listener. Second, we try to add deeper levels of listening with understanding to the couple's communication, as described next.

4C. Explain Listening with Understanding:

SUGGESTED THERAPIST SCRIPT

You both did a great job with Listening. Now we can move on to the next step. Listening with Understanding goes beyond just restating and checking the accuracy of the message received from the speaker. It shows that the listener understands the speaker at a deeper level and supports the speaker even when there is a disagreement.

The listener shows understanding of what the speaker has said by demonstrating how it makes sense to feel and think that way, given the speaker's perception of the incident, topic, or situation. Understanding is not agreeing, but rather it is understanding another person's point of view or feelings, even if they do not match your own.

Once the speaker states that the listener has gotten everything correct and there is no more they need to say, the listener can show understanding by saying:

"I can understand that" or *"It makes sense to me that you feel _____ because . . . "*

Also the listener can show more understanding by recognizing what the speaker is feeling and . saying:

"That must make you feel . . . "

Let's try discussing a new topic and incorporate both Listening and Understanding.

Therapist note: Once a couple has used the basic listening response successfully, you should move on to incorporate understanding. For those with more strained relationships, you may have to continue longer with basic listener skills until the couple becomes comfortable with practicing those new skills. If you don't feel the couple is ready to move on, then Understanding skills can be left for later sessions.

(continued)

4D. In-Session Practice of Listening with Understanding:

The process of in-session practice is the same as it was for the simpler skill of just listening. You model Listening with Understanding with one member of the couple. Then the couple practices these skills while you offer supportive and corrective feedback. When the speaker feels heard and understood, he or she switches roles and continues the conversation with a new topic.

4E. Assign Communication Session Home Practice on Listening with Understanding:

SUGGESTED THERAPIST SCRIPT

Up to now, we have discussed effective communication Dos and Don'ts, barriers, "I" Messages, and now Listening with Understanding. I would like you to have another Communication Session at home, using the "I" Message skill and Listening with Understanding. This exercise may feel awkward at first, but the idea is to learn to use the skill until it becomes second nature.

    As you both may remember, there are a few simple guidelines to help you through a Communication Session: sit face-to-face, take turns talking, and be brief (two to three sentences). Remember to pay attention to the Dos and Don'ts, as well.

    In the next week, I would like you to have three 10- to 15-minute Communication Sessions using all the skills we have discussed in this session. You can discuss positive or neutral topics and everyday problems and events but NO charged issues. We will review and practice in the next session. Do you have any questions?

- Have the couple do three Communication Sessions this week, which will include all communication skills covered to date.
- Remind the couple to practice positive nonverbal and verbal behaviors, "I" Messages, and Listening with Understanding, as discussed in the session.

5. Assign Home Practice:

→(Hand out *Home Practice Session 6 Form C.13.*)←

5A. Recovery Contract:
- Do Trust Discussion (with medication, if taking it) every day at specified time.
- Do self-help and other parts of contract.
- Mark on calendar each time Trust Discussion and other parts of contract are completed.

5B. Positive Activities—pick at least one of following to do:
- Catch and Tell—acknowledge one nice thing each day when doing Trust Discussion.
- Shared Rewarding Activity—do planned SRA; plan one for following week.
- Caring Day—give your partner a Caring Day this week.

5C. Communication Session:
- Have a Communication Session (three times for 10–15 minutes each) to practice Listening with Understanding on everyday problems and events but not charged issues, using guidelines on home practice sheet.

6. Session Closing:

6A. Answer Questions: Answer any questions about the home practice assignments.

6B. Commit to Home Practice: Get verbal commitment to do the home practice.

Checklist for BCT Session 7: Relationship Agreements

Posters Needed:	Forms Needed:
B.18. Positive Specific Requests	C.14. Positive Specific Request List
B.19. Negotiated Agreement	C.15. Negotiated Agreement
B.20. Sample Couple Requests	C.16. Home Practice Session 7

Note: B.18 refers to Poster B.18 in Appendix B, C.14 to Form C.14 in Appendix C.

Cover the following material as completely as possible. Place a checkmark next to each completed section.

1. Welcome Back

___ Review typical sequence of sessions.

___ Collect urine screen, if patient has drug problem.

___ Review urges or actual substance use in past week.

___ Review relationship problems or other concerns from past week; defer details until after review of home practice.

___ See if Promises were kept past week; commit to Promises for coming week.

2. Review Home Practice from Past Week

___ Recovery Contract

   ___ Review daily Trust Discussion (with medication, if taking it) and calendar of past week.

   ___ Couple practices Trust Discussion (with medication, if taking it) with therapist feedback.

   ___ Review self-help and other parts of Recovery Contract.

___ Positive Activities—review which of the following they chose to do:

   ___ Catch and Tell (acknowledge one nice thing partner does each day at home and best of past week in session).

   ___ Shared Rewarding Activity (do planned SRA; plan one for following week).

   ___ Caring Day (give your partner a Caring Day this week).

___ Communication Session

   ___ Review how planned Communication Session at home went.

   ___ Practice a Communication Session with coaching from therapist.

3. Deal with Current Problems/Other Support for Abstinence

(Each of the following is optional, based on couple's needs. Refer to Session 4 for details.)

___ *Problems:* Address past week or other problems directly or refer to another source of help.

___ *Exposure to substances:* Help partners decide how to deal with upcoming exposure situations.

___ *Enabling:* Help couple identify and stop enabling behaviors. →(Show *Enabling Poster B.27.*)←

(continued)

4. Relationship Agreements

___ Explain how Positive Specific Requests and Negotiation and Compromise lead to Relationship Agreements for requested changes.
→(Show *Positive Specific Requests Poster B.18.*)←
→(Show *Negotiated Agreement Poster B.19.*)←

___ Therapist models process of relationship agreements.
→(Show *Sample Couple Requests Poster B.20.*)←

___ Each person lists five requests, and therapist coaches both to be positive and specific.
→(Hand out *Positive Specific Request List Form C.14.*)←

___ Couple practices negotiation and compromise to fulfill one request each (with coaching).

___ Help partners state and record their Agreement for each to fulfill one request.
→(Hand out *Negotiated Agreement Form C.15.*)←

___ Assign home practice (do agreed-upon requests, negotiate another agreement, add requests).

5. Review Progress in Couples Counseling

___ Congratulate couple on progress made in recovery and relationship.

___ Identify what has helped the most that they would choose to continue.

___ Help couple make a list of five problems to address in upcoming BCT sessions.

___ Do not process the list. It will be a starting point for future sessions.

6. Assign Home Practice

→(Hand out *Home Practice Session 7 Form C.16.*)←

___ Recovery Contract

   ___ Do Trust Discussion (with medication, if taking it) and mark on calendar.

   ___ Do self-help and other parts of contract and mark on calendar.

___ Positive Activities—pick at least one of following to do:

   ___ Catch and Tell (acknowledge one nice thing partner does each day).

   ___ Shared Rewarding Activity (do planned SRA; plan one for following week).

   ___ Caring Day (give your partner a Caring Day this week).

___ Communication Sessions (three times for 10–15 minutes to practice Listening with Understanding on everyday problems including charged issues).

___ Agreements (do agreed-upon requests, negotiate another agreement, add to list of requests).

7. Session Closing

___ Answer questions about assignments.

___ Get commitment from each person to do home practice assignments.

BCT SESSION 7 OUTLINE
RELATIONSHIP AGREEMENTS

This session introduces Relationship Agreements to help partners effectively express what they want from the relationship and successfully negotiate agreements to initiate positive changes.

1. Welcome Back:

1A. Collect Urine Screen If Patient Has Drug Problem

1B. Review Urges or Actual Substance Use in Past Week:
Ask: "Could you tell me about times since we last met when you drank or used drugs or had an urge or temptation to do so?"

1C. Review Relationship Problems or Other Concerns from Past Week:
Ask: "How did things go between the two of you in the past week? Any arguments? Positive times? Other important issues?" This segment should give a brief overview of how the past week went. Defer any extensive discussion until after review of the home practice.

1D. Review Promises:
Review each Promise, asking each person: "Have you been able to keep these Promises since last week? Can you commit to these Promises for the upcoming week?"

2. Review Home Practice from Last Week:

2A. Recovery Contract:
1. **Repeat Assignment:** The patient and partner were to do all parts of their Recovery Contract.
2. **Rationale for Assignment:** Rebuild trust and help substance abuse patient stay abstinent.
3. **Review Assignment:** Review the calendar to see how often they did the Trust Discussion and other elements of their contract. Discuss obstacles and ways to get more benefits; for example, if going to AA, may consider getting a sponsor, joining a group.
4. **In-Session Practice of the Trust Discussion:** The partners practice the Trust Discussion (with medication, if taking it) in session, allowing for feedback and correction by therapist.

2B. Positive Activities:
1. **Repeat Assignment:** Pick at least one of following to do:
   - Catch and Tell: Acknowledge one nice thing each day when doing Trust Discussion.
   - Shared Rewarding Activity: Do planned SRA; plan one for following week.
   - Caring Day: Give your partner a Caring Day this week.
2. **Rationale for Assignment:** Increase positive activities and feelings in the relationship.
3. **Review Assignment:** Review chosen assignment(s) following instructions in Session 5.
4. **In-Session Practice:** Practice chosen assignment(s) following instructions in Session 5.

(continued)

2C. Communication Session:

1. **Repeat Assignment:** The partners were to have three Communication Sessions using general guidelines on *Communication Session Poster B.18*. Specific instructions follow:
   - Have a Communication Session (three times for 10–15 minutes each) to practice Listening with Understanding and "I" Messages on everyday problems and events but not charged issues.
   - Notice body language, tone of voice, filters, and avoid "all-talk-and-no-listen" syndrome.
2. **Rationale for Assignment:** Practicing new communication skills will help the couple learn how to resolve problems and concerns in their relationship.
3. **Review Assignment:** Ask if they completed the Communication Session following the guidelines provided. Ask for specific feedback regarding the assignment.
4. **In-Session Practice of Communication Session:** Have couple role-play a Communication Session, using skills learned up to this point. Provide feedback and correction, as necessary.

3. Deal with Current Problems/Other Support for Abstinence:

(*Each of following is optional, based on couple's needs. Refer to Session 4 for details.*)

3A. Current Problems:
Address past week or other problems directly or by referral to another source of help.

3B. Exposure to Situations Where Alcohol or Drugs Are Available:
Help couple decide how to deal with upcoming exposure situations.

3C. Spouse Enabling:
Help couple identify and stop enabling behaviors. →(Show *Enabling Poster B.27*.)←

4. Relationship Agreements:

4A. Explain How Positive Specific Requests and Negotiation Lead to Agreements for Requested Changes:
   →(Show *Positive Specific Requests Poster B.18*.)←
   →(Show *Negotiated Agreement Poster B.19*.)←

SUGGESTED THERAPIST SCRIPT

So far, we have used mostly neutral or positive topics to practice communication skills. Now we want to start working on changes you each want to see in your relationship.

No relationship is perfect. To want change from your partner or change in your relationship is normal. However, asking for and negotiating for change is difficult in almost any relationship. Often we complain in vague and unclear terms about changes we want. Or we try to coerce, browbeat, or force our partner to change.

Remember, how we send a message affects how it is received. In requesting changes, we talk about stating things in a positive fashion—saying what you want, not what you don't want—and being willing to compromise and change to make the relationship happier.

Learning to negotiate requested changes can help you resolve tough issues that have caused disagreements and hard feelings in your relationship. There are three parts to Negotiating for Requests.

The first is to make Positive Specific Requests. This is how you state changes you want: your statement is *positive*, which refers to stating what you want, not what you don't want; *specific*, stating the when, where, and what; and it is in the form of a *request*, which is not a demand and leaves an opening for compromise.

For example: *"I would like the two of us to go for a walk after dinner each night."*

(continued)

The second step is Negotiation and Compromise, meaning you can talk things through. Negotiating requests begins with each person noting which of the partner's requests they would like to fulfill, at least in part. Each person voluntarily chooses a request to address. This alone can make your relationship happier. Each of you will not feel as if everything is one-sided. To be sure you know what is being agreed to, you should discuss the following parts of the request:

Frequency: How often? (daily, weekly, monthly)

Duration: How long will this last? (a week, during summer months)

Situation: When is this agreement in effect? (at home, at a specific event)

For example: *"I can go for a walk after dinner, but only on Mondays and Thursdays."*

The final step is reaching Agreements, which are the result of successful negotiation. Once you have negotiated and reached a compromise on your specific agreement, you should each state what you have agreed to do and make a commitment to fulfill the request in the next week.

For example: *"I agree to go for walks after dinner when we are at home on Mondays and Thursdays for the months of June, July, and August."*

Perhaps the most important lesson today is that using the above formula will help you to have a request fulfilled, at least in part. It is important to recognize that partial fulfillment does not mean failure or unwillingness of your partner to make things better. Change can occur even in small steps.

What questions do you have about Negotiating for Requests before we practice it together?

4B. Therapist Models Process of *Relationship Agreements*:

→(Show *Sample Couple Requests Poster B.20.*)←

This part of the session focuses on skill practice, specifically having a Communication Session using the skills that have been discussed so far, and arriving at a Relationship Agreement. Begin by reviewing the sample of couple requests on *Poster B.20*, explaining why each is a positive specific request or not.

Next role-play the process of Relationship Agreements with the help of one of the partners. Use an example from your own experience or one that the couple suggests. Pay attention to the example: Is it specific and positive? Is it a request and not a demand? Below is a list of requests you can use to get started, if necessary:

"I would like you to . . .   give me a kiss each morning before leaving for work *or*
hold my hand while we watch TV *or*
read 20 minutes a night to the kids at bedtime *or*
plan a special date for us once a month."

Use the guidelines for a Communication Session, including sitting face-to-face, keeping sentences brief, using "I" Messages, and Listening. Negotiate and compromise until you have reached an agreement that seems workable.

4C. Couple Practices Process of Relationship Agreements (with therapist coaching).

4C.1. Positive Specific Requests—each person lists five requests:

→(Hand out *Positive Specific Request List Form C.14.*)←

SUGGESTED THERAPIST SCRIPT

We are going to try this in session. We will take it step-by-step, building in the three parts of Relationship Agreements. For our first task, I would like each of you to write down five requests on the *Positive Specific Request List* (*Form C.14.*). Remember to be positive, specific, and to request, NOT demand. For example, your request might be related to communication, money, the children, household chores, time together, or affection.

(continued)

> Now, I'd like you both to read off your Positive Specific Requests. It can be helpful to start your request with "I would like you to . . . "

Therapist note: Provide feedback to make sure that the statements are positive and specific. This process can be emotionally charged for many couples. Some think that a request for change is a criticism of the person, rather than simply a request for behavior change. Others believe that you cannot ask someone you love to change. We think requests for change are a normal part of every relationship that help two individuals meld their differences and build a stronger bond together.

4C.2. Negotiation and Compromise—each person negotiates to fulfill one request:

SUGGESTED THERAPIST SCRIPT

You have each expressed some requests. Now I want you to choose one of your partner's requests to fulfill, in full or partially, during the upcoming week.

   The partner should state the request: "I would like you to . . . " and the listener should listen carefully and respond with, "What I heard you say was . . . ", "Did I get that?" and "Is there more?"

   Be sure to discuss the specifics of the request. You should each be clear about the frequency (how often will you do this?), duration (for how long?), and situation (where, when?) involved in the request.

   Remember, this is not an all-or-nothing situation; your goal is to talk through the request, negotiating as you go. Pay attention to your verbal and nonverbal behaviors, and use your speaking and listening skills to help you in the conversation.

   Finally, ask yourself, are you being realistic and reasonable on the request and the negotiation?

   When you have reached an agreement on what you will do to fulfill your partner's request, write it down.

   Then we'll start over with the other person's list of requests. Again, you'll pick which request to address and negotiate an agreement to fulfill the request, at least in part. I will be your coach as we go along.

4C.3. Agreement—each person records their agreement to fulfill one request:
   →(Hand out *Negotiated Agreement Form C.15*.)←

SUGGESTED THERAPIST SCRIPT

Now that you have negotiated a compromise, please write down what each of you agreed to do for the other on the *Negotiated Agreement sheet* (*Form C.15*).

   In the next week, each of you should follow through with the agreed-upon request.

   It is key to remember that most requests can be fulfilled, at least in part. Negotiating or meeting each other halfway can have very positive benefits for your relationship.

4D. Assign Negotiated Agreements Home Practice:

SUGGESTED THERAPIST SCRIPT

In the next week each of you should follow through with your agreed-upon request. I would like you to continue to have three 10- to 15-minute Communication Sessions. In at least one of these sessions, I would like you each to discuss another Positive Specific Request, Negotiate and Compromise on that request, and agree to follow through with it. In the next session I will ask you how the request went that we just discussed and what new request you will fulfill.

   Do you have any questions?

(continued)

- Each person should fulfill the agreement they made in session during the upcoming week.
- Each person also should negotiate one agreement during the week and write it down on the Negotiated Agreements sheet.
- Each person also should add to their list of requests.

5. Review Progress in Couples Counseling:

If time permits: Congratulate couple on progress made in recovery and relationship. Identify what has helped the most that they would choose to continue. Have the couple make a list of five problems in their relationship, ordered from "easy" to "hard." This should take up a minimal amount of time. They are not to discuss the problems, simply to list them. Having worked with them for seven sessions, you should have a sense of their problem areas. Be sure to monitor the making of the list so it does not become a time to point out faults and create an argument. This list will be addressed in following sessions.

6. Assign Home Practice:

→(Hand out *Home Practice Session 7 Form C.16*.)←

6A. Recovery Contract:
- Do Trust Discussion (with medication, if taking it) every day at specified time.
- Do self-help and other parts of contract.
- Mark on calendar each time Trust Discussion and other parts of contract are completed.

6B. Positive Activities—pick at least one of following to do:
- Catch and Tell—acknowledge one nice thing partner does each day when doing Trust Discussion.
- Shared Rewarding Activity—do planned SRA; plan one for following week.
- Caring Day—give your partner a Caring Day this week.

6C. Communication Session:
- Have three Communication Sessions (10–15 minutes each) to practice Listening with Understanding on everyday problems and events including charged issues, using guidelines on home practice sheet. Use a Communication Session to negotiate another agreement (see next point).

6D. Relationship Agreements:
- Do the agreement they made in session during the upcoming week.
- Negotiate another agreement and write it down on the Negotiated Agreements sheet.
- Add to their list of Positive Specific Requests.

7. Session Closing:

7A. Answer Questions: Answer any questions about the home practice assignments.

7B. Commit to Home Practice: Get verbal commitment to do the home practice.

Checklist for BCT Session 8: Conflict Resolution

Posters Needed:	Forms Needed:
B.21. Responses to Conflict B.22. Time-Out	C.17. Guidelines for Managing Conflict C.18. Home Practice Session 8
Note: B.21 refers to Poster B.21 in Appendix B, C.17 to Form C.17 in Appendix C.	

Cover the following material as completely as possible. Place a checkmark next to each completed section.

1. Welcome Back

___ Review typical sequence of sessions.

___ Collect urine screen, if patient has drug problem.

___ Review urges or actual substance use in past week.

___ Review relationship problems or other concerns from past week; defer details until after review of home practice.

___ See if Promises were kept past week; commit to Promises for coming week.

2. Review Home Practice from Past Week

___ Recovery Contract

   ___ Review daily Trust Discussion (with medication, if taking it) and calendar of past week.

   ___ Couple practices Trust Discussion (with medication, if taking it) with therapist feedback.

   ___ Review self-help and other parts of Recovery Contract.

___ Positive Activities—review which of the following they chose to do:

   ___ Catch and Tell (acknowledge one nice thing partner does each day at home and best of past week in session).

   ___ Shared Rewarding Activity (do planned SRA; plan one for following week).

   ___ Caring Day (give your partner a Caring Day this week).

___ Communication Session

   ___ Review how planned Communication Session at home went.

   ___ Practice a Communication Session with coaching from therapist.

___ Relationship Agreements

   ___ Review if they did agreed-upon requests.

   ___ Help them refine new agreement they negotiated and requests to add to their lists.

(continued)

3. Deal with Current Problems/Other Support for Abstinence
(Each of the following is optional, based on couple's needs. Refer to Session 4 for details.)

___ *Problems:* Address past week or other problems directly or refer to another source of help.

___ *Exposure to substances:* Help partners decide how to deal with upcoming exposure situations.

___ *Enabling:* Help couple identify and stop enabling behaviors. →(Show *Enabling Poster B.27.*)←

4. Conflict Resolution →(Show *Responses to Conflict Poster B.21.*)←

___ Explain that conflict is normal in every relationship. It's how you handle it that counts.

___ Explain and discuss five types of responses to conflict: verbal aggression, physical aggression, flooding, avoidance and withdrawal, and verbal reasoning.

___ Review couple's usual methods of addressing conflict in the relationship.

___ Reassess risk of violence, if needed.

5. Managing and Resolving Conflict

___ Explain and discuss guidelines for managing conflict.
→(Hand out *Guidelines for Managing Conflict Form C.17.*)←

___ Explain and discuss use of Time-Out to prevent conflict from escalating.

___ Couple practices use of Time-Out in Communication Session on charged topic.
→(Show *Time-Out Poster B.22.*)←

___ Assign home practice (use a Time-Out in coming week to reduce conflict).

6. Assign Home Practice →(Hand out *Home Practice Session 8 Form C.18.*)←

___ Recovery Contract

    ___ Do Trust Discussion (with medication, if taking it) and mark on calendar.

    ___ Do self-help and other parts of contract and mark on calendar.

___ Positive Activities—pick at least one of following to do:

    ___ Catch and Tell (acknowledge one nice thing partner does each day).

    ___ Shared Rewarding Activity (do planned SRA; plan one for following week).

    ___ Caring Day (give your partner a Caring Day this week).

___ Communication Sessions (three times for 10–15 minutes each) to practice:

    ___ Listening with Understanding on everyday problems, including charged issues.

    ___ Conflict Resolution (use a Time-Out in coming week to reduce conflict).

    ___ Agreements (do agreed-upon requests and negotiate another agreement).

7. Session Closing

___ Answer questions about assignments.

___ Get commitment from each person to do home practice assignments.

BCT SESSION 8 OUTLINE
CONFLICT RESOLUTION

This session introduces Conflict Resolution to help the couple decrease negative interactions and engage in behaviors that promote dealing with problems together in an open and honest way.

1. Welcome Back:

1A. Collect Urine Screen If Patient Has Drug Problem.

1B. Review Urges or Actual Substance Use in Past Week:
Ask: "Could you tell me about times since we last met when you drank or used drugs or had an urge or temptation to do so?"

1C. Review Relationship Problems or Other Concerns from Past Week:
Ask: "How did things go between the two of you in the past week? Any arguments? Positive times? Other important issues?" This segment should give a brief overview of how the past week went. Defer any extensive discussion until after review of the home practice.

1D. Review Promises:
Review each Promise, asking each person: "Have you been able to keep these Promises since last week? Can you commit to these Promises for the upcoming week?"

2. Review Home Practice from Last Week:

2A. Recovery Contract:
1. **Repeat Assignment:** The patient and partner were to do all parts of their Recovery Contract.
2. **Rationale for Assignment:** Rebuild trust and help substance abuse patient stay abstinent.
3. **Review Assignment:** Review the calendar to see how often they did the Trust Discussion and other elements of their contract. Discuss obstacles and ways to get more benefits; for example, if going to AA, may consider getting a sponsor, joining a group.
4. **In-Session Practice of the Trust Discussion:** The partners practice the Trust Discussion (with medication, if taking it) in session, allowing for feedback and correction by therapist.

2B. Positive Activities:
1. **Repeat Assignment:** Pick at least one of following to do:
   - Catch and Tell: Acknowledge one nice thing each day when doing Trust Discussion.
   - Shared Rewarding Activity: Do planned SRA; plan one for following week.
   - Caring Day: Give your partner a Caring Day this week.
2. **Rationale for Assignment:** Increase positive activities and feelings in the relationship.
3. **Review Assignment:** Review chosen assignment(s) following instructions in Session 5.
4. **In-Session Practice:** Practice chosen assignment(s) following instructions in Session 5.

(continued)

2C. Communication Session:

1. **Repeat Assignment:** The partners were to have three Communication Sessions using general guidelines on *Communication Session Poster B.18*. Specific instructions follow:
   - Have a Communication Session (three times for 10–15 minutes each) to practice Listening with Understanding and "I" Messages on everyday problems and events but not charged issues.
   - Notice body language, tone of voice, filters, and avoid "all-talk-and-no-listen" syndrome.
2. **Rationale for Assignment:** Practicing new communication skills will help the couple learn how to resolve problems and concerns in their relationship.
3. **Review Assignment:** Ask if they completed the Communication Session following the guidelines provided. Ask for specific feedback regarding the assignment.
4. **In-Session Practice of Communication Session:** Have couple role-play a Communication Session, using skills learned up to this point. Provide feedback and correction, as necessary.

2D. Relationship Agreements:

1. **Repeat Assignment:** Do agreed-upon request from last session, negotiate one more agreement during the week, and add to their list of requests.
2. **Rationale for Assignment:** Relationship Agreements help partners effectively express what they want from the relationship and successfully initiate positive changes.
3. **Review Assignment:** Ask if they did agreement made in session last week and how it felt.
4. **In-Session Practice of Agreements:** Ask them to share new agreement they negotiated in past week. Help them specify the new agreement so both are clear and satisfied with it. Also review requests each added to their list for future negotiations. Use guidelines from Session 7.

3. Deal with Current Problems/Other Support for Abstinence:

(*Each of following is optional, based on couple's needs. Refer to Session 4 for details.*)

3A. Current Problems:
Address past week or other problems directly or by referral to another source of help.

3B. Exposure to Situations Where Alcohol or Drugs Are Available:
Help them decide how to deal with upcoming exposure situations.

3C. Spouse Enabling:
Help couple identify and stop enabling behaviors. →(Show *Enabling Poster B.27*.)←

4. Conflict Resolution:

4A. Explain that Conflict Is Normal in a Relationship—It's How You Handle It That Counts:

SUGGESTED THERAPIST SCRIPT

At some point in every relationship, partners experience conflict. Conflict comes up when one person's thoughts and beliefs about something differ from another person's. Indeed, there are times when we don't agree with something someone is doing or saying because we look at the same situation in a completely different way.

Such conflict may lead to an argument and increased tension in your relationship. In this section, we want to talk about different responses to conflict. We also will explore what your reactions to conflict look like and how they affect your relationship. Our goal is to learn how to manage and resolve conflicts successfully.

(continued)

4B. Explain and Discuss Five Types of Responses to Conflict:
→(Show *Responses to Conflict Poster B.21.*)←

SUGGESTED THERAPIST SCRIPT

First, what is Conflict Resolution? It is the positive process in which two people work together to find a solution to a problem or issue. But not all responses to conflict are positive and not all lead to resolution of the conflict. Let's start by talking about the different ways people respond to a conflict situation.

1. *Verbal Aggression* is used when a partner or both partners become very frustrated and cannot reach an agreement about something that is causing a problem. It includes blaming, name calling, and yelling. Verbal aggression is a common, highly ineffective conflict response. Someone who is using verbal aggression may think that this response is the only solution to the problem. Typically, this causes more frustration and anger and does not lead to resolution.

Examples:
• Yelling and swearing at your partner
• Calling your partner names

2. *Physical Aggression* includes slapping, hitting, biting, pushing, grabbing, hitting with an object, choking, and threatening or using a knife or gun to hurt someone. Some forms of physical aggression are more severe than others, but all forms are hurtful. Unfortunately, physical aggression by couples with a substance abuse problem is common, with the majority of couples reporting physical aggression at least once in the year before substance abuse treatment.

Examples:
• Shoving your partner when he or she doesn't agree with a choice you made
• Throwing a plate at your partner when you feel frustrated

3. *Flooding* refers to becoming "flooded" with emotions, as occurs when a car engine won't start because it's been flooded with too much gas. The person feels so overwhelmed with anxiety or frustration or anger that they cannot think clearly or speak effectively. The emotionally flooded person needs to take a Time-Out and calm down until they can think and speak effectively.

Examples:
• Suddenly feeling overwhelmed and unable to respond to your partner
• A sudden rush of emotions that causes you to feel frustrated and fed up

4. *Avoidance and Withdrawal* occurs when a person avoids discussing problems with their partner or withdraws from conflict by changing the topic or leaving the room. The person may believe that problems are unpleasant and may clear up on their own, and that discussing them directly may make matters worse. This method works sometimes, but it usually is not effective in the long run if major relationship problems are avoided and not discussed.

Examples:
• Refusing to discuss a problem that your partner wants to discuss.
• Not discussing a serious problem to avoid either of you getting upset.

(continued)

5. **Verbal Reasoning** occurs when a couple uses effective speaking and listening skills, such as those we have discussed in previous sessions, in order to resolve a conflict. Both partners get a chance to state their opinions about the situation and are able to work toward a compromise. Verbal reasoning typically leads to a mutually agreed-upon solution that leaves both partners happy. This response to conflict is the most likely to lead to conflict resolution.

Examples:
• Not avoiding the topic but having a Communication Session about the problem
• Using effective speaking and listening skills ("I" Messages, Listening, and Understanding).

4C. Review Couple's Usual Methods of Addressing Conflict in the Relationship:

SUGGESTED THERAPIST SCRIPT

We have been talking about different ways people respond to a conflict situation. Now I would like to take a few minutes to talk about how each of you addresses conflict in your relationship. I would like each of you to tell me what you normally do when an argument occurs. It may be one of the five conflict responses we just discussed, or there may be other things you do. Don't comment on each other's answers; just think about what you do. (*Therapist coaches each partner to respond.*)

Out of all of the strategies you both identified, which ones do you think are effective and which ones have been ineffective in the past? Remember, you are not labeling or attacking each other, just exploring the best ways to work out issues together. (*Therapist coaches each partner to respond.*)

4D. Reassess Risk of Violence, If Needed:

This discussion may get uncomfortable if there have been high levels of ineffective responses to conflict in the couple's relationship. Take a few minutes to assess how they are feeling. Ask if they have any concerns or comments about anything that was discussed. Determine if they are ready to move forward to talk about coping skills to manage and resolve conflicts. In some cases you will learn that verbal and physical aggression was more severe or more frequent in the relationship than the couple had reported at the start of BCT. This new information should prompt you to reassess the risk for violence. Check that they have not been hiding or minimizing verbal or physical aggression since starting BCT. At each session you have been asking them about threatened or actual violence when you reviewed the four Promises and asked about arguments or problems they had. Most couples have handled conflicts nonviolently while attending BCT; it is rare to decide a couple is not appropriate for BCT after attending this many sessions. The typical response is to move forward to examine positive methods for managing and resolving conflicts.

5. Managing and Resolving Conflict:

5A. Explain and Discuss Guidelines for Managing and Resolving Conflict:
→(Give *Guidelines for Managing Conflict Form C.17.*)←

SUGGESTED THERAPIST SCRIPT

Up to this point, we've been talking about conflict and effective and ineffective ways of dealing with it. Now let's talk about ways you can reduce the frustration that comes with a disagreement. These ways will help you stay calm so that you can communicate effectively and find solutions that benefit both of you.

Let's briefly review before we look at the guidelines. If a situation comes up in which you are arguing, use the listener and speaker skills we learned in earlier sessions. Using "I" Messages helps you state what you feel, think, or believe. Using Listening and Understanding and saying "What I heard you saying ... Is that right?" will ensure that you know what your partner is saying.

(continued)

These communication skills help slow down the conversation and also allow you to focus on each other's feelings and point of view. Remember, if you want to bring up an issue, use requests, not demands, and state what you want, not what you don't want. Allow room for negotiation and compromise. Even a partial change can have great benefits.

If you look at the *Guidelines for Managing Conflict* sheet, we can discuss these points and talk about those that you think would be most helpful to your relationship.

5B. Explain and Discuss Time-Out to Prevent Conflict from Escalating:
→(Show *Time-Out Poster B.22*.) ←

SUGGESTED THERAPIST SCRIPT

When you are unable to slow down a conversation, you may need a break from trying to solve the problem. This is when you use a Time-Out.

A Time-Out allows you to take a break and step back so that you don't rely on verbal aggression or physical aggression to solve the problem. A Time-Out allows you to compose yourself and restart the conversation later when you are able to use the communication skills that will help you work toward solving the problem.

There are four parts to a Time-Out:

1. *Before*: If either partner gets uncomfortable or frustrated while discussing a problem and thinks it may lead to increased frustration, he or she should ask the partner for a Time-Out. He or she might say, "I'm getting uncomfortable. I want to take a 15-minute Time-Out. Once the 15 minutes is up, I would like to get back together and try to discuss this again."

2. *During*: Once you both agree to take a 15-minute Time-Out, go into separate rooms, relax, and try to get your mind off the argument by taking deep breaths, listening to soothing music, or doing whatever would help you to calm down.

3. *After*: The person who requested the Time-Out should be the one who restarts the discussion. Get your partner and begin the discussion again. If things start to get tense again, ask for a second Time-Out, then postpone the discussion for an extended period of time. You might try talking again the next day or wait until your counseling session.

4. *Resolution*: One or more restarts following a Time-Out usually results in a satisfactory resolution. However, two people cannot agree about everything, so couples need to learn how to "agree to disagree" as a way to resolve those problems for which compromise is not possible.

Does this sound like something you could try?

5C. In-Session Practice of a Communication Session Using Time-Out

- Ask the couple to discuss an everyday problem using listener and speaker skills. At some point, ask if either person would like to take a Time-Out. Help partners assess feelings of frustration. If one partner feels that a Time-Out is needed, ask the partner to say "I am feeling very uncomfortable right now. Can we please have a 15-minute Time-Out?" Ask the couple to brainstorm what they would do (go to separate rooms, take a 5-minute walk, practice deep breathing).
- If time allows, have the couple practice using a more threatening or charged topic. When the conversation gets to a point where you feel a Time-Out would be helpful, intervene by saying, "I think a Time-Out would help the situation right now. Let's discuss how we would do this." Then proceed as you did with the noncharged topic to guide them through the Time-Out.

5D. Assign Time-Out Home Practice:

- Ask the couple to use a Time-Out in the coming week to reduce conflict in a real situation (perhaps an issue that arises during a Communication Session) or in a practice situation.

(continued)

6. Assign Home Practice:

→(Hand out *Home Practice Session 8 Form C.18.*)←

6A. Recovery Contract:
• Do Trust Discussion (with medication, if taking it) every day at specified time.
• Do self-help and other parts of contract.
• Mark on calendar each time Trust Discussion and other parts of contract are completed.

6B. Positive Activities—pick at least one of following to do:
• Catch and Tell: Acknowledge one nice thing each day when doing Trust Discussion.
• Shared Rewarding Activity: Do planned SRA; plan one for following week.
• Caring Day: Give your partner a Caring Day this week.

6C. Communication Sessions—have three (10–15 minutes each) to practice:
• Listening with Understanding on everyday problems, including charged issues.
• Relationship Agreements using agreement made in session and negotiating another.
• Conflict Resolution using a Time-Out in a real situation or in a practice situation.

7. Session Closing:

7A. Answer Questions: Answer any questions about the home practice assignments.

7B. Commit to Home Practice: Get verbal commitment to do the home practice.

327

Checklist for BCT Session 9: S.O.L.V.E. Problem Solving

Posters Needed:	Forms Needed:
B.23. S.O.L.V.E. Problem-Solving Model	C.19. Problem Solving Example C.20. Problem Solving Practice C.21. Home Practice Session 9

Note: B.23 refers to Poster B.23 in Appendix B, C.19 to Form C.19 in Appendix C.

Cover the following material as completely as possible. Place a checkmark next to each completed section.

1. Welcome Back

___ Review typical sequence of sessions.

___ Collect urine screen, if patient has drug problem.

___ Review urges or actual substance use in past week.

___ Review relationship problems or other concerns from past week; defer details until after review of home practice.

___ See if Promises were kept past week; commit to Promises for coming week.

2. Review Home Practice from Past Week

___ Recovery Contract

    ___ Review daily Trust Discussion (with medication, if taking it) and calendar of past week.

    ___ Couple practices Trust Discussion (with medication, if taking it) with therapist feedback.

    ___ Review self-help and other parts of Recovery Contract.

___ Positive Activities—review which of the following they chose to do:

    ___ Catch and Tell (acknowledge one nice thing partner does each day at home and best of past week in session).

    ___ Shared Rewarding Activity (do planned SRA; plan one for following week).

    ___ Caring Day (give your partner a Caring Day this week).

___ Communication Sessions (three times for 10–15 minutes each) to practice:

    ___ Listening with Understanding—on everyday problems, including charged issues.

    ___ Conflict Resolution—use a Time-Out in coming week to reduce conflict.

    ___ Relationship Agreements—do agreement made in session and negotiate another.

(continued)

3. Deal with Current Problems/Other Support for Abstinence
(Each of the following is optional, based on couple's needs. Refer to Session 4 for details.)

___ *Problems:* Address past week or other problems directly or refer to another source of help.

___ *Exposure to substances:* Help partners decide how to deal with upcoming exposure situations.

___ *Enabling:* Help couple identify and stop enabling. →(Show *Enabling Poster B.27.*)←

4. Five-Step Model of Problem Solving (S.O.L.V.E.)

___ Introduce and discuss S.O.L.V.E. problem-solving formula.
→(Show *S.O.L.V.E. Problem-Solving Model Poster B.23.*)←

___ Therapist models using S.O.L.V.E. problem solving on a sample problem.
→(Hand out *Problem-Solving Example Form C.19.*)←

___ Partners practice using S.O.L.V.E. on a problem of their own, with therapist coaching.
→(Hand out *Problem-Solving Practice Form C.20.*)←

___ Assign home practice: Partners have a 30-minute Communication Session in which they use S.O.L.V.E. with a problem chosen in session.

5. Assign Home Practice →(Hand out *Home Practice Session 9 Form C.21.*)←

___ Recovery Contract

   ___ Do Trust Discussion (with medication, if taking it) and mark on calendar.

   ___ Do self-help and other parts of contract and mark on calendar.

___ Positive Activities—pick at least one of following to do:

   ___ Catch and Tell (acknowledge one nice thing partner does each day).

   ___ Shared Rewarding Activity (do planned SRA; plan one for following week).

   ___ Caring Day (give your partner a Caring Day this week).

___ Communication Sessions—(three sessions) to practice S.O.L.V.E. plus at least one other of following:

   ___ Problem Solving using S.O.L.V.E. method on problem chosen in session.

   ___ Listening with Understanding on everyday problems, including charged issues.

   ___ Conflict Resolution using a Time-Out in a real situation or in a practice situation.

   ___ Relationship Agreements using agreement made in session and negotiating another.

6. Session Closing

___ Answer questions about assignments.

___ Get commitment from each person to do home practice assignments.

BCT SESSION 9 OUTLINE
S.O.L.V.E. PROBLEM SOLVING

This session introduces Problem Solving to help the couple learn a method they can use to work together to solve longstanding problems as well as new issues as they arise.

1. Welcome Back:

1A. Collect Urine Screen If Patient Has Drug Problem.

1B. Review Urges or Actual Substance Use in Past Week:
Ask: "Could you tell me about times since we last met when you drank or used drugs or had an urge or temptation to do so?"

1C. Review Relationship Problems or Other Concerns from Past Week:
Ask: "How did things go between the two of you in the past week? Any arguments? Positive times? Other important issues?" This segment should give a brief overview of how the past week went. Defer any extensive discussion until after review of the home practice.

1D. Review Promises:
Review each Promise, asking each person: "Have you been able to keep these Promises since last week? Can you commit to these Promises for the upcoming week?"

2. Review Home Practice from Last Week:

2A. Recovery Contract:
1. **Repeat Assignment:** The patient and partner were to do all parts of their Recovery Contract.
2. **Rationale for Assignment:** Rebuild trust and help substance abuse patient stay abstinent.
3. **Review Assignment:** Review calendar to see how often they did the Trust Discussion and other elements of their contract. Discuss obstacles and ways to get more benefits; for example, if going to AA, may consider getting a sponsor, joining a group.
4. **In-Session Practice of the Trust Discussion:** The partners practice the Trust Discussion (with medication, if taking it) in session, allowing for feedback and correction by therapist.

2B. Positive Activities:
1. **Repeat Assignment:** Pick at least one of following to do:
   - Catch and Tell: Acknowledge one nice thing each day when doing Trust Discussion.
   - Shared Rewarding Activity: Do planned SRA; plan one for following week.
   - Caring Day: Give your partner a Caring Day this week.
2. **Rationale for Assignment:** Increase positive activities and feelings in the relationship.
3. **Review Assignment:** Review chosen assignment(s) following instructions in Session 5.
4. **In-Session Practice:** Practice chosen assignment(s) following instructions in Session 5.

2C. Communication Sessions
1. **Repeat Assignment:** Have three sessions (10–15 minutes each) to practice:
   - Conflict Resolution using a Time-Out in a real situation or in a practice situation.
   - Listening with Understanding on everyday problems, including charged issues.
   - Relationship Agreements using agreement made in session and negotiating another.
2. **Rationale for Assignment:** Good communication resolves requests, conflicts, and problems.

(continued)

3. **Review Assignments:** Review assignments following instructions in Session 8.
4. **In-Session Practice:** Practice assignments following instructions in Session 8.

3. Deal with Current Problems/Other Support for Abstinence:

(*Each of following is optional, based on couple's needs. Refer to Session 4 for details.*)

3A. Current Problems:
Address past week or other problems directly or by referral to another source of help.

3B. Exposure to Situations Where Alcohol or Drugs Are Available:
Help them decide how to deal with upcoming exposure situations.

3C. Spouse Enabling:
Help couple identify and stop enabling behaviors. →(Show *Enabling Poster B.27.*)←

4. S.O.L.V.E. Problem Solving:

→(Show *S.O.L.V.E. Problem-Solving Model Poster B.23.*)←

4A. Introduce and Discuss S.O.L.V.E. Problem-Solving Formula

SUGGESTED THERAPIST SCRIPT

Many couples report that problems developed or ignored during substance abuse seem overwhelming in the early stages of recovery. Often partners disagree on solutions, or they don't know what to do, so they do nothing and try to avoid dealing with the problem. The problems remain unresolved and often get worse. Stressful, unresolved problems create a risk for relapse.

Today we will introduce a new skill, called S.O.L.V.E. This skill gives you a general problem-solving model that can help you work out a variety of problems, including finances and childrearing issues. This skill can also be used for any personal or relationship problem a family may face. S.O.L.V.E. is easy to learn and use in your daily life.

SUGGESTED THERAPIST SCRIPT

Now we are going to explain and discuss each step of the S.O.L.V.E. problem solving approach.

S—Stop, Slow Down, and See the Problem:
When we face a problem situation, we can easily be overwhelmed. You want to be sensitive to clues that tell you that a problem exists, and to use these as signals to use problem-solving skills. We can identify a problem by checking out:
   Our body: neck tension, headache, and muscle tension
   Our thoughts and feelings: feeling angry, agitated, irritated, or thinking negatively
   Our behaviors: slamming the door, avoiding someone we feel wronged us

If you begin to feel tense and overwhelmed, *stop* what you're doing, *slow down,* and take time to think about what the *problem* might be. A good way to slow down is to take a few deep breaths to help slow down and clear your mind so that you can think clearly.

   Ask yourself: What clues have I experienced that tell me there is a problem? Once you've identified that a problem exists, try to find out what it is.

   Ask yourself: Is there a problem? What exactly is the problem? If you break down the situation and identify one issue at a time, you may find it more manageable to problem solve.

(continued)

O—Outline Options:

This step requires brainstorming potential solutions for the problem.

Ask yourself: What can I do?

You want to look at all options, good and bad. Sometimes even the ideas that sound ridiculous can help you think of more helpful options. Look at the problem from different angles. Think about what you may have done in the past or in a similar situation that worked out well.

Ask yourself: What might work?

Ask someone you trust for ideas; doing so can open up choices that you may not have considered. It's important to recognize that you have choices to handle the situation.

L—Look at Consequences:

Next look at your list of options and check out the long- and short-term, as well as positive and negative, consequences for each option. This is often difficult to do. Most people tend to focus only on the short-term consequences; they are easier to see and quicker to figure out. It is important to slow down and look at the potential long-term consequences because it's often the long-term consequences that are most helpful in choosing your course of action. Making a decision based on short-term consequences alone can get you into trouble.

Ask yourself: What might really work over the long term?

V—Vote:

In this step you evaluate the consequences and eliminate those that are less effective. This is where you rank your options and pick the one that will be the most positive or helpful to you.

Ask yourself: Which choice has the most positive and the least negative consequences? Which is better for us in the long term?

E—Evaluate:

Now give your best option a fair trial. Try it out and review the results. If things don't work out, go back to your list and try another option or go through the process again. Use this step as a learning experience.

Ask yourself: How did it work? Did my choice solve the problem?

4B. Therapist Models Using S.O.L.V.E. Problem Solving on an Example Problem:

→(Hand out *S.O.L.V.E. Problem-Solving Example Form C.19*.)←

Present an example of problem situation. Work through one step at a time using the *S.O.L.V.E. Problem-Solving Model* poster, writing each step on an easel board or sheet of paper.

SUGGESTED THERAPIST SCRIPT

Here is an example of a problem situation:

It's Saturday morning and you find the OJ left on the kitchen counter. This happens a lot. It is the third day in a row that your partner has left out the OJ. You wanted some for breakfast, but you like to drink it cold, and now it's warm.

Does this, or something like it, sound familiar to you? What would you be feeling? What would be a clue that this is a problem? What's the first thing you want to do?

Yes, **S.** *Stop, slow down, and see the problem.* You want to stop and slow down before simply reacting, and you want to apply your problem-solving skills.

What exactly is the problem?

(*Continue to work through this problem, using the S.O.L.V.E. approach, encouraging participation and feedback from both partners.*)

(continued)

4C. In-Session Practice Using S.O.L.V.E. on a Problem of Their Own:

Help the couple apply the S.O.L.V.E. model to one of their own personal problem situations. To keep the task manageable, consider the following points:
- Choose a problem that is behavior-specific and not attributed to a personality factor.
- It is best if it is a recent stressor that is an external problem, not about one partner's behavior.
- Both partners should agree on the problem situation to be addressed.
- Avoid complex or emotionally charged topics at this point.
- If the situation combines several problems, break it down and problem-solve one at a time.

Allow time for the partners to practice. Encourage them to use their communication skills as part of the problem-solving process. Provide corrective feedback while highlighting strengths.

4D. Assign S.O.L.V.E. Problem-Solving Home Practice:
   →(Hand Out *S.O.L.V.E. Problem-Solving Practice Form C.20.*)←
- Before leaving the session, choose a problem on which to practice using S.O.L.V.E.
- Have a 30-minute Communication Session on this problem-solving task.
- Use the *Problem-Solving Practice* sheet and bring completed sheet to next session.

5. Assign Home Practice:

→(Hand out *Home Practice Session 9 Form C.21.*)←

5A. Recovery Contract:
- Do Trust Discussion (with medication, if taking it) every day at specified time.
- Do self-help and other parts of contract.
- Mark on calendar each time Trust Discussion and other parts of contract are completed.

5B. Positive Activities—pick at least one of following to do:
- Catch and Tell: Acknowledge one nice thing each day when doing Trust Discussion.
- Shared Rewarding Activity: Do planned SRA; plan one for following week.
- Caring Day: Give your partner a Caring Day this week.

5C. Communication Sessions (three)—to practice S.O.L.V.E. plus at least one other of following:
- Problem Solving for 30 minutes using S.O.L.V.E. method on problem chosen in session.
- Listening with Understanding on everyday problems, including charged issues.
- Relationship Agreements using agreement made in session and negotiating another.
- Conflict Resolution using a Time-Out in a real situation or in a practice situation.

Note that couple has choice regarding some assignments. This keeps assignments manageable and allows partners to choose assignments that fit their needs. Therapist should help couple choose.

6. Session Closing:

6A. Answer Questions: Answer any questions about the home practice assignments.

6B. Commit to Home Practice: Get verbal commitment to do the home practice.

Checklist for BCT Session 10: Continuing Recovery

Posters Needed:	Forms Needed:
B.24. Sample Continuing Recovery Plan	C.22. Continuing Recovery Helpful Hints C.23. My Continuing Recovery Plan C.24. Home Practice Session 10

Note: B.24 refers to Poster B.24 in Appendix B, C.22 to Form C.22 in Appendix C.

Cover the following material as completely as possible. Place a checkmark next to each completed section.

1. Welcome Back

___ Review typical sequence of sessions.

___ Collect urine screen, if patient has drug problem.

___ Review urges or actual substance use in past week.

___ Review relationship problems or other concerns from past week; defer details until after review of home practice.

___ See if Promises were kept past week; commit to Promises for coming week.

2. Review Home Practice from Past Week

___ Recovery Contract

   ___ Review daily Trust Discussion (with medication, if taking it) and calendar of past week.

   ___ Couple practices Trust Discussion (with medication, if taking it) with therapist feedback.

   ___ Review self-help and other parts of Recovery Contract.

___ Positive Activities—review which of the following they chose to do:

   ___ Catch and Tell (acknowledge one nice thing partner does each day at home and best of past week in session).

   ___ Shared Rewarding Activity (do planned SRA; plan one for following week).

   ___ Caring Day (give your partner a Caring Day this week).

___ Communication Sessions (three) to practice S.O.L.V.E. plus at least one other of following:

   ___ Problem Solving using S.O.L.V.E. method on problem chosen in session.

   ___ Listening with Understanding—on everyday problems, including charged issues.

   ___ Conflict Resolution—use a Time-Out in a real situation or in a practice situation.

   ___ Relationship Agreements—do agreement made in session and negotiate another.

(continued)

3. Deal with Current Problems/Other Support for Abstinence
(Each of the following is optional, based on couple's needs. Refer to Session 4 for details.)

___ *Problems:* Address past week or other problems directly or refer to another source of help.

___ *Exposure to substances:* Help partners decide how to deal with upcoming exposure situations.

___ *Enabling:* Help couple identify and stop enabling. →(Show *Enabling Poster B.27.*)←

4. Continuing Recovery Plan

___ Review Sample Continuing Recovery Plan to maintain abstinence and help relationship after weekly BCT ends. →(Show *Sample Continuing Recovery Plan Poster B.24*)←

___ Discuss handout on helpful hints for continuing recovery.
→(Hand out *Continuing Recovery Helpful Hints Form C.22.*)←

___ Review non-substance abusing partner's role in Continuing Recovery Plan

___ In-session practice of couple completing their own Continuing Recovery Plan.
→(Hand out *My Continuing Recovery Plan Form C.23.*)←

___ Assign home practice: Discuss and refine Continuing Recovery Plan made in session.

5. Assign Home Practice   →(Hand out *Home Practice Session 10 Form C.24.*)←

___ Recovery Contract

    ___ Do Trust Discussion (with medication, if taking it) and mark on calendar.

    ___ Do self-help and other parts of contract and mark on calendar.

___ Positive Activities—pick at least one of following to do:

    ___ Catch and Tell (acknowledge one nice thing partner does each day).

    ___ Shared Rewarding Activity (do planned SRA; plan one for following week).

    ___ Caring Day (give your partner a Caring Day this week).

___ Communication Sessions (three) to discuss continuing Recovery Plan plus at least one other of following:

    ___ Continuing Recovery Plan—discuss together, make desired changes, try to finalize.

    ___ Problem Solving—30 minutes using S.O.L.V.E. method on problem chosen in session.

    ___ Listening with Understanding—on everyday problems, including charged issues.

    ___ Conflict Resolution—use a Time-Out in a real situation or in a practice situation.

    ___ Relationship Agreements—do agreement made in session and negotiate another.

Note that couple has choice regarding some assignments. Therapist should help couple choose.

6. Session Closing

___ Answer questions about assignments.

___ Get commitment from each person to do home practice assignments.

BCT SESSION 10 OUTLINE
CONTINUING RECOVERY

This session helps the partners create a Continuing Recovery Plan of activities and tools from those they found helpful and plan to continue to use after weekly couple sessions end.

1. Welcome Back:

1A. Collect Urine Screen If Patient Has Drug Problem.

1B. Review Urges or Actual Substance Use in Past Week:
Ask: "Could you tell me about times since we last met when you drank or used drugs or had an urge or temptation to do so?"

1C. Review Relationship Problems or Other Concerns from Past Week:
Ask: "How did things go between the two of you in the past week? Any arguments? Positive times? Other important issues?" This segment should give a brief overview of how the past week went. Defer any extensive discussion until after review of the home practice.

1D. Review Promises:
Review each Promise, asking each person: "Have you been able to keep these Promises since last week? Can you commit to these Promises for the upcoming week?"

2. Review Home Practice from Last Week:

2A. Recovery Contract:
1. **Repeat Assignment:** The patient and partner were to do all parts of their *Recovery Contract*.
2. **Rationale for Assignment:** Rebuild trust and help substance abuse patient stay abstinent.
3. **Review Assignment:** Review calendar to see how often they did the Trust Discussion and other elements of their contract. Discuss obstacles and ways to get more benefits; for example, if going to AA, may consider getting a sponsor, joining a group.
4. **In-Session Practice of the Trust Discussion:** The partners practice the Trust Discussion (with medication, if taking it) in session, allowing for feedback and correction by therapist.

2B. Positive Activities:
1. **Repeat Assignment:** Pick at least one of following to do:
   - Catch and Tell: Acknowledge one nice thing each day when doing Trust Discussion.
   - Shared Rewarding Activity: Do planned SRA; plan one for following week.
   - Caring Day: Give your partner a Caring Day this week.
2. **Rationale for Assignment:** Increase positive activities and feelings in the relationship.
3. **Review Assignment:** Review chosen assignment(s) following instructions in Session 5.
4. **In-Session Practice:** Practice chosen assignment(s) following instructions in Session 5.

(continued)

2C. Communication Sessions:

1. **Repeat Assignment:** Have three sessions to practice S.O.L.V.E. plus at least one other of following:
   - Problem Solving—30 minutes using S.O.L.V.E. method on problem chosen in session.
   - Listening with Understanding—on everyday problems, including charged issues.
   - Relationship Agreements—do agreement made in session and negotiate another.
   - Conflict Resolution—use a Time-Out in a real situation or in a practice situation.
2. **Rationale for Assignment:** Good communication resolves requests, conflicts, and problems.
3. **Review Assignments:** Ask if they processed a problem using the S.O.L.V.E. model. Review solution or reasons if no solution decided. Review other chosen assignments, following instructions in Session 8.
4. **In-Session Practice:** For S.O.L.V.E., help couple finish problem from last week, and if they want to continue assignment, pick another problem to discuss in coming week. Practice other chosen assignments, following instructions in Session 8.

3. Deal with Current Problems/Other Support for Abstinence:

(*Each of following is optional, based on couple's needs. Refer to Session 4 for details.*)

3A. Current Problems:
Address past week or other problems directly or by referral to another source of help.

3B. Exposure to Situations Where Alcohol or Drugs Are Available:
Help them decide how to deal with upcoming exposure situations.

3C. Spouse Enabling:
Help couple identify and stop enabling behaviors. →(Show *Enabling Poster B.27.*)←

4. Continuing Recovery Plan:

4A. Review Sample Continuing Recovery Plan
→(Show *Sample Continuing Recovery Plan Poster B.24.*)←

SUGGESTED THERAPIST SCRIPT

Both of you have been working hard to make your lives together better. Part of your success has come from what you have learned from these couple sessions and from other recovery activities you've taken part in.

Now we are going to work on a Continuing Recovery Plan. This is basically a list of activities and tools you have found helpful and plan to continue to use after you complete this program. It is a concrete plan of activities to help you stay sober and keep your relationship happy after these weekly couple sessions end.

We'll start by looking at a sample Continuing Recovery Plan made by another couple to give you an example. It may give you some ideas for your own plan. After we review this example, then we'll have you start making your own plan here with me. At home this week you can add to the plan you started working on here.

Go over each section of the sample Continuing Recovery Plan, asking the partners to consider what they might want to do under each part of the plan, as described next.

(continued)

1. **Support for Recovery:**
   - Recovery Contract
     - Trust Discussion
     - Self-help attendance
     - Recovery medication
2. **Positive Couple Activities:**
   - Catch and Tell
   - Shared Rewarding Activity
   - Caring Day
3. **Communication Skills:**
   - Communication Sessions
     - "I" Messages
     - Listening and Understanding
   - Relationship Agreements
   - S.O.L.V.E. Problem Solving
   - Time-Out
4. **Continuing Recovery:**
   - Continuing Recovery Plan
   - Action Plan*
   - Couple checkup visits*
   - Couple relapse prevention sessions*
   (*to be introduced in Session 11)
5. **Other:**
   - See following material.

4B. Discuss Handout on Helpful Hints for Continuing Recovery
→(Hand out *Continuing Recovery Helpful Hints Form C.22*.)←

Partners can list any other rituals or routines they have found to be helpful (e.g., reading the Big Book, listening to relaxation tapes, participating in regular exercise).

SUGGESTED THERAPIST SCRIPT
Here is a handout with some helpful hints about continuing recovery that you can use. If you come across other beneficial points in your journey with recovery, you can add them to the list.

4C. Review Non-Substance-Abusing Partner's Role in Continuing Recovery Plan:

SUGGESTED THERAPIST SCRIPT
A major goal of these couple sessions has been to involve both of you in the recovery process. When both of you actively work together to improve the relationship and continue recovery, relationship satisfaction and a drug and alcohol free lifestyle are better maintained. In this section, we ask both of you to consider what the non-substance-abusing partner's role will be in the process of continuing recovery.

4D. In-Session Practice of Couple Completing Their Own Continuing Recovery Plan
→(Hand Out *My Continuing Recovery Plan Form C.23*.)←

(continued)

Discuss with the couple each item on the Continuing Recovery Plan and answer any questions. Help them work together to create a plan that is specific, reasonable, and realistic. Move slowly through each category and allow time for each person to record the items that are of particular importance on the Continuing Recovery Plan. Note areas of disagreement and possible need for negotiation and compromise. Tell the couple that they will need to reach an agreement about which skills they find helpful and can realistically continue to use. They should be specific in how often they will do the chosen activities (e.g., daily, weekly, monthly). Ask them to have a Communication Session in the coming week to discuss and try to finalize their Continuing Recovery Plan. Stress how critically important this plan is. They have made good progress so far, and they need to make a solid plan so that their progress will continue.

4E. Assign Continuing Recovery Plan Home Practice:
- Take Continuing Recovery Plan home to review together and make any desired changes.
- Bring the Continuing Recovery Plan to the next session for discussion.

5. Assign Home Practice:

→(Hand out *Home Practice Session 10 Form C.24.*)←

5A. Recovery Contract:
- Do Trust Discussion (with medication, if taking it) every day at specified time.
- Do self-help and other parts of contract.
- Mark on calendar each time Trust Discussion and other parts of contract are completed.

5B. Positive Activities—pick at least one of following to do:
- Catch and Tell: Acknowledge one nice thing each day when doing Trust Discussion.
- Shared Rewarding Activity: Do planned SRA; plan one for following week.
- Caring Day: Give your partner a Caring Day this week.

5C. Communication Sessions (three)—to discuss Continuing Recovery Plan plus at least one other of following:
- Continuing Recovery Plan—discuss together, make desired changes, try to finalize.
- Problem Solving—30 minutes using S.O.L.V.E. method on problem chosen in session.
- Listening with Understanding—on everyday problems including charged issues.
- Conflict Resolution—use a Time-Out in a real situation or in a practice situation.
- Relationship Agreements—do agreement made in session and negotiate another.

Note that couple has choice regarding some assignments. This keeps assignments manageable and allows partners to choose assignments to fit couple's needs. Therapist should help couple choose.

6. Session Closing:

6A. Answer Questions: Answer any questions about the home practice assignments.

6B. Commit to Home Practice: Get verbal commitment to do the home practice.

Checklist for BCT Session 11: Action Plan

Posters Needed:	Forms Needed:
B.25. Sample Action Plan B.26. Sample Partner's Action Plan	C.25. My Action Plan C.26. Partner's Action Plan C.27. Home Practice Session 11

Note: B.25 refers to Poster B.25 in Appendix B, C.25 to Form C.25 in Appendix C.

Cover the following material as completely as possible. Place a checkmark next to each completed section.

1. Welcome Back

___ Review typical sequence of sessions.

___ Collect urine screen, if patient has drug problem.

___ Review urges or actual substance use in past week.

___ Review relationship problems or other concerns from past week; defer details until after review of home practice.

___ See if Promises were kept past week; commit to Promises for coming week.

2. Review Home Practice from Past Week

___ Recovery Contract

    ___ Review daily Trust Discussion (with medication, if taking it) and calendar of past week.

    ___ Couple practice Trust Discussion (with medication, if taking it) with therapist feedback.

    ___ Review self-help and other parts of Recovery Contract.

___ Positive Activities—review which of the following they chose to do:

    ___ Catch and Tell (acknowledge one nice thing partner does each day at home and best of past week in session).

    ___ Shared Rewarding Activity (do planned SRA; plan one for following week).

    ___ Caring Day (give your partner a Caring Day this week).

___ Communication Sessions (three) to discuss Continuing Recovery Plan plus at least one other of following:

    ___ Continuing Recovery Plan—review in section 4 below.

    ___ Problem Solving—30 minutes using S.O.L.V.E. method on problem chosen in session.

    ___ Listening with Understanding—on everyday problems including charged issues.

    ___ Conflict Resolution—use a Time-Out in a real situation or in a practice situation.

    ___ Relationship Agreements—do agreement made in session and negotiate another.

(continued)

3. Deal with Current Problems/Other Support for Abstinence
(Each of the following is optional, based on couple's needs. Refer to Session 4 for details.)

___ *Problems:* Address past week or other problems directly or refer to another source of help.

___ *Exposure to substances:* Help partners decide how to deal with upcoming exposure situations.

___ *Enabling:* Help couple identify and stop enabling behaviors. →(Show *Enabling Poster B.27.*)←

4. Review Continuing Recovery Plan

___ Couple had agreed to discuss and refine Continuing Recovery Plan made in last session.

___ Review any changes made in plan.

___ Consider periodic couple sessions after weekly meetings end as part of plan.

___ Couple discusses Continuing Recovery Plan, with therapist coaching, until plan is finalized.

5. Action Plan
→(Show *Sample Action Plan Poster B.25*; hand out *My Action Plan Form C.25.*)←

___ Use fire drill analogy to introduce Action Plan to prevent or minimize relapse.

___ Help couple identify high-risk situations and warning signs likely in next few months and decide plan of action to deal with them.

___ Help couple decide plan of action if substance use occurs.

___ Review partner's role in Action Plan (includes safety plan to avoid violence). →(Show *Sample Partner Action Plan Poster B.26*; hand out *Partner's Action Plan Form C.26.*)←

___ Assign home practice: Discuss and refine Action Plan made in session.

6. Assign Home Practice   →(Hand out *Home Practice Session 11 Form C.27.*)←
___ Recovery Contract

   ___ Do Trust Discussion (with medication, if taking it) and mark on calendar.

   ___ Do self-help and other parts of contract and mark on calendar.

___ Positive Activities—pick at least one of following to do:

   ___ Catch and Tell (acknowledge one nice thing partner does each day).

   ___ Shared Rewarding Activity (do planned SRA; plan one for following week).

   ___ Caring Day (give your partner a Caring Day this week).

___ Communication Sessions—have three (10–15 minutes) Communication Sessions to discuss:

   ___ Action Plan (make desired changes, try to finalize, check phone numbers).

   ___ Continuing Recovery Plan (discuss checkup visits or relapse prevention sessions).

7. Session Closing
___ Answer questions about assignments.

___ Get commitment from each person to do home practice assignments.

BCT SESSION 11 OUTLINE
ACTION PLAN

This session helps the couple make an Action Plan for how they will prevent or minimize relapse when faced with high-risk situations and warning signs for relapse.

1. Welcome Back:

1A. Collect Urine Screen If Patient Has Drug Problem.

1B. Review Urges or Actual Substance Use in Past Week:
Ask: "Could you tell me about times since we last met when you drank or used drugs or had an urge or temptation to do so?"

1C. Review Relationship Problems or Other Concerns from Past Week:
Ask: "How did things go between the two of you in the past week? Any arguments? Positive times? Other important issues?" This segment should give a brief overview of how the past week went. Defer any extensive discussion until after review of the home practice.

1D. Review Promises:
Review each Promise, asking each person: "Have you been able to keep these Promises since last week? Can you commit to these Promises for the upcoming week?"

2. Review Home Practice from Last Week:

2A. Recovery Contract:
1. **Repeat Assignment:** The patient and partner were to do all parts of their Recovery Contract.
2. **Rationale for Assignment:** Rebuild trust and help substance abuse patient stay abstinent.
3. **Review Assignment:** Review calendar to see how often they did the Trust Discussion and other elements of their contract. Discuss obstacles and ways to get more benefits; for example, if going to AA, may consider getting a sponsor, joining a group.
4. **In-Session Practice of the Trust Discussion:** The partners practice the Trust Discussion (with medication, if taking it) in session, allowing for feedback and correction by therapist.

2B. Positive Activities:
1. **Repeat Assignment:** Pick at least one of following to do:
   - Catch and Tell: Acknowledge one nice thing each day when doing Trust Discussion.
   - Shared Rewarding Activity: Do planned SRA; plan one for following week.
   - Caring Day: Give your partner a Caring Day this week.
2. **Rationale for Assignment:** Increase positive activities and feelings in the relationship.
3. **Review Assignment:** Review chosen assignment(s) following instructions in Session 5.
4. **In-Session Practice:** Practice chosen assignment(s) following instructions in Session 5.

(continued)

2C. Communication Sessions:

1. **Repeat Assignment:** Have three sessions to discuss Continuing Recovery Plan plus at least one other of following:
   - Continuing Recovery Plan—covered in section 4 below.
   - Problem Solving—30 minutes using S.O.L.V.E. method on problem chosen in session.
   - Listening with Understanding—on everyday problems, including charged issues.
   - Conflict Resolution—use a Time-Out in a real situation or in a practice situation.
   - Relationship Agreements—do agreement made in session and negotiate another.
2. **Rationale for Assignment:** Good communication resolves requests, conflicts, and problems.
3. **Review Assignments:** Cover Continuing Recovery Plan in section 4 below. Review other chosen assignments, following instructions in Session 8.
4. **In-Session Practice:** Cover Continuing Recovery Plan in section 4 below. Practice other chosen assignments, following instructions in Session 8.

3. Deal with Current Problems/Other Support for Abstinence:

(Each of following is optional, based on couple's needs. Refer to Session 4 for details.)

3A. Current Problems:

Address past week or other problems directly or by referral to another source of help.

3B. Exposure to Situations Where Alcohol or Drugs Are Available:

Help couple decide how to deal with upcoming exposure situations.

3C. Spouse Enabling:

Help couple identify and stop enabling behaviors. →(Show *Enabling Poster B.27*.)←

4. Review Continuing Recovery Plan:

SUGGESTED THERAPIST SCRIPT

Last session we talked about the Continuing Recovery Plan and how it will be helpful in your continuing recovery. I asked you to take it home last week to review and make any changes you thought were needed.

Did you have a Communication Session to discuss your plan? What changes did you make in your plan? Were there things you added or removed?

Therapist note: Coach partners to consider any changes to their plan. If they did not discuss it at home, encourage them to discuss it here with you.

SUGGESTED THERAPIST SCRIPT

There is something else I would like you to think about adding to your plan. That is having periodic couple sessions with me after our weekly meetings end. Such sessions can help you stick with your continuing recovery activities.

Periodic sessions offer a more gradual phasing out of our meetings together rather than just stopping. These sessions also signify that substance abuse is a chronic health problem that benefits from active, ongoing monitoring for an extended period of time to prevent or quickly treat relapse. There are two options we frequently recommend:

(continued)

- "Checkup visits" every 2 or 3 months for 2 years, with less frequent checkups after that;
- "Relapse prevention sessions" in which we have 15 sessions in the next year, starting every 2 weeks and gradually becoming less frequent.

Let's discuss whether either of these options would be good for the two of you.

Most couples can benefit from checkup visits. Couples who have more severe problems or who had trouble during BCT may need more frequent contacts initially after weekly BCT sessions end. These couples may benefit from the relapse prevention sessions.

Consider the balance between risk factors and coping factors in deciding which, if either, format of additional couple sessions to recommend. **Risk factors** present challenges that must be addressed to maintain abstinence. Patients who have more severe, more chronic substance abuse and relationship problems, and a greater number of other problems (e.g., medical, psychiatric, job, financial, social) face higher risk factors. Similarly, those whose environments contain higher levels of ongoing stress and more frequent exposure to high-risk situations face higher risk factors. **Coping factors** reflect resources to deal with risk factors without relapsing. Those who have coped successfully with recent problems and plan to use more recovery tools after BCT ends have higher coping factors.

Couples facing more risk factors need more coping factors. For such couples, you may want to recommend that they reconsider tools they had rejected for their Continuing Recovery Plan.

Therapist note: If continued couple sessions with you are not feasible, this part can be omitted. However, the part about recommending additional tools in a Continuing Recovery Plan, if needed, applies to all couples.

5. Action Plan:

5A. Use "Fire Drill" Analogy to Introduce Action Plan to Prevent or Minimize Relapse:

SUGGESTED THERAPIST SCRIPT

Nobody plans to relapse, but we know that it does happen. So today we are going to work on an Action Plan of what you can do to prevent or minimize relapse when you face high-risk situations and warning signs for relapse.

I know that talking about relapse can be upsetting. Some couples worry that talking about relapse means that it is inevitable. Others think that such talk gives permission for drinking or drug use.

It may help to think of your Action Plan as a "relapse drill" that is similar to a fire drill to prevent or minimize fire. Taking steps to prevent a fire, for example, by removing oily rags or old paint cans stored near the furnace does not mean that a fire is inevitable. Having a fire drill to practice what to do in case of fire is meant to save lives by being prepared for quick action. Once a fire has started, the goal is to put it out as quickly as possible to minimize damage. None of these aspects of fire prevention and fire safety implies that fires are inevitable or in any way desirable. In fact, just the opposite is the case.

Does this idea of your Action Plan as a "relapse drill" to prevent or minimize a relapse make sense to you?

5B. Substance Abuser Action Plan:
→(Show *Sample Action Plan Poster B.25*; hand out *My Action Plan Form C.25*.)←

(continued)

5B.1. High-Risk Situations and Plan of Action:

SUGGESTED THERAPIST SCRIPT

Because you are both involved in this process of recovery, you will work together to come up with a plan for each of you. We will look at each section of this sample Action Plan and then decide what fits best in your own plan.

The first step is to write down high-risk situations you expect to face in the next 6 months. High-risk situations are people, places, moods, and physical or emotional signs that are possible triggers to a lapse or relapse. A high-risk situation affects your thoughts and feelings so that chances increase that you will drink or use drugs. A high-risk situation might involve driving by an old neighborhood where you used to use, or stopping by the bar you used to hang out in to "just get a soda," or having an argument with your partner. Other examples could be a friend's wedding, a change in income, or an anniversary of abstinence. These situations put you at risk for drinking or using because alcohol or drugs are easily available or may be an escape from the pain and frustration of an argument. If you can identify high-risk situations and make a plan of how to avoid them, you will increase your chances of staying drug and alcohol free.

This does not mean that these triggers will directly lead you to a lapse or relapse. Rather, it means you've done your homework and made your own plan to increase your awareness of high-risk situations. When your plan is complete, you will be better prepared to identify these situations and make choices that will help you continue in your recovery.

Next, write down how you plan to either avoid these situations or how you will cope once you find yourself in a high-risk situation. For example, you could call your partner to pick you up from the bar, be aware of the neighborhoods to avoid, and so forth.

(Be sure the partner gives his or her input to this and the rest of the Action Plan process.)

5B.2. Warning Signs and Plan of Action:

SUGGESTED THERAPIST SCRIPT

Let's talk about warning signs of relapse next. These signs don't necessarily mean you are going to use, but they can warn of changes you are experiencing that may eventually lead to use. Examples of warning signs are:

- *Behavior changes*: include skipping self-help meetings, smoking or eating more because of feeling stressed out, stopping in a bar to have a soda.
- *Attitude changes*: include slipping into a negative attitude or not caring about your recovery.
- *Changes in feelings and moods*: include strong feelings such as anger, depression, frustration, or sudden feelings of euphoria.
- *Changes in thoughts*: include thinking about using alcohol or drugs, believing that one drink won't hurt, or remembering only the fun times connected with using.

In this section write down what warning signs have led you to use in the past and which ones you think could cause you to use in the future.

Next, write down specific ways in which you can try to prevent relapse. For example, you could call your sponsor, have a Communication Session with your partner, go to a meeting, etc.

(continued)

5B.3. Action Plan If Drinking or Drug Use Occurs:

> **SUGGESTED THERAPIST SCRIPT**
>
> An important part of your Action Plan is to decide ahead of time what you will do to deal with any drinking or drug use that might occur. The goal is to keep the length and negative effects of any lapse or relapse to a minimum. We have three suggestions for your plan.
>
> The first suggestion is that you **act quickly** if use occurs. Consider again how a relapse is like a fire. A small fire gets bigger if it is not put out. Counting on a fire to burn itself out is risky. The fire may just keep on raging, gaining strength as it goes along. Or it may burn itself out, but only after destroying what was in its path. So unless you want to be back to where you started, it is better to nip a relapse in the bud. Getting substance use stopped quickly should be a top priority. Now, write down on your plan what you will do to *act quickly*.

> **SUGGESTED THERAPIST SCRIPT**
>
> The next suggestion is to **get help**. It can be hard for a person to think clearly and act sensibly when faced with substance use, especially after they have worked hard to stay abstinent. Talking to someone else who is more objective and not immediately affected can help. Calling me or a sponsor is the most common action plan that couples choose for getting help.
>
> Both of you need to agree on this plan in advance. This way, the partner feels they have the substance abuser's permission to call someone. The Action Plan reduces feelings that such a call is an act of disloyalty or sharing problems with an outsider. Now, write down on your plan what you will do to *get help*.

> **SUGGESTED THERAPIST SCRIPT**
>
> The third suggestion, to **stay safe**, refers to the fact that many couples tend to argue when the substance abuser drinks or uses drugs. However, arguing with an intoxicated person can lead to conflict and possible violence. Therefore, we encourage all couples to plan to avoid arguing when the substance abuser is under the influence of alcohol or drugs. Now, write down on your plan what you will do to *stay safe*.

5B.4. Support Network of Persons to Call for an Urge or a Lapse:

> **SUGGESTED THERAPIST SCRIPT**
>
> Having people in your life who support your decision to be drug and alcohol free is essential to your recovery. When facing a high-risk situation or urges to use or a lapse, your best line of defense is to have someone you can call on for help. This person should be someone you would call in an emergency. They need to be able to listen and encourage you to avoid using, or to stop using if you have already started.
>
> In this section write down the names and numbers of people in your support group. This list could include sponsors, group members, therapists, friends, or family. You need more than one person you can call in case someone cannot be reached when you need them. These need to be people who support your recovery and are willing to be called.

5B.5. Other Helpful Activities for Action Plan:

List other activities that were helpful in the past in dealing with urges and cravings. Examples include listening to relaxing music, taking a hot bath, going for a walk, and so forth.

(continued)

5C. Partner Action Plan:
→(Show *Sample Partner's Action Plan Poster B.26.*)←
→(Hand out *Partner's Action Plan Form C.26.*)←

SUGGESTED THERAPIST SCRIPT

It can be difficult to think about what would happen if your partner began using substances again. But like a fire drill, your own Action Plan can prepare you to prevent or minimize a relapse. Let's look at this sample Partner's Action Plan and decide what fits best in your plan.

5C.1. Warning Signs and the Partner's Plan of Action:

SUGGESTED THERAPIST SCRIPT

Please write down some typical warning signs that may suggest your partner is on the path to relapse. Think in terms of changes in behavior, attitude, moods, and mindset.

Now what could you do, if you notice these warning signs, to help your partner? Some examples may be to talk to your partner about the changes you've noticed, call your partner's sponsor, attend an Al-Anon meeting, etc. Let's get your ideas first. Then we can ask your partner what they would suggest you do.

5C.2. Partner's Action Plan If Use Occurs:

SUGGESTED THERAPIST SCRIPT

If substance use occurs, you need a plan to keep yourself safe. Arguing with someone who is intoxicated is a recipe for trouble. Tempers flare, which increases the chances of someone acting out in violence and getting hurt. Some examples of what you may want to write here are "I will avoid getting into an argument with him if he comes home drunk"; or "If an argument starts, I will leave the house. I can go to my sister's house and stay there until he sobers up"; or "I will try not to confront him about his use when he is drunk."

Let's also talk about what you can do to act quickly to get help.

Therapist note: This section needs to be treated delicately. Pose these questions as a way to keep both partners safe and free from unwanted conflict.

5C.3. Partner's Support Network:

SUGGESTED THERAPIST SCRIPT

Finally, list some people you can contact when you are feeling overwhelmed, in need of some friendly support, or in the event that your partner has used. Think of a family member, close friend, someone from a support group, etc. Write their name and phone number on your plan.

(continued)

Congratulations! You have created two Action Plans, which will help you in your recovery and in your relationship. We've talked about high-risk events, how to minimize risk for use and conflict, and access to individual support. I encourage both of you to keep your plans handy, review them often, and update them as necessary.

Where do you think you will keep your plan?

5D. Assign *Action Plan* Home Practice:
- Take Action Plans home to review together and make any desired changes.
- Make sure that they have accurate phone numbers for their support contacts.
- Bring Action Plans and Continuing Recovery Plan to next session for discussion.

6. Assign Home Practice:

→(Hand out *Home Practice Session 11 Form C.27.*)←

6A. Recovery Contract:
- Do Trust Discussion (with medication, if taking it) every day at specified time.
- Do self-help and other parts of contract.
- Mark on calendar each time Trust Discussion and other parts of contract are completed.

6B. Positive Activities—pick at least one of following to do:
- Catch and Tell: Acknowledge one nice thing each day when doing Trust Discussion.
- Shared Rewarding Activity: Do planned SRA; plan one for following week.
- Caring Day: Give your partner a Caring Day this week.

6C. Communication Sessions—have three (10–15 minutes) Communication Sessions to discuss:
- Action Plan—discuss together, make desired changes, try to finalize.
- Continuing Recovery Plan—discuss checkup visits or relapse prevention sessions.
- Bring Action Plans and Continuing Recovery Plan to next session to finalize.

7. Session Closing:

7A. Answer Questions: Answer any questions about the home practice assignments.

7B. Commit to Home Practice: Get verbal commitment to do the home practice.

Checklist for BCT Session 12:
Wrap-Up and Goodbye (until We Meet Again)

Posters Needed:	Forms Needed
None	None

Cover the following material as completely as possible. Place a checkmark next to each completed section.

1. Welcome Back

___ Review typical sequence of sessions.

___ Collect urine screen, if patient has drug problem.

___ Review urges or actual substance use in past week.

___ Review relationship problems or other concerns from past week; defer details until after review of home practice.

___ See if Promises were kept past week.

2. Review Home Practice from Past Week

___ Recovery Contract

    ___ Review daily Trust Discussion (with medication, if taking it) and calendar of past week.

    ___ Couple practices Trust Discussion (with medication, if taking it) with therapist feedback.

    ___ Review self-help and other parts of Recovery Contract.

___ Positive Activities—review which of the following they chose to do:

    ___ Catch and Tell (acknowledge one nice thing partner does each day at home and best of past week in session).

    ___ Shared Rewarding Activity (do planned SRA; plan one for following week).

    ___ Caring Day (give your partner a Caring Day this week).

___ Communication Sessions—have three (10–15 minutes) Communication Sessions to discuss:

    ___ Action Plan—review in next section.

    ___ Continuing Recovery Plan—review in next section.

(continued)

3. Review and Finalize Action Plan and Continuing Recovery Plan

___ Couple had agreed to discuss and refine Action Plan made in last session.

___ Review any changes made in plan.

___ Couple discusses Action Plan with therapist coaching until plan is finalized.

___ Discuss how hard it is to ask for help and how to do it.

___ Role-play asking for help as part of Action Plan (e.g., from sponsor, spouse, or friend).

___ Review and finalize Continuing Recovery Plan.

4. Review the Four Major Parts of BCT

___ BCT covered (1) support for recovery, (2) positive activities, (3) communication skills, and (4) continuing recovery.

___ Recognize the couple's gains in each of these areas.

___ Discuss what aspects of their recovery and relationship they want to continue improving.

5. Wrap-up and Goodbye

___ End on a positive note, emphasizing the couple's progress to date and hope for the future.

___ When will they contact you? Based on their Continuing Recovery Plan, this could be "as needed" or as planned contacts (set time and date now) for regular checkups or relapse prevention sessions.

BCT SESSION 12 OUTLINE
WRAP-UP AND GOODBYE

This session finalizes the couple's Action Plans and Continuing Recovery Plan. It also recaps the BCT program and prepares the couple for a smooth transition as weekly couple sessions end.

1. Welcome Back:

1A. Collect Urine Screen If Patient Has Drug Problem.

1B. Review Urges or Actual Substance Use in Past Week:
Ask: "Could you tell me about times since we last met when you drank or used drugs or had an urge or temptation to do so?"

1C. Review Relationship Problems or Other Concerns from Past Week:
Ask: "How did things go between the two of you in the past week? Any arguments? Positive times? Other important issues?" This segment should give a brief overview of how the past week went. Defer any extensive discussion until after review of the home practice.

1D. Review Promises:
Review each Promise, asking each person: "Have you been able to keep these Promises since last week?"

2. Review Home Practice from Last Week:

2A. Recovery Contract:
1. **Repeat Assignment:** The patient and partner were to do all parts of their Recovery Contract.
2. **Rationale for Assignment:** Rebuild trust and help substance abuse patient stay abstinent.
3. **Review Assignment:** Review calendar to see how often they did the Trust Discussion and other elements of their contract. Discuss obstacles and ways to get more benefits; for example, if going to AA, may consider getting a sponsor, joining a group.
4. **In-Session Practice of the Trust Discussion:** The partners practice the Trust Discussion (with medication, if taking it) in session, allowing for feedback and correction by therapist.

2B. Positive Activities:
1. **Repeat Assignment:** Pick at least one of following to do:
   - Catch and Tell: Acknowledge one nice thing each day when doing Trust Discussion.
   - Shared Rewarding Activity: Do planned SRA; plan one for following week.
   - Caring Day: Give your partner a Caring Day this week.
2. **Rationale for Assignment:** Increase positive activities and feelings in the relationship.
3. **Review Assignment:** Review chosen assignment(s) following instructions in Session 5.
4. **In-Session Practice:** Practice chosen assignment(s) following instructions in Session 5.

(continued)

2C. Communication Sessions:
1. **Repeat Assignment:** Have three (10–15 minutes) Communication Sessions to discuss:
   - Action Plan—cover in next section.
   - Continuing Recovery Plan—cover in next section.
2. **Rationale for Assignment:** Good communication resolves requests, conflicts, and problems.
3. **Review Assignments:** Cover in next section.
4. **In-Session Practice:** Cover in next section.

---

3. Review and Finalize Action Plans and Continuing Recovery Plan:

3A. Review and Finalize Action Plans:

SUGGESTED THERAPIST SCRIPT

Last session we talked about your Action Plan for dealing with warning signs and high-risk situations to prevent a relapse or keep it to a minimum. I asked you to take it home last week to review and make any changes you thought were needed.

Did you have a Communication Session to discuss your plan? What changes did you make in your plan? Were there things you added or removed?

Therapist note: Coach them to consider any changes to their plan. If they did not discuss the plan at home, encourage them to discuss it here with you.

SUGGESTED THERAPIST SCRIPT

You have completed the Action Plan. Now let's talk about where you intend to keep your plan and how often you hope to update it in order to address potential high-risk events?

3B. Asking for Help and Support:
Asking for help and support to deal with high-risk events is part of an Action Plan, but it may be hard for many people to follow through and actually ask for help and support when they need it.

3B.1. Discuss How Hard It Is to Ask for Help and How To Do It:

SUGGESTED THERAPIST SCRIPT

Couples dealing with substance abuse problems are often afraid and embarrassed to ask for help and support from others, even those they feel closest to. You may think that asking for support is a good thing to do, but if you lack skill and comfort doing it, you may not follow through and ask for help when you need it. So I'm going to ask you to practice asking for help and support.

Before you practice asking for support, let's discuss your ideas about asking for help from others. Do you choose someone who listens, someone who can help financially, or someone who gives you advice?

(continued)

3B.2. In-Session Practice Role-Playing Asking for Help as Part of Action Plan:

SUGGESTED THERAPIST SCRIPT

First, I would like for you to practice asking for support from each other. While practicing, use your communication skills, especially "I" Messages and Listening with Understanding. Be specific about what kind of help and support you want: for example, "I just want you to listen," or "I could use your help in figuring out some options," or "I need a hug." OK, let's think of a time when you would have liked to ask for help from your partner. Practice asking for help now.
    (First model asking for support. Then partners alternate asking for support from each other.)
    Now that you have practiced asking for help from each other, choose a support person you listed in your Action Plan. With your partner pretending to be that individual, practice asking for help and support. Keep in mind the skills and guidelines we just discussed.

3C. Review and Finalize Continuing Recovery Plan:

SUGGESTED THERAPIST SCRIPT

Last session we talked about the possibility of your having periodic couple sessions with me after our weekly meetings end today. Such sessions can help you stick with your Continuing Recovery Plan. The sessions also signify that substance abuse is a chronic health problem that benefits from active, ongoing monitoring for an extended period of time to prevent or quickly treat relapse. There were two options we discussed:
• "Checkup visits" every 2 or 3 months for the next few years;
• "Relapse prevention sessions" in which we have 15 sessions spread out over the next year.
    Your assignment was to have a Communication Session to discuss whether you wanted to continue with periodic couple sessions. What did you decide?
    (If partners agree to either of these options, then schedule their next appointment. If they refuse both options try the following. Most couples will agree to a checkup visit if they do not feel it obligates them beyond that visit.)
    So you're not sure if you really need more couple sessions. I can understand that. Why don't we just schedule a checkup visit for 2 months from now? At that time we can decide whether you want any further visits after that. If that's OK with you, then let's set up an appointment now. My office will give you a reminder call a few days before the appointment.

4. Review the Four Major Parts of BCT:

Because this is the last BCT session, an overview of all the skills learned, the progress the partners have made, and any future issues that may arise should be covered. Briefly review the four major parts of the BCT program:

1. Support for Recovery
2. Positive Activities
3. Communication Skills
4. Continuing Recovery

Refer to their completed Continuing Recovery Plan to review each area of BCT, noting what they learned and plan to continue using.

(continued)

353

4A. Recognize Gains and Improvements Couple Has Made:

SUGGESTED THERAPIST SCRIPT

You've both put a lot of effort into these sessions. Thanks for being a part of this. I've noticed . . . [specific comments on skills and partners' progress]. Is there anything further you can think of that you'd like to discuss at this time?

4B. What Do They Want to Continue to Improve after BCT Ends?

SUGGESTED THERAPIST SCRIPT

We've also talked about many different areas of your recovery and relationship. Which of these areas stand out for you as areas to continue to work on?

5. Wrap-up and Goodbye:

- Ask couple to discuss their feelings about the completion of treatment and offer feedback.
- End on a positive note, emphasizing their progress to date and hope for the future.
- When will they contact you next? Based on their Continuing Recovery Plan, this could be "as needed" or as a planned contact (set time and date now) for regular checkups or relapse prevention sessions.

APPENDIX B

Posters Used in BCT

Why BCT?

	Active Drinking and Drug Use	Recovery	BCT
Alcohol or Drug Use	Alcohol and drug use become main focus of relationship	Gone but not forgotten Tension, nagging, arguments, fear, distrust	✓ Recovery Contract ✓ Continuing Recovery Plan
Love and Daily Caring	Anger and resentment replace love and caring; take over relationship	Anger and resentment continue; hard to remember what relationship was like without drugs and alcohol	Caring Behaviors ✓ Catch and Tell ✓ Caring Days
Fun Together	Time spent drinking, using drugs, arguing, or doing things without one another	Time spent trying to solve problems caused by drinking and drugging instead of doing things together	Shared Rewarding Activities
Problems	Too many problems caused by substance use (bills, job losses, etc.) Everyday relationship problems and differences pile up Problems go unresolved and often unrecognized	Problems caused by substance use can still be overwhelming and even worse Relationship problems becoming obvious Blame game: No good will or skills to solve problems and differences	Communication Skills Training ✓ Effective listening ✓ Effective speaking ✓ Communication sessions ✓ Problem solving ✓ Relationship agreements ✓ Conflict resolution

Promises

➢ No Threats of Divorce or Separation

➢ No Violence or Threats of Violence (no angry touching)

➢ Focus on the Present and Future—Not on the Past

➢ Actively Participate in All Sessions and Do Homework Assignments

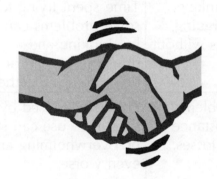

Typical Sequence of Sessions

✓ Urine Screen If There Is a Drug Problem

✓ Review of Use/Urges to Use That Occurred
in the Past Week

✓ Review of Relationship Problems or Significant
Issues Experienced in Past Week

✓ Review of Promises

✓ Review of Last Session and Home Practice
(Perform Trust Discussion in Session)

✓ Cover New Material (Instruction, Therapist Model,
and In-Session Practice)

✓ Assign Home Practice for Next Week

Daily Trust Discussion Formula

Client

"I have been drug and alcohol free for the last 24 hours and plan to remain drug and alcohol free for the next 24 hours. Thank you for listening and being supportive of my effort to be drug and alcohol free."

Partner

"Thank you for staying drug and alcohol free for the last 24 hours. I appreciate the effort you are making to stay clean and sober."

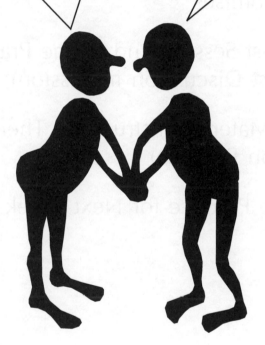

Sample Recovery Contract Calendar

☒ ✓ = Trust Discussion Done   ☐ N = Al-Anon or Nar-Anon

☐ Ⓥ = Trust Discussion with   ☒ D = Drug Urine + or −
    Medication (_____)

☒ A = AA or NA Meeting   ☒ O = Other
                                          (*Group Therapy*)

Mo & Yr: *September, 20xx*

S	M	T	W	T	F	S
						A 1
2	✓ O 3	✓ 4	✓ D− 5	✓ 6	7	A 8
9	✓ O 10	✓ 11	✓ D− 12	✓ A 13	✓ 14	A 15
16	✓ O 17	✓ 18	✓ D+ 19	✓ A 20	✓ 21	A 22
✓ 23	✓ O 24	✓ A 25	✓ D− 26	✓ A 27	✓ 28	✓ A 29
✓ 30						

Sample Caring Behaviors

Paid the bills

Went to work to earn money

Helped with shopping

Packed a lunch for me

Cooked dinner

Did the dishes

Straightened up the house

Set the table

Did the yard work

Played with the children

Changed the baby's diaper

Gave the kids a bath

Helped kids with homework

Let me sleep in

Hugged or kissed me

Cuddled close to me in bed

Brought me a cup of coffee, tea, etc.

Complimented me on my appearance

Thanked me for doing something

Called to tell me where he or she was

Catch Your Partner Doing Something Nice

Each day, notice at least one nice thing that your partner does and note it on the following chart. It is ALWAYS POSSIBLE to notice at least one CARING BEHAVIOR—even if you do not see your partner for an entire day. Don't share your list with your partner yet!

Day	Date	Caring Behavior
Mon.	4/6	Waited to have dinner with me because I had to stay late at work. Made me feel good.
Tues.	4/7	Told me she loved me.
Wed.	4/8	Cooked a delicious Italian dinner and afterwards we had a very romantic evening.
Thurs.	4/9	Was patient with me when I came home tired and moody from work.
Fri.	4/10	Enjoyed a walk together around the neighborhood.
Sat.	4/11	Woke me gently and rubbed my back.
Sun.	4/12	She asked me how my day was and listened to me talk.

Acknowledging Caring Behaviors

What you say:
- "I liked it when you . . . ."
- "It made me feel . . ."
- *(Leave out the negative)*

How to say it:
- Look at the other person
- Use pleasant tone of voice
- Smile
- Be sincere

Possible Shared Activities

As a couple:
- Pop popcorn and rent a movie
- Go out to our favorite restaurant
- Go out to the movies
- Go bowling
- Do a project at home together

With other couples:
- Have a cookout for our families
- Hike with my sister and her boyfriend
- Invite sponsor and his wife for dinner
- Go to church supper with neighbors
- Invite couples to our house after high school concert

With the kids:
- Have a picnic by the river
- Go to Jimmy's T-ball game
- Play board games—no TV
- Go camping
- Play miniature golf as a family

Caring Day!

♥ A day when you plan ahead to do some special things to show you care for your partner. Make it a surprise.

♥ You can do a number of little things throughout the day or a bigger, special gesture of caring.

Examples:

♥ *"I left work early to cook a lasagna dinner with strawberry shortcake for dessert. Also gave him a card to let him know I love him."*

♥ *"I picked up a new bike for my wife. Picked up her medication. Cut the lawn and cleaned the shed. Took her for an ice cream."*

Message Intended = Message Received

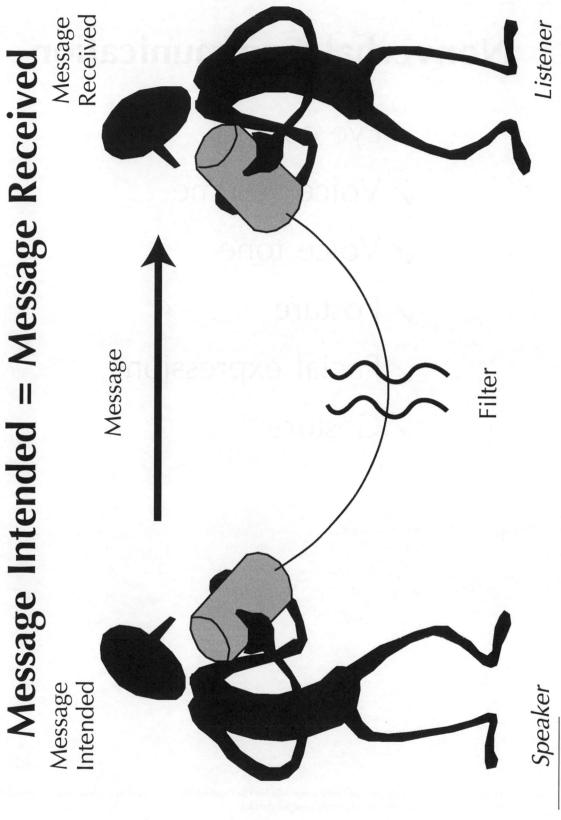

Nonverbal Communication

✓ Eye contact

✓ Voice volume

✓ Voice tone

✓ Posture

✓ Facial expression

✓ Gesture

Barriers to Communication

- Filters

- "All-Talk-and-No-Listen" Syndrome

- Blaming and Shaming

- Individual Communication Styles

  - Passive

  - Aggressive

  - Assertive

Direct and Indirect Communication

Direct Communication:

⇒ Taking responsibility for your feelings

⇒ Not waiting to share your feelings

⇒ Actively expressing yourself

⇒ Being assertive

Indirect Communication:

∅ Accusing and blaming the other person

∅ Delaying

∅ Passively withdrawing

∅ Sulking or aggressing

∅ Mind reading

Communication Session

➤ Sit down face to face.

➤ Plan time and place ahead so that you will have privacy.

➤ Do not allow distractions, such as TV.

➤ Schedule 10–15 minutes.

➤ Use communication skills learned in couples therapy.

➤ Discuss concerns and problems.

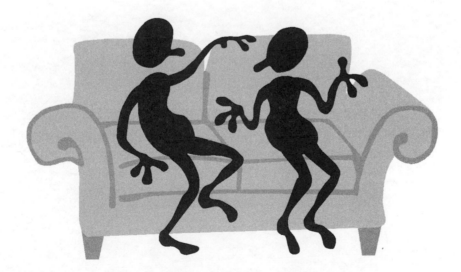

Expressing Feelings Directly Using "I" Messages

"I feel _____ [emotion]

when you _____ [behavior]."

"I feel _____ [emotion]

when you _____ [behavior]

because _____ [specific reason]."

Listening and Understanding

Listening

- Restate message received.
  "What I heard you say was. . . ."

- Ask if you heard correctly.
  "Did I get that right?"

- Get more information
  "Is there more?"

Understanding

- *"It makes sense that you feel the way you do."*

- *"That must make you feel. . . ."*

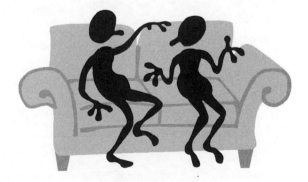

Positive Specific Requests

- <u>Positive</u>—what you want, not what you don't want.

- <u>Specific</u>—what, where, and when.

- <u>Requests</u>—not demands (which use force and threats), but rather requests, which have possibility for negotiation and compromise.

Negotiated Agreement

I agreed to (be specific: what, when, how many times):

My partner agreed to:

Did I follow through with my agreement? (describe):

Sample Couple Requests

I would like my partner to:

1. Kiss me when I come home from work.
2. Help out more around the house.
3. Tell me about his or her workday at dinner-time.
4. Stop bugging me so much.
5. Do the dishes on nights that I go to class.
6. Appreciate me more.
7. Stop watching sports on TV all the time.
8. Hold my hand while we watch TV.
9. Put his or her dirty clothes in the hamper.
10. Spend more time with our kids.

Items 1, 3, 5, 8, and 9 are positive specific requests.
Items 4 and 7 are negative.
Items 2, 6, and 10 are not specific.

Responses to Conflict

Verbal Aggression: Commonly used when couple is frustrated and can't reach agreement; highly ineffective; causes more frustration and anger; doesn't lead to resolution.

Examples: blaming, name calling, swearing, yelling

Physical Aggression: Ineffective coping behaviors that hurt victim and relationship; common among couples with substance abuse.

Examples: slapping, hitting, biting, pushing, grabbing, shoving

Flooding: Person becomes overwhelmed with emotion and can't think clearly or speak effectively—like a car engine that won't start because it's been flooded with too much gas.

Avoidance and Withdrawal: Avoids discussing problems with his or her partner or withdraws from conflict by changing topic or leaving room; usually not effective if major relationship problems are not discussed.

Verbal Reasoning: Couple uses effective speaking and listening communication skills to resolve a conflict; both partners state their opinions; able to reach a compromise; typically leads to mutually agreed-upon solution.

Time Out

Before: When discomfort or frustration in discussion first begins.

During: A "Time-Out" is requested. Couple separates to calm down and clear thoughts.

After: The "Time-Out" is over and discussion restarts.

Resolution: A "Time-Out" increases chances of successful resolution.

S O L V E

S **STOP, SLOW DOWN, AND SEE THE PROBLEM**
✓ Is there a problem?
✓ What <u>exactly</u> is the problem?

O **OUTLINE OPTIONS**
✓ Brainstorm: What can I do?
✓ What might work?

L **LOOK AT CONSEQUENCES**
✓ Look at long- and short-term consequences.
✓ Look at positive and negative consequences.
✓ What will happen if I do this?

V **VOTE**
✓ Evaluate consequences and eliminate bad choices.
✓ Which solutions have the most positive and least negative consequences?

E **EVALUATE**
✓ How did it work?
✓ Did my choice solve the problem?

SAMPLE CONTINUING RECOVERY PLAN

As part of my Continuing Recovery, I have checked the tools, activities, and skills I will practice and use to maintain sobriety and to continue to improve my relationship after weekly couples therapy ends.

1. Recovery Contract:

_X_ Trust Discussion (daily)

_X_ Take medication (_Antabuse_) during Trust Discussion

_X_ Regular support meetings

Tuesday 7 p.m. AA meeting—church

Friday 8 p.m. AA meeting—church

Saturday 9 a.m. NA meeting—treatment center

2. Positive Activities:

____ Catch and Tell

_X_ Shared Rewarding Activities (_1_ x/week)

____ Caring Day (____ x/week)

3. Communication Skills:

_X_ Communication Sessions (_1_ x/week)

____ Listening and Understanding

____ "I" Messages

_X_ Relationship Agreements (_review bills together weekly_)

____ Problem Solving

____ Time-Out

4. Continuing Recovery Tools:

_X_ Continuing Recovery Plan

_X_ Action Plan to prevent or minimize relapse

_X_ Couple checkup visits (every 2 months for 2 years)

____ Couple relapse prevention sessions (15 sessions in next year)

5. Other: _I will read from the Big Book before bed and go to gym 3x/wk._

We will focus on present and future and avoid arguments about past.

6. Partner's Role (completed by partner): _I will_

a. Practice above skills with my partner to help our relationship.

b. Take care of the kids on nights my partner goes to meetings.

c. Go to Al-Anon 1x/wk on Monday 8 p.m. at church.

SAMPLE ACTION PLAN

1. High-Risk Situations and My Plan of Action:

High Risk Situation	Action
Court date	Attend a meeting before and after court.
Pay day	Arrange for direct deposit or have my partner deposit my check.
Family wedding	Remind friends and family I can't drink or use drugs (even "just this once").

2. Warning Signs and My Plan of Action:

Warning Signs	Action
Sleeping too much	Get back on regular schedule by attending morning meetings.
Thinking one drink won't hurt	Remember that my last relapse started this way. Call my sponsor.

3. Action Plan If Use Occurs:

Goal	Action
Stay Safe →	I will try not to argue with Nancy if I am under the influence.
Act Quickly →	I will call someone within 48 hours if I drink or use.
Get Help →	I will call my AA sponsor or Sally, my BCT counselor.

4. Support Network—If I Feel an Urge or Have a Lapse, I Will Call:

Name	Phone #	Other Phone #
My sponsor	555-1234	555-2468 (cell)
Sally (my BCT counselor	555-4321	
AA local central office	853-0388	

5. Other Helpful Activities: _Go for a ride in the country._

Ride my bike or take a walk when I feel stressed out.

SAMPLE PARTNER'S ACTION PLAN

1. Warning Signs:

Partner isolates.
Partner starts losing his temper a lot.

2. Action I Will Take If I Notice Warning Signs:

Ask to go to a meeting with my partner.
Ask for a Communication Session with my partner to tell him my concerns.
Plan a Shared Rewarding Activity to reduce stress.

3. Action Plan If Use Occurs:

Goal	Action
Stay Safe →	*I will avoid getting into an argument if my partner comes home drunk. If an argument starts, I will leave the house. I can go to my sister's house until it is safe to return home. I will not confront my partner about his use while he is drunk or high.*
Act Quickly →	*I will wait no more than 48 hours to call someone if he drinks.*
Get Help →	*I will call Sally, my BCT counselor, or my Al-Anon sponsor.*

4. Support Network:

Name	Phone #	Other Phone #
My sponsor	*555-1234*	*555-2468 (cell)*
Sally (my BCT counselor)	*555-4321*	
Al-Anon	*567-8342*	

Enabling

- Spouses try many ways to cope with their partner's substance abuse. Some coping behaviors unintentionally trigger or reward substance use.

- Enabling by spouse
  - Rewards partner's drinking or drug use directly.
  - Protects partner from the consequences of his or her drinking or drug use.

- Enabling often has short-term benefit.
  - It may avoid conflict or protect family from legal or economic problems.
  - *But* enabling increases chance of future substance use.

Examples of spouse's enabling of substance-abusing partner:
- Bought alcohol or drugs for partner.
- Gave partner money to buy alcohol or drugs.
- Drank or used drugs with partner.
- Took over partner's neglected duties when partner was drinking or drugging.
- Lied or made excuses to family, friends, or others to cover for partner.
- Helped nurse partner through a hangover or helped partner to bed when drunk.
- Borrowed money to pay bills caused by partner's drinking or drug use.
- Cancelled family plans or social activities because partner was impaired.
- Paid lawyer or court fees or bailed partner out of jail due to substance use.
- Cleaned up (vomit, urine, etc.) after partner got sick.
- Asked family members to be silent about partner's drinking or drug use.
- Helped conceal partner's drinking or drug use from employers or coworkers (e.g., called in sick for partner; lied to supervisors or customers).
- Reassured partner that his or her drinking or drug use wasn't that bad.
- Lied or told a half-truth to a physician, counselor, probation officer, judge, or police officer about partner's substance drug use or about partner's participation (or nonparticipation) in treatment/recovery programs.

These examples of enabling behaviors are from "Enabling Behavior in a Clinical Sample of Alcohol Dependent Clients and Their Partners," by R. J. Rotunda, L. West, and T. J. O'Farrell, 2004, *Journal of Substance Abuse Treatment*, 26, p. 272. Copyright 2004 by Elsevier Inc. Adapted with permission.

APPENDIX C

Forms Used in BCT

RECOVERY CONTRACT

In order to help (patient) _____ with his/her recovery and to bring peace of mind to (partner) _____, we commit to the following.

Patient's Responsibilities	Partner's Responsibilities
□ DAILY TRUST DISCUSSION	
(with medication _____ if taking it)	
• States his or her intention to stay substance free that day (and takes medication if applicable).	• Records that the intention was shared (and medication taken, if applicable) on calendar.
• Thanks partner for supporting his or her recovery.	• Thanks patient for his or her recovery efforts.
□ FOCUS ON PRESENT AND FUTURE, NOT PAST	
• If necessary, requests that partner not mention past or possible future substance abuse outside of counseling sessions.	• Agrees not to mention past substance abuse or fears of future substance abuse outside of counseling sessions.
□ WEEKLY SELF-HELP MEETINGS	
• Commitment to 12-step meetings: _____ _____ _____	• Commitment to 12-step meetings: _____ _____ _____
□ URINE DRUG SCREENS	
• Urine Drug Screens: _____ _____	
□ OTHER RECOVERY SUPPORT	
• _____	• _____

EARLY WARNING SYSTEM

If, at any time, the Trust Discussion (with medication, if taking it) does not take place for 2 days in a row, we will contact (therapist/phone #: _____) immediately.

LENGTH OF CONTRACT

This agreement covers the time from today until the end of weekly therapy sessions, when it can be renewed. It cannot be changed unless all of those signing below discuss the changes together.

_____
Patient

_____
Partner

_____
Therapist

___ / ___ / ___
Date

RECOVERY CONTRACT CALENDAR

□ ✓ = Trust Discussion Done
□ ⊘ = Trust Discussion with
　　　Medication (＿＿＿＿＿)
□ A = AA or NA Meeting

□ N = Al-Anon or Nar-Anon
□ D = Drug Urine + or –
□ O = Other
　　　(＿＿＿＿＿)

Mo & Yr: ＿＿＿＿＿

S	M	T	W	T	F	S

Mo & Yr: ＿＿＿＿＿

S	M	T	W	T	F	S

CATCH YOUR PARTNER
DOING SOMETHING NICE WORKSHEET

Name: _____

Date: ___ / ___ / ___

A satisfying relationship is based on each partner giving and receiving caring behaviors. The first step in enhancing caring behaviors in a relationship is noticing them when you get them. This is the purpose of "Catch Your Partner Doing Something Nice."

Day	Date	Caring Behavior

TARGET: Each day, notice at least one nice thing that your partner does and write it on the above chart. It is ALWAYS POSSIBLE to notice at least one CARING BEHAVIOR—even if you don't see your partner for an entire day. Don't share your list with your partner!

HOME PRACTICE SESSION 1

1. RECOVERY CONTRACT

A. Choose a specific time and place to do the Trust Discussion (i.e., during breakfast, right before bed, etc.).

B. Do the daily Trust Discussion (with medication, if taking it):

Patient: "I have been drug and alcohol free for the last 24 hours and plan to remain drug and alcohol free for the next 24 hours. I want to thank you for listening and being supportive of my effort to be drug and alcohol free."
Partner: "Thank you for all your hard work. Let me know if there is anything I can do to help you."

C. Mark on the calendar each day you do the Trust Discussion, attend a self-help meeting, complete a urine drug screen, or do any other part of your Recovery Contract.

D. Review the Recovery Contract and bring it back to next session.

2. CATCH YOUR PARTNER DOING SOMETHING NICE

In any relationship, each partner's needs are met *negatively* by punishment, threats, annoyances, and arguments, or *positively* by the mutual giving and receiving of CARING BEHAVIORS. One of the major ideas behind BCT is that a satisfying relationship is based on each partner giving and receiving caring behaviors. We think partners can each *say* and *do* certain things that will bring them greater happiness in their relationship.

This *first step* in learning to give and receive caring behaviors is to *notice* them when they occur . . . instead of taking your partner for granted. This is the purpose of Catch Your Partner Doing Something Nice.

Assignment: Each day notice one nice thing your partner did and write it on the *Catch Your Partner Worksheet*. But do not tell each other what you wrote down. Bring this sheet to the next session.

CATCH YOUR PARTNER DOING SOMETHING NICE
AND TELL HIM OR HER
(CATCH AND TELL)

Name: _____   Date: ___ / ___ / ___

A satisfying relationship is based on each person giving and receiving caring behaviors. The first step in building caring behaviors in a relationship is noticing them when you get them. The second step is to TELL your partner how you felt when he or she did something nice. This is the purpose of the Catch and Tell homework.

Day	Date	Caring Behavior	Tell*

TARGET: Each day, notice one nice thing your partner did and write it on the above chart. Then TELL your partner you liked what they did and how it made you feel.

*Check (✓) under "TELL" if you told your partner you liked the behavior you wrote down today.

HOME PRACTICE SESSION 2

1. RECOVERY CONTRACT

A. Do Trust Discussion (with medication, if taking it) every day at specified time.

B. Do self-help and other parts of contract.

C. Mark on calendar when Trust Discussion and other parts of contract are completed.

2. CATCH YOUR PARTNER DOING SOMETHING NICE AND TELL HIM OR HER

Last week you learned to recognize when your partner is doing something CARING for you. If you want your partner to continue doing those CARING things, you have to acknowledge or reward him or her. This homework is designed to give you practice in both *recognizing* and *acknowledging* your partner for the CARING BEHAVIORS he or she gives you.

With a small word, gesture, or token of appreciation you can make your partner feel very good and want to do even more for you. Or you can take your partner for granted. It's your choice!

ACKNOWLEDGING CARING BEHAVIORS

What You Say	*How You Say It*
"I like it when you . . . "	Look at the other person.
"It made me feel . . . "	Use pleasant tone of voice
(Leave out the negative)	Smile. Be sincere.

Catch and Tell assignment: Notice and acknowledge one nice thing your partner does each day and write it on the *Catch and Tell Worksheet.* Bring this sheet to the next session.

HOME PRACTICE SESSION 6

1. RECOVERY CONTRACT

Continue to do all parts of the Recovery Contract and mark on calendar when they are completed.

2. POSITIVE ACTIVITIES—pick at least one of the following to do:

☐ **Catch and Tell:** Acknowledge one nice thing your partner does each day; consider adding this as a "daily compliment" to the end of your Trust Discussion.

☐ **Shared Rewarding Activity:** Do planned activity together; plan one for following week.

☐ **Caring Day:** Surprise your partner with a Caring Day on which you plan ahead to do some special things to show you care.

3. COMMUNICATION SESSION (*to Practice Listening with Understanding*)

In a Communication Session you plan ahead to talk privately, face-to-face, without distractions, each giving the other full attention. This week use your Communication Sessions to practice listening and showing your partner that you truly understand his or her point of view.

1. Have three Communication Sessions of 5 to 15 minutes this week. Below write the time you plan to have the session and make a checkmark once you've had the session
2. Start by acknowledging the Caring Behavior you noticed that day, then continue talking about everyday problems and events but not charged issues.
3. **Speaker:** Starts statements with "I" Messages, owns up to his or her feelings, doesn't accuse the other person, and speaks only for him- or herself.
4. **Listener:** Restates the Message Received to see if he or she understood correctly ("**What I heard you say was. . . . Did I get that?**"), then he or she becomes the speaker.

	Planned time	Check (✓) after session completed
MONDAY	_____	_____
TUESDAY	_____	_____
WEDNESDAY	_____	_____
THURSDAY	_____	_____
FRIDAY	_____	_____
SATURDAY	_____	_____
SUNDAY	_____	_____

POSITIVE SPECIFIC REQUEST LIST

It is not unusual for couples to talk about what is wrong and what they are **not** getting from a relationship. However, we are often vague and unclear when it comes to talking about what we **do** want. "Positive specific requests" is a technique that helps us effectively express our wants and desires to our partner.

Positive—say what you want, not what you don't want.
Specific—what, where, and when.
Requests—not demands, which use force or threats, but requests, which have the possibility for negotiation and compromise.

Make a list of Positive Specific Requests. Requests might include things that would make you happier in your relationship and would make your life easier. Some areas to consider are communication, childrearing, money, leisure time and social activities, household responsibilities, sex, job, and independence.

_____

_____

_____

_____

_____

_____

_____

_____

_____

_____

_____

_____

_____

_____

_____

_____

_____

_____

_____

_____

_____

_____

NEGOTIATED AGREEMENT

During the session you negotiated one agreement to fulfill during the week. For this agreement, each of you *volunteered* to fulfill one of your partner's requests, either in full or in part. Remember, this is voluntary on your part, out of the "goodness of your heart." This agreement is not a matter of "I'll do mine only if you do your part" but instead reflects two people each doing something to help the other of their own free will.

_____(name) agreed to [be specific: what, when, how many times]: _____

_____

_____(name) agreed to: _____

_____

Did each of you follow through with your agreement? (describe): _____

_____

Home Practice: During your Communication Session this week, *negotiate another agreement at home.* If possible, pick an item off your partner's list of requests that you would be willing to fulfill in full or part. Remember to use the Listening and Understanding techniques ("What I heard you say was. . . . Did I get that?"). Write what you agreed to below.

_____(name) agreed to [be specific: what, when, how many times]: _____

_____

_____(name) agreed to: _____

_____

Did each of you follow through with your agreement? [describe]: _____

_____

HOME PRACTICE SESSION 7

1. RECOVERY CONTRACT

Continue to do all parts of the Recovery Contract and mark on calendar when they are completed.

2. POSITIVE ACTIVITIES—pick at least one of the following to do:

☐ **Catch and Tell:** Acknowledge one nice thing your partner does each day; consider adding this as a "daily compliment" to the end of your Trust Discussion.

☐ **Shared Rewarding Activity:** Do planned activity together; plan one for following week.

☐ **Caring Day:** Surprise your partner with a Caring Day on which you plan ahead to do some special things to show you care.

3. COMMUNICATION SESSION (to Practice Listening with Understanding)

In a Communication Session you plan ahead to talk privately, face-to-face, without distractions, each giving the other full attention. This week use your Communication Sessions to practice listening and showing your partner that you truly understand his or her point of view.

1. Have three Communication Sessions of 5 to 15 minutes this week. Below write the time you plan to have the session and make a checkmark once you've had the session.
2. Start by acknowledging the Caring Behavior you noticed that day, then continue talking about everyday problems and events including charged issues.
3. **Speaker:** Starts statements with "I" Messages, owns up to his or her feelings, doesn't accuse the other person, and speaks only for him- or herself.
4. **Listener:** Restates the Message Received to see if he or she understood correctly ("**What I heard you say was. . . . Did I get that?**"), then he or she becomes the speaker.

Planned time   Check (✓) after session completed

_____   _____

_____   _____

_____   _____

_____   _____

4. RELATIONSHIP AGREEMENTS

- Each of you should do the agreement you made in session during the upcoming week.
- Use one of your Communication Sessions to negotiate another agreement and write it down on the *Negotiated Agreements* sheet.
- Add to your list of *Positive Specific Requests*, but do not share the list with your partner.

GUIDELINES FOR MANAGING CONFLICT

- Keep discussions respectful, even when feeling frustrated or hurt. Avoid using put-downs, name calling, or swearing . . . also known as verbal aggression.

- Maintain emotional control, even when feeling angry. Control emotions to avoid yelling. Take a **Time-Out** if you cannot control your emotions.

- Keep interactions on "hot topics" within a structured process. Make **Positive Specific Requests** for such issues. Using a planned negotiation, mediation, or other formalized process. **Negotiation and Compromise** help focus and balance communication.

- Show a willingness to understand. Use **Listening and Understanding** to help your partner feel understood and acknowledged.

- Communicate honestly and openly, using **"I" Messages**. Holding back will only delay or complicate the resolution process.

- Be as objective as possible; avoid speculation, rumors, and assumptions.

- Express concerns in a constructive manner. Again, use **Positive Specific Requests**, because these are typically better received than demanding changes.

- Focus on future solutions rather than past blame. Keep in mind the **Promises** that you made at the beginning of couples counseling.

- Look for solutions that meet both people's needs.

HOME PRACTICE SESSION 8

1. RECOVERY CONTRACT

Continue to do all parts of the Recovery Contract and mark on calendar when they are completed.

2. POSITIVE ACTIVITIES—pick at least one of the following to do:

☐ **Catch and Tell:** Acknowledge one nice thing your partner does each day; consider adding this as a "daily compliment" to the end of your Trust Discussion.

☐ **Shared Rewarding Activity:** Do planned activity together; plan one for following week.

☐ **Caring Day:** Surprise your partner with a Caring Day on which you plan ahead to do some special things to show you care.

3. COMMUNICATION SESSION

In a Communication Session you plan ahead to talk privately, face-to-face, without distractions, each giving the other full attention. Use the following guidelines.

1. Start by acknowledging the Caring Behavior you noticed that day. At the bottom write the time you plan to have the session and make a checkmark once you've had the session.
2. **Speaker:** Starts statements with "I" Messages, owns up to his or her feelings, doesn't accuse the other person, and speaks only for him- or herself.
3. **Listener:** Restates the Message Received to see if he or she understood correctly (**"What I heard you say was. . . . Did I get that?"**), then he or she becomes the Speaker.
4. **Have three Communication Sessions of at least 10–15 minutes this week to practice each of the following:**

   ☐ **Listening with Understanding**—on everyday problems, *including charged issues.*

   ☐ **Relationship Agreements**—do agreement made in session and negotiate another.

   ☐ **Conflict Resolution**—use a *Time-Out* in a real situation or in a practice situation.

Planned time	Check (✓) after session completed
_____	_____
_____	_____
_____	_____
_____	_____

PROBLEM-SOLVING EXAMPLE

S: Stop, Slow Down, and See the Problem

- Is there a problem?
- What exactly is the problem?

  Husband left OJ out 3 days in a row. Wife wanted some for breakfast, but she likes it cold,
  and now it is warm

O: Outline Options

- Brainstorm: What can I do?
- What might work?

  1. Put ice in the glass and not tell husband that you were upset.
  2. Ask husband to put the OJ away from now on.

L: Look at Consequences

- What are the positive and negative consequences in the short run and long term?
- What will happen if I do each of the options?

  1. Husband will keep leaving OJ out. Wife may get too angry, end up yelling.
  2. Husband would know wife likes the OJ cold. He can change his behavior.

V: Vote

- Evaluate consequences and eliminate bad choices.
- Which solutions have the most positive and least negative consequences?

  The second option seems better because it would bring positive results and display effective
  communication.

E: Evaluate

- How did it work?
- Did my choice solve the problem?

  Husband now puts OJ away so wife feels satisfied. Also, wife is proud she used effective communication
  by letting husband know how she was feeling.

PROBLEM-SOLVING PRACTICE

S: Stop, Slow Down, and See the Problem

- Is there a problem?
- What exactly is the problem?

_____

_____

_____

O: Outline Options

- Brainstorm: What can I do?
- What might work?

_____

_____

_____

L: Look at Consequences

- What are the positive and negative consequences in the short run and long term?
- What will happen if I do each of the options?

_____

_____

_____

V: Vote

- Evaluate consequences and eliminate bad choices.
- Which solutions have the most positive and least negative consequences?

_____

_____

_____

E: Evaluate

- How did it work?
- Did my choice solve the problem?

_____

_____

_____

HOME PRACTICE SESSION 9

1. RECOVERY CONTRACT

Continue to do all parts of the Recovery Contract and mark on calendar when they are completed.

2. POSITIVE ACTIVITIES—pick at least one of the following to do:

☐ **Catch and Tell:** Acknowledge one nice thing your partner does each day; consider adding this as a "daily compliment" to the end of your Trust Discussion.

☐ **Shared Rewarding Activity:** Do planned activity together; plan one for following week.

☐ **Caring Day:** Surprise your partner with a Caring Day on which you plan ahead to do some special things to show you care.

3. COMMUNICATION SESSION

In a Communication Session you plan ahead to talk privately, face-to-face, without distractions, each giving the other full attention. Use the following guidelines.

1. Start by acknowledging the Caring Behavior you noticed that day. At the bottom write the time you plan to have the session and make a checkmark once you've had the session.
2. **Speaker:** Starts statements with "I" Messages, owns up to his or her feelings, doesn't accuse the other person, and speaks only for him- or herself.
3. **Listener:** Restates the message received to see if he or she understood correctly ("**What I heard you say was. . . . Did I get that?**"), then he or she becomes the speaker.
4. **Have three Communication Sessions of at least 10–15 minutes this week to practice Problem Solving plus at least one other of the following:**

   ☐ **Problem Solving**—use S.O.L.V.E. method for 30 minutes on problem chosen in session.

   ☐ **Listening with Understanding**—on everyday problems, *including charged issues.*

   ☐ **Relationship Agreements**—do agreement made in session and negotiate another.

   ☐ **Conflict Resolution**—use a *Time-Out* in a real situation or in a practice situation.

Planned time	Check (✓) after session completed
_____	_____
_____	_____
_____	_____
_____	_____

CONTINUING RECOVERY HELPFUL HINTS

☞ Continuing recovery is a process. It can change. You can change. You can add ideas as you learn and grow.

☞ You are in a different place now. You bring with you new skills and experiences to deal with high-risk situations.

☞ Reach out and call someone from your support network. Plan to deal with any effects of the lapse.

☞ Remember to do your regular daily inventory to check for high-risk factors.

☞ Be alert for high-risk factors and plan to take action to reverse the effects.

☞ Make a commitment to be active in your recovery.

☞ A lapse or relapse tells you that there is a hole in your Continuing Recovery Plan. Go back and check it out. Add to it. Make it more specific.

☞ A lapse can be part of the learning process. Learn more about your high-risk factors. Decide what coping skills you will use next time to cope without using.

☞ When you can, avoid a particular high-risk factor, and if not, use one of your coping strategies.

☞ Don't just plan—act. Do it. Try it.

☞ Your confidence will increase when you successfully cope with high-risk situations.

MY CONTINUING RECOVERY PLAN

As part of my Continuing Recovery, I have checked the tools, activities, and skills I will practice and use to maintain sobriety and to continue to improve my relationship after weekly couples therapy ends.

1. Recovery Contract:

_____ Trust Discussion (daily)

_____ Take medication (_____) during Trust Discussion

_____ Regular support meetings

_____

_____

_____

2. Positive Activities:

_____ Catch and Tell

_____ Shared Rewarding Activities (____ x/week)

_____ Caring Day (____ x/week)

3. Communication Skills:

_____ Communication Sessions (____ x/week)

_____ Listening and Understanding

_____ "I" Messages

_____ Relationship Agreements (specify: _____)

_____ Problem Solving

_____ Time-Out

4. Continuing Recovery Tools:

_____ Continuing Recovery Plan

_____ Action Plan to prevent or minimize relapse

_____ Couple checkup visits (every 2 months for 2 years)

_____ Couple relapse prevention sessions (15 sessions in next year)

5. Other: _____

_____

6. Partner's role (completed by partner): _____

_____

_____

_____

HOME PRACTICE SESSION 10

1. RECOVERY CONTRACT

Continue to do all parts of the Recovery Contract and mark on calendar when they are completed.

2. POSITIVE ACTIVITIES—pick at least one of the following to do:

☐ **Catch and Tell:** Acknowledge one nice thing your partner does each day; consider adding this as a "daily compliment" to the end of your Trust Discussion.

☐ **Shared Rewarding Activity**: Do planned activity together; plan one for following week.

☐ **Caring Day**: Surprise your partner with a Caring Day on which you plan ahead to do some special things to show you care.

3. COMMUNICATION SESSION

In a Communication Session you plan ahead to talk privately, face-to-face, without distractions, each giving the other full attention. Use the following guidelines.

1. Start by acknowledging the Caring Behavior you noticed that day. At the bottom write the time you plan to have the session and make a checkmark once you've had the session.
2. **Speaker:** Starts statements with "I" Messages, owns up to his or her feelings, doesn't accuse the other person, and speaks only for him- or herself.
3. **Listener:** Restates the Message Received to see if he or she understood correctly ("**What I heard you say was. . . . Did I get that?**"), then he or she becomes the speaker.
4. **Have three Communication Sessions of at least 10–15 minutes this week to discuss your Continuing Recovery Plan plus at least one other of the following:**

   ☐ <u>Continuing Recovery Plan</u>—discuss together, make desired changes, try to finalize.

   ☐ **Problem Solving**—use S.O.L.V.E. method for 30 minutes on problem chosen in session.

   ☐ **Listening with Understanding**—on everyday problems, *including charged issues*.

   ☐ **Relationship Agreements**—do agreement made in session and negotiate another.

   ☐ **Conflict Resolution**—use a *Time-Out* in a real situation or in a practice situation.

Planned time	Check (✓) after session completed
_____	_____
_____	_____
_____	_____
_____	_____

MY ACTION PLAN

1. High-Risk Situations and My Plan of Action:

High-Risk Situation	Action

2. Warning Signs and My Plan of Action:

Warning Signs	Action

3. Action Plan If Use Occurs:

Goal	Action
Stay Safe →	
Act Quickly →	
Get Help →	

4. Support Network—If I Feel an Urge or Have a Lapse, I Will Call:

Name	Phone #	Other Phone #

5. Other Helpful Activities: _____

_____

_____

PARTNER'S ACTION PLAN

1. Warning Signs:

2. Action I Will Take If I Notice Warning Signs:

3. Action Plan If Use Occurs:

Goal	Action
Stay Safe →	
Act Quickly →	
Get Help →	

4. Support Network:

Name	Phone #	Other Phone #

HOME PRACTICE SESSION 11

1. RECOVERY CONTRACT

Continue to do all parts of the Recovery Contract and mark on calendar when they are completed.

2. POSITIVE ACTIVITIES—pick at least one of the following to do:

☐ **Catch and Tell**: Acknowledge one nice thing your partner does each day; consider adding this as a "daily compliment" to the end of your Trust Discussion.

☐ **Shared Rewarding Activity**: Do planned activity together; plan one for following week.

☐ **Caring Day**: Surprise your partner with a Caring Day on which you plan ahead to do some special things to show you care.

3. COMMUNICATION SESSION

In a Communication Session you plan ahead to talk privately, face-to-face, without distractions, each giving the other full attention. Use the following guidelines.

1. Start by acknowledging the Caring Behavior you noticed that day. At the bottom write the time you plan to have the session and make a checkmark once you've had the session.
2. **Speaker:** Starts statements with "I" Messages, owns up to his or her feelings, doesn't accuse the other person, and speaks only for him- or herself.
3. **Listener:** Restates the Message Received to see if he or she understood correctly ("**What I heard you say was. . . . Did I get that?**"), then he or she becomes the speaker.
4. **Have three Communication Sessions of at least 10–15 minutes this week to discuss:**

☐ *Action Plan*—discuss together, make desired changes, try to finalize.

☐ *Continuing Recovery Plan*—discuss checkup visits (every few months) or relapse prevention sessions (15 spread over next year).

☐ Bring *Action Plan* and *Continuing Recovery Plan* to next session to finalize.

Planned time	Check (✓) after session completed
_____	_____
_____	_____
_____	_____
_____	_____

DUAL RECOVERY CONTRACT

In order to help with their recoveries _____ and _____ agree to the following.

_____'s Responsibilities	_____'s Responsibilities
□ DAILY TRUST DISCUSSION	
• States intention to stay substance free that day (takes medication _____, if applicable). • Thanks partner for recovery efforts and support. • Records these actions on calendar.	• States intention to stay substance free that day (takes medication _____, if applicable). • Thanks partner for recovery efforts and support. • Records these actions on calendar.
□ FOCUS ON PRESENT AND FUTURE, NOT PAST	
• Agrees not to mention partner's past substance abuse or fear about future use outside of counseling session.	• Agrees not to mention partner's past substance abuse or fear about future use outside of counseling session.
□ WEEKLY SELF-HELP MEETINGS	
• Commitment to 12-step meetings: _____ _____ _____	• Commitment to 12-step meetings: _____ _____ _____
□ URINE DRUG SCREENS	
• Urine drug screens: _____ _____	• Urine drug screens: _____ _____
□ OTHER RECOVERY SUPPORT	
• _____	• _____

EARLY WARNING SYSTEM
If, at any time, the Trust Discussion (with medication, if taking it) does not take place for 2 days in a row, we will contact (therapist/phone #: _____) immediately.

LENGTH OF CONTRACT
This agreement covers the time from today until the end of weekly therapy sessions, when it can be renewed. It cannot be changed unless all of those signing below discuss the changes together.

_____   _____

_____   ___ / ___ / ___
                Therapist   Date

414

DUAL RECOVERY CONTRACT CALENDAR

☐ ✔ = Trust Discussion Done
☐ ⊘ = Trust Discussion with
       Medication ( )
☐ A = AA or NA Meeting

☐ N = Al-Anon or Nar-Anon
☐ D = Drug Urine + or –
☐ O = Other ( )

_____'s Calendar

Mo & Yr: _____

S	M	T	W	T	F	S

_____'s Calendar

Mo & Yr: _____

S	M	T	W	T	F	S

THOUGHTS OF HAVING A DRINK OR DRUG
(IF NONE, WRITE "NONE")

Time & Day	Situation (where, with whom, doing what, your mood)	How Strong (1–10)

RECOVERY CONTRACT PREPARATION

1. Write down any positive reasons for the two of you to be involved in a Recovery Contract together.

Patient	Partner

2. Write down any questions or concerns you have about the contract:

Patient	Partner

3. Discuss the following together and write your decisions in the space provided:

   a. Best time of day to do the daily Trust Discussion

   _____

   _____

   b. Best place to keep the calendar (hint—near where you will do the Trust Discussion so that you won't forget to mark it)

   _____

   _____

   c. Situations likely to interrupt the daily Trust Discussion (such as times apart, being angry)

   _____

   _____

APPENDIX D

Suggested Resources

REFERENCES

The following texts provide supplemental information that you might find helpful. Although some focus on treating a specific substance such as cocaine or alcohol, each text is widely applicable to most abused substances.

Daley, D. C., Mercer, D., & Carpenter, G. (2002). *Group drug counseling for cocaine dependence: The Collaborative Cocaine Treatment Study Model* (NIDA Therapy Manuals for Drug Addiction, Manual 4). Rockville, MD: National Institute on Drug Abuse.

Mercer, D., & Woody, G. (1999). *An individual drug counseling approach to treat cocaine addiction: The Collaborative Cocaine Treatment Study* Model (NIDA Therapy Manuals for Drug Abuse, Manual 3, NIH Publication No. 99-4380). Rockville, MD: National Institute on Drug Abuse.

Meyers, R. J., & Wolfe, B. L. (2004). *Get your loved one sober: Alternatives to nagging, pleading, and threatening.* Center City, MN: Hazelden.

Monti, P. M., Kadden, R. M., Rohsenow, D. J., Cooney, N. L., & Abrams, D. B. (2002). *Treating alcohol dependence: A coping skills training guide* (2nd ed.). New York: Guilford Press.

Nowinski, J. K. (1999). *Family recovery and substance abuse: A twelve-step guide for treatment.* Thousand Oaks, CA: Sage.

O'Farrell, T. J. (Ed.). (1993). *Treating alcohol problems: Marital and family interventions.* New York: Guilford Press.

Smith, J. E., & Meyers, R. J. (2004). *Motivating substance abusers to enter treatment: Working with family members.* New York: Guilford Press.

INFORMATION ON TRAINING

Timothy J. O'Farrell, PhD
Families and Addiction Program
Harvard Medical School Department of Psychiatry
  at the VA Boston Healthcare System
940 Belmont St. (VAMC-116B1)
Brockton, MA 02301
Phone: (508) 583-4500 ext. 63493
Email: timothy_ofarrell@hms.harvard.edu

William Fals-Stewart, PhD
RTI International
3040 Cornwallis Road, Hobbs Building
P.O. Box 12194
Research Triangle Park, NC 27709-2194
Phone: (919) 990-8460
Email: wstewart@rti.org

For a listing of planned BCT training events and other BCT materials,
visit www.addictionandfamily.org

For a Web-based distance learning course on BCT for alcoholism and drug abuse,
visit www.neattc.org/training.htm

References

Al-Anon Family Groups. (1981). *This is Al-Anon*. New York: Author.

Alberti, R. E., & Emmons, M. L. (2001). *Your perfect right: Assertiveness and equality in your life and relationships* (8th ed.). Atascadero, CA: Impact.

American Psychological Association. (1992). Ethical principles of psychologists and code of conduct. *American Psychologist, 47*, 1597–1611.

Azrin, N. H. (1976). Improvements in the community-reinforcement approach to alcoholism. *Behaviour Research and Therapy, 14*, 330–348.

Azrin, N. H., Sisson, R. W., Meyers, R., & Godley, M. (1982). Alcoholism treatment by disulfiram and community reinforcement therapy. *Journal of Behavior Therapy and Experimental Psychiatry, 13*, 105–112.

Birchler, G. R., & Fals-Stewart, W. (1994). The Response to Conflict Scale: Psychometric properties. *Assessment, 1*, 335–344.

Birchler, G. R., & Fals-Stewart, W. (2001, November). *Use of behavioral couples therapy with alcoholic couples: Effects on maladaptive responses to conflict during treatment*. Poster presented at the annual meeting of the Association for Advancement of Behavior Therapy, Philadelphia.

Birchler, G. R., & Fals-Stewart, W. (2003). Does reduced conflict during treatment mediate the effect of BCT on partner violence after treatment among male alcoholics? In T. J. O'Farrell (Chair), *Behavioral couples therapy for alcoholism and drug abuse: Recent advances*. Symposium conducted at the annual meeting of the Association for the Advancement of Behavior Therapy, Boston.

Blumstein, P., & Schwartz, P. (1983). *American couples: Money, work, and sex*. New York: Morrow.

Bowen, M. (1985). *Family therapy in clinical practice*. Northvale, NJ: Jason Aronson.

Bowers, T. G., & Al-Redha, M. R. (1990). A comparison of outcome with group/marital and standard/individual therapies with alcoholics. *Journal of Studies on Alcohol, 51*, 301–309.

Brown, E. D., O'Farrell, T. J., Maisto, S. A., Boies, K., & Suchinsky, R. (Eds.). (1997). *Accreditation guide for substance abuse treatment programs*. Newbury Park, CA: Sage.

Burke, B. L., Arkowitz, H., & Dunn, C. (2002). The efficacy of motivational interviewing and its adaptations: What we know so far. In W. R. Miller & S. Rollnick, *Motivational interviewing: Preparing people for change* (2nd ed., pp. 217–250). New York: Guilford Press.

Busby, D. M., Crane, D. R., Larson, J. H., & Christensen, C. (1995). A revision of the Dyadic Adjustment Scale for use with distressed and nondistressed couples: Construct hierarchy and multidimensional scales. *Journal of Marital and Family Therapy, 21*, 289–308.

Carise, D., McLellan, A. T., Gifford, L. S., & Kleber, H. D. (1999). Developing a national addiction treatment information system: An introduction to the drug evaluation network system. *Journal of Substance Abuse Treatment, 17*, 67–77.

Carpenter, L. M., Mayer, K. H., Stein, M. D., Leibman, B. D., Fisher, A., & Fiore, T. (1991). Human immunodeficiency virus infection in North American women: Experience with 200 cases and a review of the literature. *Medicine, 70*, 307–325.

Carroll, K. M., Fenton, L. R., Ball, S. A., Nich, C., Frankforter, T. L., Shi, J., et al. (2004). Efficacy of disulfiram and cognitive behavior therapy in cocaine-dependent outpatients. *Archives of General Psychiatry, 61*, 264–272.

Carroll, K. M., Nich, C., Ball, S., McCance, E., Frankforter, T. L., & Rounsaville, B. J. (2000).

One-year follow-up of disulfiram and psychotherapy for cocaine-alcohol users: Sustained effects of treatment. *Addiction, 95,* 1335–1349.

Cascardi, M., Langhinrichsen, J., & Vivian, D. (1992). Marital aggression: Impact, injury, and health correlates for husbands and wives. *Archives of Internal Medicine, 152,* 1178–1184.

Catalano, R. F., Gainey, R. R., & Fleming, C. B. (1999). An experimental intervention with families of substance abusers: One-year follow-up of the focus on families project. *Addiction, 94*(2), 241–254.

Catania, J. A., Coates, T. J., Stall R., Turner, H. A., Peterson, J., Hearst, N., et al. (1992). Prevalence of AIDS-related risk factors and condom use in the United States. *Science, 258,* 1101–1106.

Centers for Disease Control and Prevention. (1999). *HIV/AIDS surveillance report.* Atlanta, GA: Author.

Centers for Disease Control and Prevention. (2002). *HIV/AIDS surveillance report.* Atlanta, GA: Author.

Chamberlain, P., Reid, J. B., Ray, J., Capaldi, D. M., & Fisher, P. (1997). Parent inadequate discipline (PID). In T. A. Widiger, A. J. Frances, H. A. Pincus, R. Ross, M. B. First, & W. Davis (Eds.), *DSM-IV sourcebook* (Vol. 3, pp. 569–629). Washington, DC: American Psychiatric Association.

Chase, K., O'Farrell, T. J., Murphy, C. M., Fals-Stewart, W., & Murphy, M. (2003). Factors associated with partner violence among female alcoholic patients and their male partners. *Journal of Studies on Alcohol, 64,* 137–149.

Chick, J., Anton, R., Checinski, K., Crop, R., Drummond, D. C., Farmer, R., et al. (2000). A multicentre, randomized, double-blind, placebo-controlled trial of naltrexone in the treatment of alcohol dependence or abuse. *Journal of Alcohol and Alcoholism, 35,* 587–593.

Chick, J., Gough, K., Falkowski, W., Kershaw, P., Hore, B., Mehta, B., et al. (1992). Disulfiram treatment of alcoholism. *British Journal of Psychiatry, 161,* 84–89.

Choi, K., Catania, J. A., & Dolcini, M. M. (1994). Extramarital sex and HIV risk behavior among U.S. adults: Results from the National AIDS Behavior Survey. *American Journal of Public Health, 84,* 2003–2007.

Clark, H. W. (2003). Office-based practice and opioid-use disorders. *New England Journal of Medicine, 39*(10), 928–930.

Cooke, C. G., Kelley, M. L., Fals-Stewart, W., & Golden, J. (2004). An examination of the psychosocial functioning of children with drug- or alcohol-abusing fathers. *American Journal of Drug and Alcohol Abuse, 130,* 695–710.

Cordova, J. V., Warren, L. Z., & Gee, C. B. (2001). Motivational interviewing with couples: An intervention for at-risk couples. *Journal of Marital and Family Therapy, 27,* 315–326.

Crits-Christoph, P., Siqueland, L., Blaine, J., Frank, A., Luborsky, L., Onken, L. S., et al. (1999). Psychosocial treatments for cocaine dependence: Results of the National Institute on Drug Abuse Collaborative Cocaine Treatment Study. *Archives of General Psychiatry, 56,* 493–502.

Daley, D. C., & Marlatt, G. A. (1997). *Therapist's guide for managing your alcohol or drug problem.* San Antonio, TX: Psychological Corporation.

Daley, D. C., Mercer, D., & Carpenter, G. (2002). *Group drug counseling for cocaine dependence: The Collaborative Cocaine Treatment Study model* (NIDA Therapy Manuals for Drug Addiction, Manual 4). Rockville, MD: National Institute on Drug Abuse.

Dittrich, J. E. (1993). A group program for wives of treatment-resistant alcoholics. In T. J. O'Farrell (Ed.), *Treating alcohol problems: Marital and family interventions* (pp. 78–114). New York: Guilford Press.

el-Guebaly, N., Richard, R., Currie, S., & Hudson, V. (2004, November). *Behavioral couple therapy (BCT) individual and group interventions.* Paper presented at the World Psychiatric Association International Congress, Madrid, Spain.

Epstein, E. E., & McCrady, B. S. (1998). Behavioral couples treatment of alcohol and drug use disorders: Current status and innovations. *Clinical Psychology Review, 18,* 689–711.

Fals-Stewart, W. (2004, April). *Substance abuse and domestic violence: Many issues, some answers.* Invited address presented at the conference on Substance Abuse and Antisocial Behavior Across the Lifespan: Research Findings and Clinical Implications, Toronto.

Fals-Stewart, W., & Birchler, G. R. (1998). Marital interactions of drug-abusing patients and their partners: Comparisons to distressed couples and relationship to drug-using behavior. *Psychology of Addictive Behaviors, 12,* 28–38.

Fals-Stewart, W., & Birchler, G. R. (2001). A national survey of the use of couples therapy in substance abuse treatment. *Journal of Substance Abuse Treatment, 20,* 277–283.

Fals-Stewart, W., & Birchler, G. R. (2002). Behavioral couples therapy for alcoholic men and their intimate partners: The comparative effectiveness of master's- and bachelor's-level counselors. *Behavior Therapy, 33,* 123–147.

Fals-Stewart, W., Birchler, G. R., & Ellis, L. (1999). Procedures for evaluating the dyadic adjustment of drug-abusing patients and their intimate partners: A multimethod assessment approach. *Journal of Substance Abuse Treatment, 16,* 5–16.

Fals-Stewart, W., Birchler, G. R., Hoebbel, C., Kashdan, T. B., Golden, J., & Parks, K. (2003). An examination of indirect risk of exposure to HIV among wives of substance-abusing men. *Drug and Alcohol Dependence, 70,* 65–76.

Fals-Stewart, W., Birchler, G. R., & Kelley, M. (in press). Learning sobriety together: A randomized clinical trial examining behavioral couples therapy with female alcoholic patients. *Journal of Consulting and Clinical Psychology*.

Fals-Stewart, W., Birchler, G. R., & O'Farrell, T. J. (1996). Behavioral couples therapy for male substance-abusing patients: Effects on relationship adjustment and drug-using behavior. *Journal of Consulting and Clinical Psychology*, *64*, 959–972.

Fals-Stewart, W., Birchler, G. R., & O'Farrell, T. J. (1999). Drug abusing patients and their partners: Dyadic adjustment, relationship stability, and substance use. *Journal of Abnormal Psychology*, *108*, 11–23.

Fals-Stewart, W., Kashdan, T. B., O'Farrell, T. J., & Birchler, G. R. (2002). Behavioral couples therapy for drug abusing patients: Effects on partner violence. *Journal of Substance Abuse Treatment*, *22*, 87–96.

Fals-Stewart, W., Kelley, M. L., Cooke, C. G., & Golden, J. C. (2003). Predictors of the psychosocial adjustment of children living in households of parents in which fathers abuse drugs: The effects of postnatal parental exposure. *Addictive Behaviors*, *28*(6), 1013–1031.

Fals-Stewart, W., Kelley, M. L., Fincham, F., & Golden, J. (2004). Substance-abusing parents' attitudes toward allowing their custodial children to participate in treatment: A comparison of mothers versus fathers. *Journal of Family Psychology*, *18*, 666–671.

Fals-Stewart, W., Kelley, M. L., Fincham, F. D., Golden, J., & Logsdon, T. (2004). Emotional and behavioral problems of children living with drug-abusing fathers: Comparisons with children living with alcohol-abusing and non-substance-abusing fathers. *Journal of Family Psychology*, *18*, 319–330.

Fals-Stewart, W., & Kennedy, C. (2005). Addressing intimate partner violence in substance-abuse treatment. *Journal of Substance Abuse Treatment*, *29*, 5–17.

Fals-Stewart, W., Klosterman, K., Yates, B. T., O'Farrell, T. J., & Birchler, G. R. (2005). Brief relationship therapy for alcoholism: A randomized clinical trial examining clinical efficacy and cost-effectiveness. *Psychology of Addictive Behaviors*, *19*(4), 363–371.

Fals-Stewart, W., Logsdon, T., & Birchler, G. R. (2004). Dissemination of empirically supported treatments for substance abuse: An organization autopsy of technology transfer success and failure. *Clinical Psychology: Science and Practice*, *11*, 177–182.

Fals-Stewart, W., & O'Farrell, T. J. (2002). *Behavioral couples therapy increases compliance with naltrexone among male alcoholic patients*. Unpublished data, Research Institute on Addiction, Buffalo, NY.

Fals-Stewart, W., & O'Farrell, T. J. (2003). Behavioral family counseling and naltrexone for male opioid dependent patients. *Journal of Consulting and Clinical Psychology*, *71*, 432–442.

Fals-Stewart, W., O'Farrell, T. J., & Birchler, G. R. (1995). *Domestic violence among drug abusing couples*. Poster presented at the annual convention of the Association for Advancement of Behavior Therapy, Washington, DC.

Fals-Stewart, W., O'Farrell, T. J., & Birchler, G. R. (1997). Behavioral couples therapy for male substance abusing patients: A cost outcomes analysis. *Journal of Consulting and Clinical Psychology*, *65*, 789–802.

Fals-Stewart, W., O'Farrell, T. J., & Birchler, G. R. (2001a). Behavioral couples therapy for male methadone maintenance patients: Effects on drug-using behavior and relationship adjustment. *Behavior Therapy*, *32*, 391–411.

Fals-Stewart, W., O'Farrell, T. J., & Birchler, G. R. (2001b). Use of abbreviated couples therapy in substance abuse. In J. V. Cordova (Chair), *Approaches to brief couples therapy: Application and efficiency*. Symposium conducted at the World Congress of Behavioral and Cognitive Therapies, Vancouver, British Columbia.

Fals-Stewart, W., O'Farrell, T. J., & Birchler, G. R. (2003a). Behavioral couples therapy for drug-abusing couples: Effects on HIV-risk. In T. J. O'Farrell (Chair), *Behavioral couples therapy for alcoholism and drug abuse: Recent advances*. Symposium conducted at the annual meeting of the Association for Advancement of Behavior Therapy, Boston.

Fals-Stewart, W., O'Farrell, T. J., & Birchler, G. R. (2003b). Couples therapy for substance use disorders. In M. A. Whisman & D. K. Snyder (Chairs), *Couple therapy for mental and physical health problems*. Symposium conducted at the annual meeting of the Association for Advancement of Behavior Therapy, Boston.

Fals-Stewart, W., O'Farrell, T. J., & Birchler, G. R. (2004). Behavioral couples therapy for substance abuse: Rationale, methods, and findings. *Science and Practice Perspectives*, *2*, 30–41.

Fals-Stewart, W., O'Farrell, T. J., Birchler, G. R., & Gorman, C. (2004a). *Behavioral couples therapy for drug abuse and alcoholism: A 12-session manual* (Addiction and Families Research Group Manual Series, Manual 1). Buffalo, NY: Addiction and Families Research Group.

Fals-Stewart, W., O'Farrell, T. J., Birchler, G. R., & Gorman, C. (2004b). *Brief behavioral couples therapy for drug abuse and alcoholism: A 6-session manual* (Addiction and Families Research Group Manual Series, Manual 2). Buffalo, NY: Addiction and Families Research Group.

Fals-Stewart, W., O'Farrell, T. J., Feehan, M., Birchler, G. R., Tiller, S., & McFarlin, S. K. (2000). Behavioral couples therapy versus individual-based treatment for male substance abusing patients: An evaluation of significant individual change and comparison of improvement rates. *Journal of Substance Abuse Treatment, 18,* 249–254.

Fals-Stewart, W., O'Farrell, T. J., Freitas, T. T., McFarlin, S. K., & Rutigliano, P. (2000). The Timeline Followback reports of psychoactive substance use by drug-abusing patients: Psychometric properties. *Journal of Consulting and Clinical Psychology, 68,* 134–144.

Fals-Stewart, W., O'Farrell, T. J., Golden, J., & Birchler, G. R. (2004). *Group behavioral couples therapy for drug abuse and alcoholism: A 10-session rotation manual (1 Introductory session and 9 group sessions)* (Addiction and Families Research Group Manual Series, Manual 3). Buffalo, NY: Addiction and Families Research Group.

Fals-Stewart, W., O'Farrell, T. J., & Martin, J. (2002, March). *Using behavioral family counseling to enhance HIV-medication compliance among HIV-infected male drug abusing patients.* Paper presented at conference on Treating Addictions in Special Populations, Binghamton, NY.

Fudala, P. J., Bridge, P., Herbert, S., Williford, W. O., Chiang, C. N., Jones, K., et al. (2003). Office-based treatment of opiate addiction with a sublingual-tablet formulation of buprenorphine and naloxone. *New England Journal of Medicine, 39*(10), 949–958.

Gee, C. B., Scott, R. L., Castellani, A. M., & Cordova, J. V. (2002). Predicting 2-year marital satisfaction from partners' reaction to a marriage checkup. *Journal of Marital and Family Therapy, 28,* 399–408.

Gorman, C., Klostermann, K., Fals-Stewart, W., Birchler, G. R., & O'Farrell, T. J. (2004). *Treatment for dual drug-abusing couples: The effectiveness of contingency management plus couples therapy.* Poster presented at the 38th annual meeting of the Association for Advancement of Behavior Therapy, New Orleans.

Gottman, J., Notarius, C., Gonso, J., & Markman, H. (1976). *A couple's guide to communication.* Champaign, IL: Research Press.

Graham, A. W., Schultz, T. K., Mayo-Smith, M. F., Ries, R. K., & Wilford, B. B. (Eds.). (2003). *Principles of addiction medicine* (3rd ed.). Chevy Chase, MD: American Society of Addiction Medicine.

Grant, B. F. (2000). Estimates of U.S. children exposed to alcohol abuse and dependence in the family. *American Journal of Public Health, 90,* 112–115.

Hader, S. L., Smith, D. K., Moore, J. S., & Holmberg, S. D. (2001). HIV infection in women in the United States: Status at the millennium. *Journal of the American Medical Association, 285,* 1186–1193.

Hall, J., Fals-Stewart, W., & Fincham, F. (2004). Risk of exposure to STDS among wives of alcoholic men. *Alcoholism: Clinical and Experimental Research, 28*(5, Suppl.), 31A.

Hedberg, A. G., & Campbell, L. (1974). A comparison of four behavioral treatments of alcoholism. *Journal of Behavior Therapy and Experimental Psychiatry, 5,* 251–256.

Help for children of addicted parents. (2003, Spring). *Substance Abuse and Mental Health Services News, 11*(2). Retrieved November 3, 2004, from http://www.samhsa.gov/SAMHSA_News/VolumeXI_2/text_only/article5txt.htm

Hequembourg, A., Hoebbel, C., Fals-Stewart, W., O'Farrell, T. J., & Birchler, G. R. (2004). *Behavioral couples therapy for gay and lesbian substance-abusing couples.* Poster presented at the annual meeting of the Association for the Advancement of Behavior Therapy, New Orleans.

Higgins, S. T., Heil, S., & Lussier, J. P. (2004). Clinical implications of reinforcement as a determinant of substance use disorders. *Annual Review of Psychology, 55,* 431–461.

Hoebbel, C., & Fals-Stewart, W. (2003, June). *The effect of behavioral couples therapy on the degree of HIV risk exposure among wives of drug-abusing men.* Poster presented at the annual meeting of the College of Problems on Drug Dependence, Bal Harbor, FL.

Jackson, J. K. (1955). The adjustment of the family to the crisis of alcoholism. *Quarterly Journal of Studies on Alcohol, 15,* 562–586.

Jacob, T., & Bremer, D. A. (1986). Assortative mating among men and women alcoholics. *Journal of Studies on Alcohol, 47,* 219–222.

Jellinek, E. M. (1960). *The disease concept of alcoholism.* New Brunswick, NJ: Hillhouse.

Johnson, M. P. (1995). Patriarchal terrorism and common couple violence: Two forms of violence against women in U.S. families. *Journal of Marriage and the Family, 57,* 283–294.

Joint United Nations Programme on HIV/AIDS. (2004). *Q & A II: Basic facts about the AIDS epidemic and its impact, UNAIDS questions and answers.* Retrieved from www.unaids.org.

Kadden, R., Carroll, K., Donovan, D., Cooney, N., Monti, P., Abrams, D., et al. (1992). *Cognitive-behavioral coping skills therapy manual: A clinical research guide for therapists treating individuals with alcohol abuse and dependence* (NIAAA Project MATCH Monograph Series, Vol. 3, DHHS Publication No. ADM 92-1895). Washington, DC: U.S. Government Printing Office.

Kazdin, A. E. (1995). *Conduct disorders in childhood and adolescence* (2nd ed.). Thousand Oaks, CA: Sage.

Keller, J. (Ed.). (1974). Trends in treatment of alcoholism. In *Second special report to the U.S. Congress on alcohol and health* (pp. 145–167). Washington, DC: Department of Health, Education, and Welfare.

Kelley, M. L., & Fals-Stewart, W. (2002). Couples versus individual-based therapy for alcoholism and drug abuse: Effects on children's psychosocial functioning. *Journal of Consulting and Clinical Psychology, 70,* 417–427.

Kelley, M. L., & Fals-Stewart, W. (2003). Adding parent skills training to behavioral couples therapy for drug-abusing couples: Effects on children. In T. J. O'Farrell (Chair), *Behavioral couples therapy for alcoholism and drug abuse: Recent advances.* Symposium conducted at the annual meeting of the Association for Advancement of Behavior Therapy, Boston.

Kelley, M. L., & Fals-Stewart, W. (2004). Psychiatric disorders of children living with drug-abusing, alcohol-abusing, and non-substance-abusing fathers. *Journal of the American Academy of Child and Adolescent Psychiatry, 43*(5), 621–628.

Kelly, J., & Kalichman, S. (2002). Behavioral research in HIV/AIDS and secondary prevention: Recent advances and future directions. *Journal of Consulting and Clinical Psychology, 70,* 626–639.

Kinsey, A. C., Pomeroy, W. B., & Martin, C. E. (1948). *Sexual behavior in the human male.* Philadelphia: Saunders.

Kleber, H. D., & Kosten, T. R. (1984). Naltrexone induction: Psychologic and pharmacologic strategies. *Journal of Clinical Psychiatry, 45,* 29–38.

Kost, K., & Forrest, J. D. (1992). American women's sexual behavior and exposure to risk of sexually transmitted diseases. *Family Planning Perspectives, 24,* 244–254.

Kosten, T. R., & Kleber, H. D. (1984). Strategies to improve compliance with narcotic antagonists. *American Journal of Drug and Alcohol Abuse, 10,* 249–266.

Kranzler, H. R., & Van Kirk, J. (2001). Efficacy of naltrexone and acamprosate for alcoholism treatment: A meta-analysis. *Alcoholism: Clinical and Experimental Research, 25,* 335–341.

Ku, L., Sonnenstein, F. L., & Pleck, H. H. (1994). The dynamics of young men's condom use during and across relationships. *Family Planning and Perspectives, 26,* 246–251.

Kumpfer, K. L., Molgaard, V., & Spoth, R. (1996).The Strengthening Families Program for the prevention of delinquency and drug use. In R. D. Peters & R. J. McMahon (Eds.), *Preventing childhood disorders, substance abuse, and delinquency* (pp. 241–267). Thousand Oaks, CA: Sage.

Kwiatkowski, C. F., Stober, D. R., Booth, R. E., & Zhang, Y. (1999). Predictors of increased condom use following HIV intervention with heterosexually active drug users. *Drug and Alcohol Dependence, 54,* 57–62.

Laumann, E. O., Gagnon, J. H., Michael, R. T., & Michaels, S. (1994). *The social organization of sexuality: Sexual practices in the United States.* Chicago: University of Chicago Press.

Laundergan, J. C., & Williams, T. (1993). The Hazelden Residential Family Program: A combined systems and disease model approach. In T. J. O'Farrell (Ed.),

Treating alcohol problems: Marital and family interventions (pp. 145–169). New York: Guilford Press.

Legal Action Center. (2003). *Confidentiality and communication: A guide to the federal alcohol and drug confidentiality law and HIPAA* (rev. ed.). New York: Author.

Liberman, R. P., Wheeler, E. G., DeVisser, L. A., Keuhnel, J., & Keuhnel, T. (1980). *Handbook of marital therapy: A positive approach to helping troubled relationships.* New York: Plenum Press.

Maisto, S. A., McKay, J. R., & O'Farrell, T. J. (1995). Relapse precipitants and behavioral marital therapy. *Addictive Behaviors, 20,* 383–393.

Maisto, S. A., O'Farrell, T. J., Connors, G. J., McKay, J., & Pelcovits, M. A. (1988). Alcoholics' attributions of factors affecting their relapse to drinking and reasons for terminating relapse episodes. *Addictive Behaviors, 13,* 79–82.

Margolin, G. (1998). Effects of domestic violence on children. In P. K. Trickett & C. J. Schellenbach (Eds.), *Violence against children in the family and the community* (pp. 57–101). Washington, DC: American Psychological Association.

Margolin, G., Talovic, S., & Weinstein, C. D. (1983). Areas of Changes Questionnaire: A practical approach to marital assessment. *Journal of Consulting and Clinical Psychology, 51,* 920–931.

Markman, H. J., Renick, M. J., Floyd, F. J., Stanley, S. M., & Clements, M. (1993). Preventing marital distress through communication and conflict management training: A 4- and 5-year follow-up. *Journal of Consulting and Clinical Psychology, 61,* 70–77.

Marlatt, G. A., & Gordon, J. R. (Eds.). (1985). *Relapse prevention: Maintenance strategies in the treatment of addictive behaviors.* New York: Guilford Press.

Massachusetts Guidelines and Standards for Certification of Batterers' Treatment Programs. (1995, March revision). Boston: Massachusetts Department of Public Health.

Mayes, L., & Truman, S. D. (2002). Substance abuse and parenting. In M. H. Bornstein (Ed.), *Handbook of parenting: Vol. 4. Social conditions and applied parenting* (2nd ed., pp. 329–359). Mahwah, NJ: Erlbaum.

McCarthy, B., & McCarthy, E. (2002). *Sexual awareness: Couple sexuality for the twenty-first century.* New York: Carroll & Graf.

McCarthy, B., & McCarthy, E. (2003). *Rekindling desire: A step-by-step program to help low-sex and no-sex marriages.* New York: Brunner/Routledge.

McCoy, C. B., & Inciardi, J. (1993). Women and AIDS: Social determinants of sex-related activities. *Women Health, 20,* 69–86.

McCrady, B. S. (1983). Marital dysfunction: Alcoholism and marriage. In E. M. Pattison & E. Kaufman (Eds.), *Encyclopedic handbook of alcoholism* (pp. 673–685). New York: Gardner Press.

McCrady, B., Stout, R., Noel, N., Abrams, D., & Nelson,

H. (1991). Comparative effectiveness of three types of spouse involved alcohol treatment: Outcomes 18 months after treatment. *British Journal of Addiction, 86,* 1415–1424.

McLellan, A. T., Hagan, T. A., Levine, M., Gould, F., Meyers, K., Bencivengo, M., et al. (1998). Supplemental social services improve outcome in public addiction treatment. *Addiction, 93,* 1489–1499.

McLellan, A. T., Hagan, T. A., Levine, M., Meyers, K., Gould, F., Bencivengo, M., et al. (1998). Does clinical case management improve outpatient addiction treatment? *Drug and Alcohol Dependence, 55,* 91–103.

McLellan, A. T., Luborsky, L., Cacciola, J., Griffith, J., Evans, F., Barr, H. L., et al. (1985). New data from the Addiction Severity Index: Reliability and validity in three centers. *Journal of Nervous and Mental Disease, 173,* 412–423.

Mercer, D., & Woody, G. (1999). *An individual drug counseling approach to treat cocaine addiction: The Collaborative Cocaine Treatment Study Model.* (NIDA Therapy Manuals for Drug Abuse, Manual 3, NIH Publication No. 99-4380). Rockville, MD: National Institute of Drug Abuse.

Miller, P. M. (1976). *Behavioral treatment of alcoholism.* New York: Pergamon Press.

Miller, P. M., & Hersen, M. (1975). *Modification of marital interaction patterns between an alcoholic and his wife.* Unpublished manuscript. (Available from Peter Miller, Medical University of South Carolina, 114 Doughty Street, Room 113, Box 250772, Charleston, SC 29425.)

Miller, W. R., & Rollnick, S. (2002). *Motivational interviewing: Preparing people for change* (2nd ed.). New York: Guilford Press.

Miller, W. R., Tonigan, J. S., & Longabaugh, R. (1995). *The Drinker Inventory of Consequences (DRINC): An instrument for assessing adverse consequences of alcohol abuse.* Rockville, MD: National Institute on Alcohol Abuse and Alcoholism.

Moos, R. H., Bromet, E., Tsu, V., & Moos, B. (1979). Family characteristics and the outcome of treatment for alcoholism. *Journal of Studies on Alcohol, 40,* 78–88.

Moos, R. H., Finney, J. W., & Cronkite, R. C. (1990). *Alcoholism treatment: Context, process, and outcome.* New York: Oxford University Press.

Mrazek, P. J., & Haggerty, R. J. (Eds.). (1994). *Reducing risks for mental disorders: Frontiers for preventive intervention research.* Washington, DC: National Academies Press.

Newman, S., Sarin, P., Kumarasamy, N., Amalraj, E., Rogers, M., Madhivanan, M., et al. (2000). Marriage, monogamy, and HIV: A profile of HIV infected women in south India. *International Journal of Studies on AIDS, 11,* 250–253.

Noel, N. E., & McCrady, B. S. (1993). Alcohol-focused spouse involvement with behavioral marital ther-

apy. In T. J. O'Farrell (Ed.), *Treating alcohol problems: Marital and family interventions* (pp. 210–235). New York: Guilford Press.

Nowinski, J. K. (1999). *Family recovery and substance abuse: A twelve-step guide for treatment.* Thousand Oaks, CA: Sage.

Nowinski, J. K., Baker, S., & Carroll, K. (1992). *Twelve step facilitation therapy manual: A clinical research guide for therapists treating individuals with alcohol abuse and dependence* (NIAAA Project MATCH Monograph Series, Vol. 1, DHHS Publication No. ADM 92-1893). Washington, DC: U.S. Government Printing Office.

O'Brien, C. P. (1994). Opioids: Antagonists and partial agonists. In M. Galanter & H. Kleber (Eds.) *American Psychiatric Press textbook of substance abuse treatment* (pp. 223–236). Washington, DC: American Psychiatric Press.

O'Farrell, T. J. (1993a). A behavioral marital therapy couples group program for alcoholics and their spouses. In T. J. O'Farrell (Ed.), *Treating alcohol problems: Marital and family interventions* (pp. 170–209). New York: Guilford Press.

O'Farrell, T. J. (1993b). Couples relapse prevention sessions after a behavioral marital therapy couples group program. In T. J. O'Farrell (Ed.), *Treating alcohol problems: Marital and family interventions* (pp. 305–326). New York: Guilford Press.

O'Farrell, T. J., Allen, J. P., & Litten, R. Z. (1995). Disulfiram (Antabuse) contracts in treatment of alcoholism. In J. D. Blaine & L. Onken (Eds.), *Integrating behavior therapies with medications in the treatment of drug dependence* (NIDA Research Monograph 150, pp. 65–91). Washington, DC: National Institute on Drug Abuse.

O'Farrell, T. J., & Birchler, G. R. (1987). Marital relationships of alcoholic, conflicted, and nonconflicted couples. *Journal of Marital and Family Therapy, 13,* 259–274.

O'Farrell, T. J., Choquette, K. A., & Cutter, H. S. G. (1998). Couples relapse prevention sessions after behavioral marital therapy for male alcoholics: Outcomes during the three years after starting treatment. *Journal of Studies on Alcohol, 59,* 357–370.

O'Farrell, T. J., Choquette, K. A., Cutter, H. S. G., & Birchler, G. R. (1997). Sexual satisfaction and dysfunction among alcoholic, maritally conflicted and nonconflicted couples. *Journal of Studies on Alcohol, 58,* 91–99.

O'Farrell, T. J., Choquette, K. A., Cutter, H. S. G., Brown, E. D., Bayog, R., McCourt, W., et al. (1996). Cost-benefit and cost-effectiveness analyses of behavioral marital therapy with and without relapse prevention sessions for alcoholics and their spouses. *Behavior Therapy, 27,* 7–24.

O'Farrell, T. J., Choquette, K. A., Cutter, H. S. G., Brown, E. D., & McCourt, W. F. (1993). Behavioral marital therapy with and without additional couples relapse prevention sessions for alcoholics and their wives. *Journal of Studies on Alcohol, 54,* 652–666.

O'Farrell, T. J., Choquette, K. A., Cutter, H. S. G., Floyd, F. J., Bayog, R. D., Brown, E. D., et al. (1996). Cost-benefit and cost-effectiveness analyses of behavioral marital therapy as an addition to outpatient alcoholism treatment. *Journal of Substance Abuse, 8,* 145–166.

O'Farrell, T. J., & Cutter, H. S. G. (1977a). *Behavioral marital therapy (BMT) for alcoholics and their wives: Review of the literature and a proposed research program.* Paper presented at the NATO International Conference on Experimental and Behavioral Approaches to Alcoholism, Bergen, Norway.

O'Farrell, T. J., & Cutter, H. S. G. (1977b). *Wanted: A behavioral couples group model for alcoholics and their wives.* Paper presented at the Eighth Annual Brockton Symposium on Behavior Therapy, Brockton, MA.

O'Farrell, T. J., & Cutter, H. S. G. (1984a). Behavioral marital therapy for alcoholics: Clinical procedures from a treatment outcome study in progress. *American Journal of Family Therapy, 12,* 33–46.

O'Farrell, T. J., & Cutter, H. S. G. (1984b). Behavioral marital therapy couples groups for male alcoholics and their wives. *Journal of Substance Abuse Treatment, 1,* 191–204.

O'Farrell, T. J., Cutter, H. S. G., Choquette, K. A., Floyd, F. J., & Bayog, R. D. (1992). Behavioral marital therapy for male alcoholics: Marital and drinking adjustment during the two years after treatment. *Behavior Therapy, 23,* 529–549.

O'Farrell, T. J., & Fals-Stewart, W. (2000). Behavioral couples therapy for alcoholism and drug abuse. *Journal of Substance Abuse Treatment, 18,* 51–54.

O'Farrell, T. J., & Fals-Stewart, W. (2001). Family-involved alcoholism treatment: An update. In M. Galanter (Ed.), *Recent developments in alcoholism: Vol. 15. Services research in the era of managed care* (pp. 329–356). New York: Plenum Press.

O'Farrell, T. J., & Fals-Stewart, W. (2003). Alcohol abuse. *Journal of Marital and Family Therapy, 29,* 121–146.

O'Farrell, T. J., Fals-Stewart, W., & Murphy, M. (2003). Do outcomes for behavioral couples therapy differ based on gender of the alcoholic patient? In T. J. O'Farrell (Chair), *Behavioral couples therapy for alcoholism and drug abuse: Recent advances.* Symposium conducted at the annual meeting of the Association for the Advancement of Behavior Therapy, Boston.

O'Farrell, T. J., Fals-Stewart, W., Murphy, M., Alter, J., Sepulveda, I., & Chan, A. (2004). A randomized study of a brief family intervention to promote aftercare among substance abusing patients in inpatient detoxification. *Alcoholism: Clinical and Experimental Research, 28*(5, Suppl.), 76A.

O'Farrell, T. J., Fals-Stewart, W., Murphy, M., & Murphy, C. M. (2003). Partner violence before and after individually based alcoholism treatment for male alcoholic patients. *Journal of Consulting and Clinical Psychology, 71,* 92–102.

O'Farrell, T. J., Feehan, M., Murphy, C. M., & Fals-Stewart, W. (1999, November). *Male-to-female domestic violence among women alcoholic patients and their male partners.* Paper presented at the annual meeting of the Association for Advancement of Behavior Therapy, Toronto.

O'Farrell, T. J., Harrison, R. H., Schulmeister, C. A., & Cutter, H. S. G. (1981). A Closeness to Divorce Scale for wives of alcoholics. *Drug and Alcohol Dependence, 7,* 319–324.

O'Farrell, T. J., Kleinke, C. L., & Cutter, H. S. G. (1997). A Sexual Adjustment Questionnaire for use in therapy and research with alcoholics and their spouses. *Journal of Substance Abuse Treatment, 14,* 259–268.

O'Farrell, T. J., & Murphy, C. M. (1995). Marital violence before and after alcoholism treatment. *Journal of Consulting and Clinical Psychology, 63,* 256–262.

O'Farrell, T. J., & Murphy, C. M. (2002). Behavioral couples therapy for alcoholism and drug abuse: Encountering the problem of domestic violence. In C. Wekerle & A. M. Wall (Eds.), *The violence and addiction equation: Theoretical and clinical issues in substance abuse and relationship violence* (pp. 293–303). New York: Brunner/Routledge.

O'Farrell, T. J., Murphy, C. M., Stephan, S. H., Fals-Stewart, W., & Murphy, M. (2004). Partner violence before and after couples-based alcoholism treatment for male alcoholic patients: The role of treatment involvement and abstinence. *Journal of Consulting and Clinical Psychology, 72,* 202–217.

O'Farrell, T. J., Van Hutton, V., & Murphy, C. M. (1999). Domestic violence after alcoholism treatment: A two-year longitudinal study. *Journal of Studies on Alcohol, 60,* 317–321.

O'Leary, A. (2000). Women at risk for HIV from a primary partner: Balancing risk and intimacy. *Annual Review of Sex Research, 11,* 191–243.

Peterson, K. A., Swindle, R. W., Phibbs, C. S., Recine, B., & Moos, R. H. (1994). Determinants of readmission following inpatient substance abuse treatment: A national study of VA programs. *Medical Care, 32,* 535–550.

Petry, N. M., & Simcic, F. (2002). Recent advances in the dissemination of contingency management techniques: Clinical and research perspectives. *Journal of Substance Abuse Treatment, 23,* 81–86.

Project MATCH Research Group. (1997). Matching alcoholism treatments to client heterogeneity: Project MATCH posttreatment drinking outcomes. *Journal of Studies on Alcohol, 58,* 7–29.

Rotunda, R., Alter, J., & O'Farrell, T. J. (2001). Behavioral couples therapy for comorbid substance abuse and psychiatric problems. In M. M. MacFarlane (Ed.), *Family therapy and mental health: Innovations in theory and practice* (pp. 289–309). Binghamton, NY: Haworth Press.

Rotunda, R. J., West, L., & O'Farrell, T. J. (2004). Enabling behavior in a clinical sample of alcohol dependent clients and their partners. *Journal of Substance Abuse Treatment, 26,* 269–276.

Rychtarik, R. G., & McGillicuddy, N. B. (2005). Coping skills training and 12-step facilitation for women whose partner has alcoholism: Effects on depression, the partner's drinking, and partner physical violence. *Journal of Consulting and Clinical Psychology, 73,* 249–261.

Schumacher, J. A., Fals-Stewart, W., & Leonard, K. E. (2003). Domestic violence treatment referrals for men seeking alcohol treatment. *Journal of Substance Abuse Treatment, 24,* 279–283.

Schumm, J. A., O'Farrell, T. J., Murphy, M., & Fals-Stewart, W. (2006). *Outcomes following behavioral couples therapy for couples in which both partners have alcoholism versus couples in which only one partner has alcoholism.* Poster presented at the annual meeting of the Association for the Advancement of Behavior Therapy, Chicago.

Shadish, W. R., & Baldwin, S. A. (2005). Effects of behavioral marital therapy: A meta-analysis of randomized controlled trials. *Journal of Consulting and Clinical Psychology, 73,* 6–14.

Sobell, L. C., & Sobell, M. B. (1996). *Time-Line Follow-Back: A calendar method for assessing alcohol and drug use (User's Guide).* Toronto: Addiction Research Foundation.

Spanier, G. (1976). Measuring dyadic adjustment: New scales for assessing the quality of marriage and similar dyads. *Journal of Marriage and the Family, 38,* 15–30.

Stanton, M. D., & Shadish, W. R. (1997). Outcome, attrition, and family–couple treatment for drug abuse: A meta-analysis and review of the controlled, comparative studies. *Psychological Bulletin, 122,* 170–191.

Stanton, M. D., Todd, T. C., and Associates (1982). *The family therapy of drug abuse and addiction.* New York: Guilford Press.

Steinglass, P., Bennett, L., Wolin, S., & Reiss, D. (1987). *The alcoholic family.* New York: Basic Books.

Stets, J. E., & Straus, M. A. (1990). Gender differences in reporting marital violence and its medical and psychological consequences. In M. A. Straus & R. J. Gelles (Eds.), *Physical violence in American families* (pp. 151–165). New Brunswick, NJ: Transaction.

Straus, M. A. (1979). Measuring intrafamily conflict and violence: The Conflict Tactics Scales. *Journal of Marriage and the Family, 41,* 75–88.

Straus, M. A. (1990). The Conflict Tactics Scale and its critics: An evaluation and new data on validity and reliability. In M. A. Straus & R. J. Gelles (Eds.), *Physical violence in American families* (pp. 49–73). New Brunswick, NJ: Transaction.

Straus, M. A., Hamby, S. L., Boney-McCoy, S., & Sugarman, D. B. (1996). The Revised Conflict Tactics Scale (CTS2). *Journal of Family Issues, 17,* 283–316.

Stuart, R. B. (1980). *Helping couples change: A social learning approach to marital therapy.* New York: Guilford Press.

Tracy, S. W., Kelly, J. F., & Moos, R. H. (2005). The influence of partner status, relationship quality and relationship stability on outcomes following intensive substance-use disorder treatment. *Journal of Studies on Alcohol, 66,* 497–505.

U.S. Department of Health and Human Services. (1994). *Substance abuse among women and parents.* Washington, DC: National Institute on Drug Abuse and the Office of the Assistant Secretary for Planning and Evaluation.

Verebey, K., & Turner, C. E. (1991). Laboratory testing. In R. J. Frances & S. I. Miller (Eds.), *Clinical textbook of addictive disorders* (pp. 221–236). New York: Guilford Press.

Volpicelli, J. R., Rhines, K. C., Rhines, J. S., Volpicelli, J. A., Alterman, A. I., & O'Brien, C. P. (1997). Naltrexone and alcohol dependence. *Archives of General Psychiatry, 54,* 737–742.

Weiss, R. L., & Birchler, G. R. (1975). *Areas of Change Questionnaire.* Unpublished manuscript, University of Oregon.

Weiss, R. L., Birchler, G. R., & Vincent, J. P. (1974). Contractual models for negotiation training in marital dyads. *Journal of Marriage and the Family, 36,* 321–331.

Weiss, R. L., & Cerreto, M. C. (1980). The Marital Status Inventory: Development of a measure of dissolution potential. *American Journal of Family Therapy, 8,* 80–85.

Whisman, M. A. (1990). The efficacy of booster maintenance sessions in behavior therapy: Review and methodology critique. *Clinical Psychology Review, 10,* 155–170.

Wilsnack, S. C., & Beckman, L. J. (1984). *Alcohol problems in women.* New York: Guilford Press.

Winters, J., Fals-Stewart, W., O'Farrell, T. J., Birchler, G. R., & Kelley, M. L. (2002). Behavioral couples therapy for female substance-abusing patients: Effects on substance use and relationship adjustment. *Journal of Consulting and Clinical Psychology, 70,* 344–355.

Zubretsky, T. M., & Knights, C. L. (2001). *Basic information about domestic violence.* Rensselaer, NY: New York State Office for the Prevention of Domestic Violence.

Index

Page numbers followed by *f* indicate figure, *n* indicate note, and *t* indicate table